A Comprehensive Approach to Complementary and Alternative Medicine

A Comprehensive Approach to Complementary and Alternative Medicine

Brett Harris

MURPHY & MOORE
www.murphy-moorepublishing.com

Published by Murphy & Moore Publishing,
1 Rockefeller Plaza,
New York City, NY 10020, USA
www.murphy-moorepublishing.com

A Comprehensive Approach to Complementary and Alternative Medicine
Brett Harris

International Standard Book Number: 978-1-63987-000-4 (Hardback)

Cataloging-in-Publication Data

A comprehensive approach to complementary and alternative medicine / Brett Harris.
p. cm.
Includes bibliographical references and index.
ISBN 978-1-63987-000-4
1. Alternative medicine. 2. Integrative medicine. 3. Medicine. I. Harris, Brett.
R733 .C66 2022
615.5--dc23

TABLE OF CONTENTS

PREFACE

Complementary and alternative medicines refer to all those healthcare practices and medical products which are not a part of standard medical care and procedures. Complementary medicine can be administered with conventional medicine, while alternative medicine tends to replace the conventional medical procedures. Some of their prominent examples are acupressure, ayurvedic medicine, homeopathy, chiropractic medicine, naturopathy, herbalism, and traditional Chinese medicine. It often uses natural substances such as herbs, foods, animal and fungal products, non-vitamin supplements, minerals, and megavitamins. Complementary and alternative medicine procedures are being extensively used worldwide to treat various medical conditions such as anxiety, depression, sleep disorders, infertility, back pain, allergies, etc. The book studies and analyzes the different facets of complementary and alternative medicine, and its significance in modern times. It elucidates the concepts and innovative models around prospective developments with respect to this field. This book will provide comprehensive knowledge to the readers.

To facilitate a deeper understanding of the contents of this book a short introduction of every chapter is written below:

Chapter 1- Complementary and alternative medicine refers to the various practices that are intended to maintain or improve human health. These practices are not a part of conventional medicine. This is an introductory chapter which will briefly introduce all the significant aspects of complementary and alternative medicine such as its history and economics.

Chapter 2- Traditional medicine practices include the utilization of skills, practices and knowledge based on theories and experiences of different cultures to prevent, diagnose and treat physical and mental illness. There are different forms of traditional medicine such as traditional Mongolian medicine, traditional Chinese medicine, Iranian traditional medicine, etc. This chapter has been carefully written to provide an easy understanding of the varied facets of these traditional medicine practices.

Chapter 3- Ayurveda is a form of alternative medicine having roots in the Indian subcontinent. Various topics studied under Ayurveda are history and eight branches of Ayurveda, Dosha in Ayurveda, Ayurvedic herbs, Ayurvedic acupressure, Dincharyah and Rasa Shastra. All these topics have been carefully analyzed in this chapter.

Chapter 4- Some of the important alternative therapies are acupuncture, acupressure, apitherapy, hydrotherapy, halotherapy and animal assisted therapy. Acupuncture is practiced to attempt pain relief and involves inserting thin needles into the body. The topics elaborated in this chapter will help in gaining a better perspective about these various alternative therapies.

Chapter 5- A form of alternative medicine that makes use of an array of pseudoscientific practices that are natural and promote self-healing is termed as naturopathy. There are various types of treatments in naturopathy such as fasting therapy, mud therapy, masso therapy and magnet therapy. This chapter discusses in detail these significant types of treatments in naturopathy.

Chapter 6- A form of alternative medicine that deals with the diagnosis and treatment of diseases related to the musculoskeletal system is referred to as chiropractic treatment. Some of the significant topics studied under chiropractic treatment are chiropractic treatment techniques, chiropractic criticism, spinal adjustment, etc. This chapter elaborates these topics in detail.

Chapter 7- Osteopathy is a type of alternative medicine that is concerned with the physical manipulation of the bones and muscle tissues of the body. It is attempted to diagnose and treat somatic dysfunction by manipulating the muscles and bones of the person. The topics explained in this chapter are crucial for a complete understanding of osteopathy.

Finally, I would like to thank the entire team involved in the inception of this book for their valuable time and contribution. This book would not have been possible without their efforts. I would also like to thank my friends and family for their constant support.

Brett Harris

Chapter 1

Basics of Complementary and Alternative Medicine

Complementary and alternative medicine refers to the various practices that are intended to maintain or improve human health. These practices are not a part of conventional medicine. This is an introductory chapter which will briefly introduce all the significant aspects of complementary and alternative medicine such as its history and economics.

The origins of medicine are deeply rooted in a civilization's culture and religious beliefs. Often, educated priests practiced medicine. Early medicine dealt with experiences, observations, and reflections of the self and one's surroundings. There was no separation of mind and body. In the 1600s, Rene Descartes, in an attempt to protect the spirit from science, separated the mind from the body. This set the stage for the current state of the Western style mind–body split and evidence-based medicine versus nonconventional or complementary medicine. This was the beginning of the reductionistic movement with the goal of understanding the parts to gain a larger understanding of the whole. Only within the past few decades, has there been an attempt to reunite the medical systems of curing (technological, microscopic, and disease-based) with healing (nonphysical, holistic, and relationship-based). The following is a brief history of important and relevant world cultures that have contributed to the field of medicine, conventionally and unconventionally.

Mesopotamia and Egypt

It is believed that the oldest civilizations were in the areas of present-day Egypt and Iraq (Mesopotamia). Given that medicine is so often culturally based, it undoubtedly follows that the first medicine came from these civilizations. Thoth was an Egyptian god who was the inventor of art in general. He is believed to have been the author of the oldest Egyptian medical work with the contents engraved upon pillars of stone. His words formed a part of the Hermetic Books (cited by Bass) used by the physicians of the day. Interestingly, Egyptian medicine was divided into two degrees. The Science of higher degree consisted of conjurations, dissolving the charms of gods by prayer, and interpretations of revelations received by the sick person during incubations in temples. The highest class of priest performed as the physicians of the higher Science. The Science of the lower degree was "ordinary medical practice" and was practiced by the lowest grade of priests. They studied anatomy, pathology, pharmacology, ophthalmology, and gynecology. It is interesting, therefore, that the higher order of Science dealt with areas, which today some people have called "Voodoo" medicine.

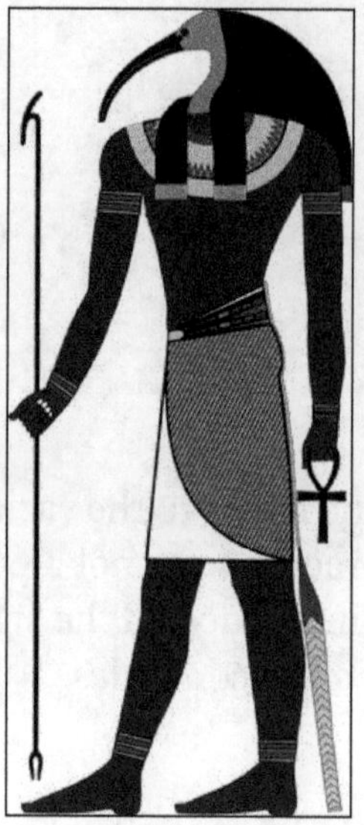

Figure: Thoth, ancient Egyptian god often depicted as an ibis-headed man.
Based on New Kingdom tomb painting.

The Egyptians developed a system of specialties described as "physicians in Egypt for each part of the body." In fact, there were priestly physicians who followed the army and were employed by the state. In Outlines of the History of Medicine and the Medical Profession, it is stated: "This specialism is per se an evidence of a civilization of high development, indeed of one tending towards its downfall, and in Egypt it attained a perfection which our own system, with all its completeness, has not yet reached." Current day Western biomedicine continues to pursue scientific inquiry with specialization and microscopic divisions.

Thus, could our system of intense specialization be a portent of our health care system's downfall if it is continued without deviation? Aromatherapy began in ancient Egypt. The Egyptians excelled in the use of oils, salts, alabasters, and creams for all kinds of diseases and for preservation of the dead. Nefertum was the god of perfumes, incense, and fragrant oils. His mother, Sekmer, was the goddess of healing and alchemical distillation. The use of fragrance was the means of communication between the gods and humanity, offering health to the living and assisting the dead in the next life. The Egyptians believed that the body could heal itself and used reflexology to restore balance and the natural equilibrium.

India in 2500 BC

Unlike many civilizations that imported systems of other outside cultures, Indian medicine was derived in India and had interwoven systems of other cultures, predominately Greek, as part of India's own system, but this interweaving occurred only at a later time period. The ancient Indians wrote about medicine in their sacred books, known as the Vedas. The Vedas are believed to be of divine origin and were passed down through oral traditions until the sixteenth century ad. One of the Vedas, the Atharvaveda, is a collection of spells, hymns, and incantations for magical curing of diseases, and is thought to have been the origin of the traditional Indian medicine system known as Ayurveda. Ayurveda is based on the concepts of longevity and the nourishment of life. Later commentaries on the Vedas, known as the Brahmanas and the Upanishads, explained these texts and speculated about the nature of the universe as well as the human condition.

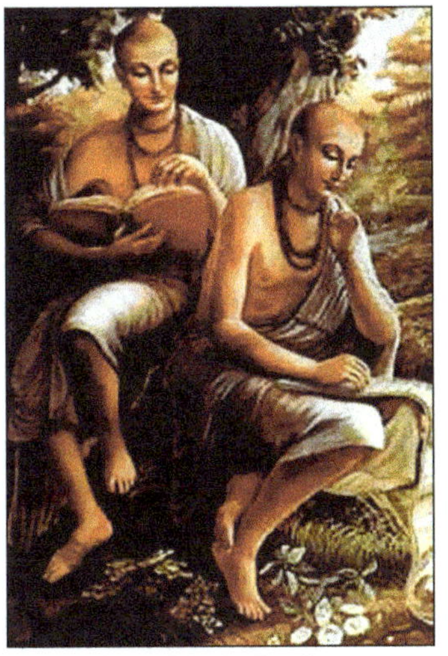

Figure: The Recording of the Vedas in Ancient India. This is the front cover of the book "The Nectar of Instruction 1st edition" by A.C. Bhaktivedanta Swami, Founder of the International Society of Krishna Consciousness.

Yoga, a term derived from the Sanskrit word yug—was a theological practice that was believed to lead to the unification of self with the Divine. Yoga's origins are believed to date back to pre-Vedic traditions. Yoga is a practice that was considered to be given directly from God. The foundation is based on the suppression of all activities so that one can identify and separate the self from the body, mind, and will. In doing so, one attains spiritual liberation. Yoga, when practiced in the true Indian tradition, is more than a physical exercise program. It has a meditative and spiritual core, and offers a meaningful purpose for life and living.

Buddhism originated in India in the sixth century BC under the teachings of the Buddha. These teachings were in protest of the strict stratification of the Hindu society as well as the religious control of the Brahmanic priests. Buddha emphasized universal love, service, and peace of mind brought about through abandonment of desire. Unani medicine, a lesser-known India medicine subtype, is based on the theory of the Four Elements of the human body (i.e., Fire, Water, Earth and Air). Different fluids represent these elements. When the fluids are balanced, there is health; when the fluids are imbalanced there is illness.

An esoteric form of alternative medicine described in Indian literature is the healing practice of Uropathy. This is a method of healing with the use of one's own urine. It is referred to as Shivambu or "holy liquid." In the Tantric Yoga culture, it is termed Amroli. Amroli is derived from the word Amar, which means undying. Hence, Amroli was a spiritual practice that was beneficial to the mind, body, and spirit for the attainment of immortality. It is believed that hundreds of ailments can be cured by urine therapy. Uropathy is not widely practiced today; however, there are World Congresses on the subject, numerous books and articles on this topic. Finally, Indian medicine was weakest in the area of anatomy because of a prohibition against living people having physical contact with dead people.

China in 1600 BC

It is widely believed that Traditional Chinese Medicine (TCM) has a 3000–4000-year history. TCM was embedded in the "philosophy of Confucius who called for the ideal family ties and the promotion of social and ethical standards of societies." The oldest Chinese medical texts are thought to be on herbal medicine. The Yellow Emperor, Huang Di, wrote about acupuncture, the concept of Yin and Yang, and the Five Phases in his book, The Yellow Emperor's Inner Classic.

TCM spread across Asia throughout the centuries and came eventually into the Western world in the sixteenth to the twentieth centuries AD. However, only fragments of TCM are practiced in the West. Nonetheless, TCM has influenced the delivery of Western-style health care. Likewise, TCM has not remained stagnant in practice either. Concepts have come and gone and returned over time, depending on current societal perspectives and political environments. Unlike the West, in which an incomplete theory or unacceptable concept is rejected and then disappears, TCM may reject a theory but it does not disappear. It may fade in practice, but it continues to exist and may return at a later time. In the West, it is often thought that something is "either this or that." However, in TCM, opposing theories can exist. An example of this is the concept of Yin and Yang. Although Yin and Yang oppose each other, they are also complementary to each other.

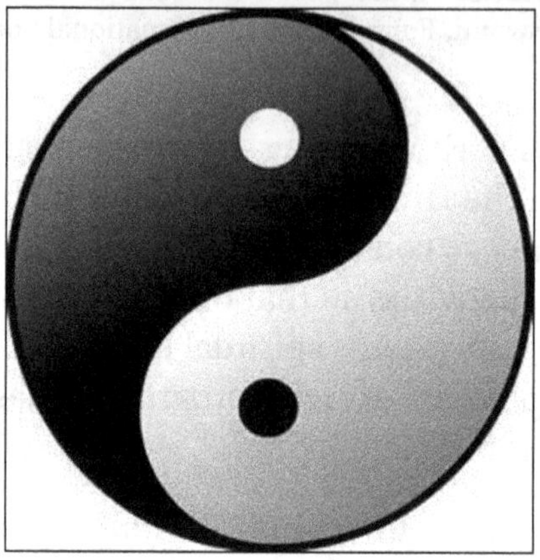

Figure: Yin Yang Symbol.

TCM is the overreaching umbrella for many disciplines. Acupuncture is one of those disciplines. The mythological basis of acupuncture suggests that the Chinese speared human bodies to rid towns and villages of demons and evil spirits. Acupuncture evolved over time. The practice of acupuncture was influenced significantly by the reorganized text of the Yellow Emperor's Inner Classic and other earlier texts into the text Systematic Text of Acupuncture circa the third century CE. TCM was primarily a system for the Chinese elite rather than for the population of the entire nation. Much of the country's population was illiterate, and, as such, little is known about the population. It is believed that the illiterate people's traditions were based on folk superstitions, legends, and survival.

The true history of acupuncture may never be known. Despite the fact that classical texts on acupuncture exist, these texts often do not describe the clinical practices. The theories and concepts of Chinese acupuncture do not always translate well and, therefore, the meaning and significance of both have been lost. Throughout history, TCM and acupuncture have been subject to religious, cultural, and political pressures. During the late nineteenth and early twentieth centuries, TCM was politically under attack to make way for a new and more modern China. In 1822, acupuncture was banned from the Imperial Medical Academy after nearly 1200 years of basic Imperial medical education. There was a significant movement to move toward scientifically based medicine. Many of the scientifically trained physicians were concentrated in only three major cities, leaving voids in the other urban and in all rural areas. Thus, the ban undercut the health care system of the common people, because much of their care was solely based one TCM.

Only after 1954, did acupuncture become reinvented. Chairman Mao ordered all Western medicine practitioners to study acupuncture. This resulted in organization of the TCM practitioners to provide health care. However, it is not clear if this new acupuncture actually resembled the true acupuncture of the millennia before. Other TCM practices include movement of invisible energies (Feng Shui), dietary/herbal therapies ("we are what we eat"), and kinesiology (t'ai chi, Qigong). This system of exercise was known as the "Frolics of Five Animals." Similar to Indian medicine, TCM supports the holistic view of treating the mind, body, and spirit, and the individual's experience of the disease. TCM has been practiced in the United States since the mid nineteenth century. Bache was the first American physician to use acupuncture in his practice (in 1826). In 1901, Ah Fong Chuck was the first licensed practitioner of TCM.

Greece in 800 BC

The ancient traditions of Greece have provided the foundations of Western philosophy, science, and medicine. However, history shows that the Greeks went to Egypt for their medical training. Greek medicine was comprised of magic and legendary beliefs. Like what occurred in preceding cultures, Greek medicine was strongly embedded with priests, seers, and god figures. Apollo, the most powerful god–physician, would cause epidemics as punishments. Yet, he would also revive and heal wounded people.

Pythagoras, well-known for his mathematical formulas, was the first Greek philosopher interested in medicine. Mathematics influenced the concept of opposite quantities. The balancing of these opposites was important to health and disease. Hippocrates is considered to be the father of Western medicine. He established "medicine as an art, science and a profession of profound value and dignity." Medicine was no longer a part of philosophy.

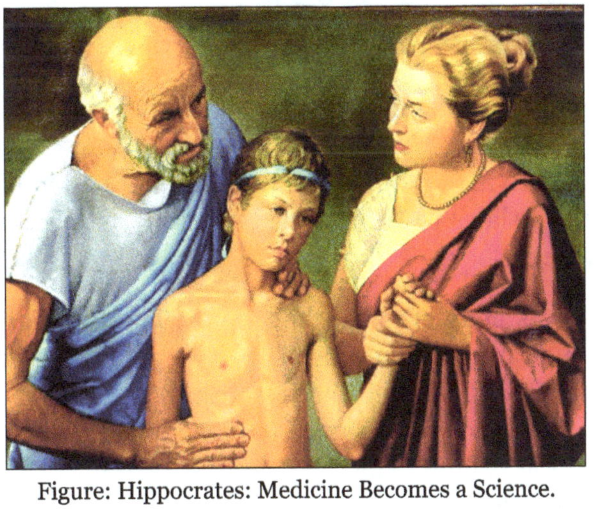

Figure: Hippocrates: Medicine Becomes a Science.

The life of Hippocrates is not well-documented, and it is argued by some scholars that Hippocrates was not an individual person. Nonetheless, he is credited with the theory of the Four Humors to mirror the earth's four elements. These humors, with their associated qualities (hot, cold, moist, and dry), formed the human microcosm, which was reflective of the larger universal macrocosm.

Health was achieved through a balance and blending of the humors. Hippocrates believed that dietetics was the basis for the art of healing. Thus, food could be used to achieve health and healing.

Current standard herbal textbooks are based on the herbal medicine book written by the Greek physician Dioscorides (cited by Oumeish). The term medica comes from the Greek mythological story of Medea, sorcerer of the seventh century and the land Media. Media is the area of current northwestern Iran and southwestern Turkey. The plants of Media were known as "median herbs" and their ointments, medicamentum, the root for our current term medications, could be used to heal or poison. This implied that medications could be used for healing or harming.

Rome in 27 BC

In the early days of Christianity, the system of medicine had a strong overlay of mysticism. The Christians believed that disease was the result of sinful behaviors and cure was achieved through grace or suffering. Often, the ability to touch a "holy relic" was a promise of healing. Some of the relics noted to have these healing properties included the "finger of the Holy Ghost," rays of the Star which led the Wise Men to the birthplace of Jesus," and a rib of the Word made flesh."

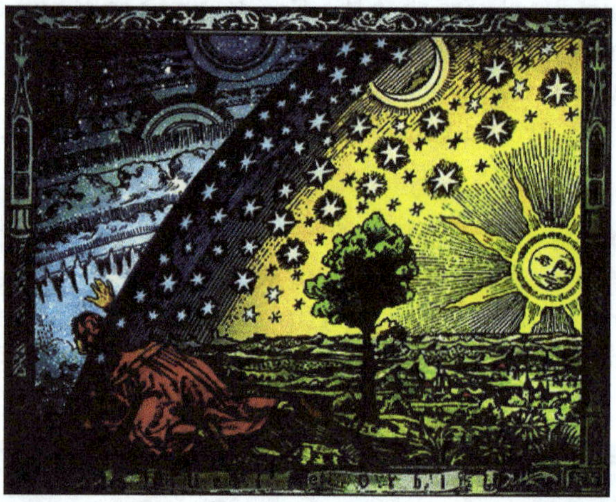

The Flammarion engraving is a wood engraving by an unknown artist that first appeared in Camille Flammarion's L'atmosphère: météorologie populaire. The image depicts a man crawling under the edge of the sky, depicted as if it were a solid hemisphere, to look at the mysterious Empyrean beyond. The caption translates to "A medieval missionary tells that he has found the point where heaven and Earth meet".

Much of Roman medicine was adapted from the Greeks. The Romans improved aromatherapy with their spas, saunas, and baths. Roman medicine was greatly influenced by the work of the prominent physician Galen. It was believed that imbalance in the four humors led to diseases, a belief that was originated by Hippocrates. After Galen's death, medicine in Rome began to stagnate. There was distrust in the system, which is now considered to be greedy, incompetent, and dishonest. The public sought new means of treatment from their own gardens, a principle known as Euporista. Books on the subject began to replace physicians. It was believed that nature provided remedies. In the late Roman period, individuals could practice medicine without training. Organized medicine was replaced by supernatural principles and home remedies. Public beliefs overran scientific principles.

Islamic Golden Age

During the Islamic Golden Age, Persian physicians contributed to medicine in two phases. The first was a period of translations (750–900 BC). The philosophers, Gerber (721 BC), Al-Kindi (801 BC), Rhazes (865 BC), Al-Farabi (872 BC), Avicenna (980 BC), and Averroës (1126 AD) had profound effect on the Dark Ages of Europe. The Dark Ages comprised a period of time when there was little advancement in the field of medicine.

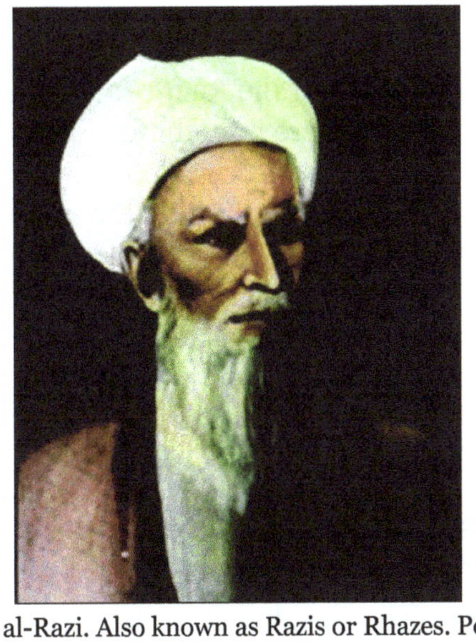

Figure: Muhammed ibn Zakariya al-Razi. Also known as Razis or Rhazes. Persian philosopher and physician.

The previous civilizations' medical knowledge, especially the Greek knowledge, was preserved, which enabled its passage to Europe upon that region's emergence from the Dark Ages period. Moir, a Scottish physician states that "medicine is incalculably indebted to the Saracens," [a generic term for Muslim during the later medieval era] "for the preservation of the Greek writers; as it was only after the return of the French, Italian and English from the Crusades that these came to be known in Europe, through translations from the Arabic."

The second period was a period of observations and expansion. (900–1100 BC). During the time of Mohammed, the culture promoted learning, arts, and sciences for intellectual development. The region established great medical colleges with strict admission guidelines. The schools followed rigorous scientific principles, and understood the use of anesthetics and hygiene. Their ancient materia medica rivals that of Western medical textbooks today.

Arabic medicine was practiced within the context of Islam's system of ethnics. It became known as Prophetic Medicine. It was believed that true medical knowledge came from revelations from the Prophet. It was supernatural, and esoteric, and filled with unconventional imagery; however, this medicine suited the majority of the people, was inexpensive, and was widely accepted. Arabic medicine was linked to philosophy and tied to numerical and astrological symbolism. Magicoreligious thoughts had significant influences on the system. Some of the practices included fortune telling, exorcisms, inspirations, amulets, healing gems and crystals, charms and spells, and cupping. The physician stressed treating the early symptoms by unconventional means to expose disease early treatable stages. These physicians often used herbals for such treatments. Although the Arabic physicians copied much from other civilizations, these physicians did expand their knowledge of medicine. They divided medicine into three distinct professions: physic; pharmacy; and surgery. In the areas of aromatics and purgatives, Arabic physicians added their knowledge to botanical and materia medicas extensively. Rhazes wrote the first treatise on the diseases of children. The Arabs raised the dignity of the medical profession from one of a menial calling to a learned profession with examinations and licensing.

The Renaissance to the Modern Era

The emergence of the Dark Ages into that of the Renaissance was largely the result of the Arabic period of translation. The ancient works were brought forward to the modern era through translation into the common language of the time: Latin. This was followed by an expansion in experimental investigation, particularly in dissection of the human body. As a result, human anatomy and neurology had significant advancements. Famous theories and principles were criticized and often debunked. Science began to replace mysticism. New publications spurred excitement and interest. Anatomical dissection theaters flourished, attracting artists, students, and scientists. University medical training began in Salerno and then later in Padua and Bologna, Italy, followed by France and England. However, this training was primarily academic with little clinical experience. Medicine began its descriptive phase.

During the next several centuries, medicine expanded in its scientific knowledge base exponentially. Technological advances contributed and enabled a deeper range of observations, interactions, and interventions. Generalities became specific. Specialization occurred at an unprecedented rate and to the point that there was subspecialization for treating minute portions of organ systems. As such, medicine became compartmentalized with some people stating that medicine had become depersonalized as well. This trend was advanced and complemented by economic, political, and military powers of the times. Powerful cultures colonized older, less-powerful cultures, so that Western medicine became global.

Shamans, Medicine Men and Curanderos

The term shaman comes from the Tungas language of Central Siberia. A shaman is an individual who enters altered states of consciousness in order to acquire knowledge and power and to help patients. Shamans use drums to call upon spirit allies. The repetitive sound of the drum facilitates the trance states in shamanistic practices. These drums are likened to a canoe or horse that transports the shaman into “the Lowerworld or Upperworld.” Shamanism cannot be learned, but rather, shamans are born into the life. This calling is that of a healer. Shamanism represents “the most widespread and ancient methodological system of healing known to humanity.”

During the practice of shamanism, both the shaman and the patient travel on the journey together. There is a deep level of connectedness between the two; something that is often lacking in today’s doctor–patient relationship. Despite the significant differences in the cultures and the separation by distances, shamanistic practices across the world are similar. Thus, “the basic uniformity of shamanic methods suggests that, through trial and error, people arrived at the same conclusions. In many regions of the world, the shaman is seen as “the great specialist of the human soul: he alone ‘sees’ it, for he knows its ‘form’ and its destiny.” Names such as witch, magic man, witchdoctor, seer, sorcerer and medicine man have been used interchangeably for shamans.

Shamanistic practices are very prevalent in traditional Native American practices of today. These shamans are often known as medicine men. Most of the pre-Columbian practices were not recorded or did not survive. The early European settlers provided the earliest accounts. Native Americans were not a homogenous population and, as such, neither were their practices. However, a common thread of the medicine men was that all aspects of life were intimately connected to good health and well-being. Life was a circle, and the healing included all aspects of an individual's life, family, and community. The medicine man practiced a highly advanced medicine that was effective for combating diseases that were common to their day. Some herbal-based treatments included echinacea (*Echinacea spp.*), ephedrine (*Ephedraceae spp.*) and cacao (*Theobroma cacao*) which are widely used in contemporary medicine and society.

Cacao was cultivated in the Mesoamerica region (current day central Mexico) dating back to 1900 BC. Cacao was so revered, that "all subjects in service to the Aztec emperor were required to bring several bags of cacao in tribute." The Aztecs mixed cacao with other ingredients such as chili (*Capsicum annuum*), black pepper (*Piper nigrum*), cornmeal or plantains to make the traditional drink chocolatl. Sugar was not added until 1528, when Columbus introduced cacao to the Spaniards. Cacao was used for a multitude of illnesses (weight gain, invigoration of the nervous system of the apathetic, exhausted or weak, improvement of digestion and bowel function and stimulation of kidney) as well as a flavoring for other medicines, especially those for children. In addition to the cacao bean, the leaves, flowers, bark and oil had medicinal properties that were used to treat burns, cuts and skin irritations.

The term curanderismo describes a broad healing tradition of Latin America. The word is derived from the Spanish verb curar, which means "to heal." There are seven pillars or cultural and historical roots of curanderismo. These represent the blending of ancient civilizations with the native populations of Latin America. The construct of curanderismo is based on the duality of natural and supernatural causes. Natural causes can be treated with herbal remedies, whereas the supernatural causes require treatment only by the supernatural manipulations performed by curanderos. Supernatural causes of illness are the result of either espiritos malos (evil spirits) or brujos. Brujos are individuals who practice maligning magic. The supernatural manipulations consist of several types of rituals such as sweeping, incensing, or conjuring, which lead to removal of negative forces. Curanderismo practices often provide better healing for chronic mental health conditions as well as for alcohol and drug addiction than interventions of Western psychiatry and psychology.

Economics of CAM

We refer to medical practices that evolved with indigenous peoples and that they have introduced to other countries through emigration as traditional medicine. We refer to approaches that emerged primarily in Western, industrial countries during the past two centuries as scientific or Western medicine, although we acknowledge that not all Western medicine is based on scientifically proven knowledge. The terms complementary and alternative describe practices and products that people choose as adjuncts to or as alternatives to Western medical approaches. Increasingly, the terms CAM and TM are being used interchangeably. Endless varieties of practices are scientifically unproven and poorly accepted by medical authorities. For the sake of organizing an agenda for research into these approaches, the U.S. National Institutes of Health has grouped them into five somewhat overlapping domains as follows:

- Biologically based practices: These include use of a vast array of vitamins and mineral supplements, natural products such as chondroitin sulfate, which is derived from bovine or shark cartilage; herbals, such as ginkgo biloba and echinacea; and unconventional diets, such as the low-carbohydrate approach to weight loss.
- Manipulative and body-based approaches: These kinds of approaches, which include massage, have been used throughout history. In the 19th century, additional formal manipulative disciplines emerged in the United States: chiropractic medicine and osteopathic medicine. Both originated in an attempt to relieve structural forces on vertebrae and spinal nerve roots that practitioners perceived as evoking a panoply of illnesses beyond mere musculoskeletal pain.
- Mind-body medicine: Many ancient cultures assumed that the mind exerts powerful influences on bodily functions and vice versa. Attempts to reassert proper harmony between these bodily systems led to the development of mind-body medicine, an array of approaches that incorporate spiritual, meditative, and relaxation techniques.
- Alternative medical systems: Whereas the ancient Greeks postulated that health requires a balance of vital humors, Asian cultures considered that health depends on the balance and flow of vital energies through the body. This latter theory underlies the practice of acupuncture, for example, which asserts that vital energy flow can be restored by placing needles at critical body points.
- Energy medicine: This approach uses therapies that involve the use of energy—either biofield- or bioelectromagnetic based interventions. An example of the former is Reiki therapy, which aims to realign and strengthen healthful energies through the intervention of energies radiating from the hands of a master healer.

Alternative systems of medicine use elements from each of these CAM and TM domains. For example, traditional Chinese medicine incorporates acupuncture, herbal medicines, special diets, and meditative exercises such as tai chi. Ayurveda in India similarly uses the meditative exercises of yoga, purifying diets, and natural products. In the West, homeopathic medicine and naturopathic medicine each arose in the late 19th century as reactions to the largely ineffectual and toxic conventional approaches of the day: purging, bleeding, and treatments with heavy metals such as mercury and arsenicals.

Demography use Toxicity and Efficacy

The use of CAM and TM varies widely between and within countries. The World Health Organization (WHO) has published and summarized numerous surveys of use. In developing nations, TM is the sole source of health care for all but the privileged few. By contrast, in affluent countries individuals select CAM approaches according to their specific beliefs. For example, as many as 60 percent of those living in France, Germany and the United Kingdom consume homeopathic or herbal products. Only 1 to 2 percent of Americans use homeopathy, but 10 percent of adults use herbal medicines, 8 percent visit chiropractors, and 1 to 2 percent undergo acupuncture every year. Use of CAM and TM among patients with chronic, painful, debilitating, or fatal conditions, such as HIV/AIDS and cancer, is far higher, ranging from 50 to 90 percent.

Table: Estimated use of CAM and TM by patients and practitioners worldwide.

Region or Country	Extent of Use
Africa	Used by 80 percent of the population for primary health care.
Australia	Used by 49 percent of adults.
China	Accounts for 30 to 50 percent of total health care. Fully integrated into the health system 95 percent of Chinese hospitals have TM units.
India	Widely used 2,860 hospitals provide TM.
Indonesia	Used by 40 percent of the entire population. Used by 70 percent of the rural population.
Japan	72 percent of physicians practice TM.
Thailand	TM integrated into 1,120 health centers.
Vietnam	Fully integrated into the health care system. 30 percent of the population is treated with TM.
Western countries	CAM and TM not strongly integrated into the health care system.
	France: at least 75 percent of the population has used CAM at least once.
	Germany: 77 percent of pain clinics provide acupuncture United States: 29 to 42 percent of population uses CAM.

There is remarkably little correlation between the use of CAM and TM approaches and scientific evidence that they are safe or effective. For many CAM and TM practices, the only evidence of their safety and efficacy is embodied in folklore. Beginning more than 1,500 years ago, data on the use of thousands of natural products were assembled into impressive monographs in China, India, and Korea, but these compendiums—and similar texts from Arabic, Egyptian, Greek, and Persian sources and their major European derivatives—are merely catalogs of products and their use rather than formal analyses of safety and efficacy.

Table: Some natural products that may alter drug actions.

Herbal Product	Class of Drug
Ephedra	Alpha and beta adrenergics.
Garlic	Anticoagulants; some HIV protease inhibitors.
Ginkgo biloba extract	Anticoagulants.
Glucosamine	Antidiabetics.
Saw palmetto	Androgens.
St. John's wort	HIV protease inhibitors; some chemotherapy drugs; cyclosporine A; birth control.
Valerian	Sedatives.

Many people who today choose herbal products in lieu of prescription medications assume that because these products are natural, they must be safe, even when the evidence for this assertion is essentially anecdotal. Recent studies have shown that herbals are highly variable in quality and composition, with many marketed products containing little of the intended ingredients and containing unintended contaminants, such as heavy metals and prescription drugs. A few herbals are banned outright in several countries. Comfrey and kava have been associated with liver failure, aristolochia with genitourinary cancer, and ephedra with heart attacks and strokes. More important, herbals contain ingredients that can accelerate or inhibit the metabolism of prescription drugs. The most notorious of these is St. John's wort, which affects the metabolism of nearly 50 percent of all prescription drugs. The cumulative data on the pharmacological and potential adverse effects of herbal supplements now dictate that patients discuss their use of supplements with knowledgeable practitioners before initiating treatment.

As to evidence of the efficacy of CAM and TM approaches, thousands of small studies and case series have been reported over the past 50 years. Few were rigorous enough to be at all compelling, but they are sufficient to generate hypotheses that are now being tested in robust clinical trials. The existing body of data already shows that some approaches are useless, that for many the evidence is positive but weak, and that a few are highly encouraging.

Economics of Complementary and Alternative Medicine and Traditional Medicine

Although social, medical, and cultural reasons may account for why people in a given country prefer CAM and TM to conventional (Western) medicine, economic forces are also at play. Much of this evidence is from industrial countries; few studies have been conducted in or are applicable to low- and middle-income countries. This caveat is important for two reasons. First, the CAM and TM modalities discussed in this section may not be used in many developing countries. Second, the limited data on cost-effectiveness may not be applicable in the case of those countries. Nevertheless, the data give a rough picture of the relative cost-effectiveness of a number of CAM and TM practices.

Economic Factors that Influence the use of Complementary and Alternative Medicine and Traditional Medicine

Users of CAM and TM approaches choose health practices that resonate with their beliefs about health. Although economic factors play a role in this choice, the underlying incentives are not always predictable. For instance, a common misconception is that patients opt for CAM and TM services because they are cheaper alternatives to conventional medical care. Even though there are certainly instances when the cost of treatment using CAM or TM is much cheaper than the cost of accessing a conventional medical service, several studies have found that CAM and TM cost the same or more than conventional treatments for the same conditions.

At least one study has shown that financial considerations are rarely the primary factor in choosing a traditional healer, ranking behind such reasons as confidence in the treatment, ease of access, and convenience. In the United States, the average cost of a single visit to a Navajo healer was US$388, and the average annual cost of using a traditional healer represented roughly a fifth of the reported annual income of respondents in a survey. The high cost of using a healer was cited as the most common barrier to seeking care from this source. In Kenya, the average charge per patient per visit to a TM practitioner was K Sh 46 (US$4 in 1981), which was significantly greater than the average charge per visit even in private health care facilities. Finally, a survey in Zimbabwe reported that the median cost of consulting an herbalist was Z$23 per visit, compared with Z$1 for a government clinic and Z$29 for a private doctor. The same survey found that outcomes tended to be better when patients went to government clinics (67.3 percent of visits resulted in a good outcome) than when patients consulted herbalists (50 percent of visits resulted in a good outcome).

TM is not always more expensive than conventional medicine. People in Ghana reported that the cost of malaria treatment at a health clinic ranged from ¢1,900 to ¢3,000 (US$1.30 to US$2.00 in 1997), treatment at home using drugs bought from pharmacies or health care workers ranged between ¢200 and ¢1,000 (US$0.10 to US$0.70), and treatment by an herbalist was virtually free.

Table: Levels of evidence for the efficacy of selected CAM and TM approaches.

CAM or TM Approach	Potential Use	Study Outcome	Level of Evidence
Artemisia annua	Treating drug-resistant malaria.	Positive	A
Black cohosh	Controlling menopausal symptoms.	Mixed	B
Cranberry	Preventing urinary tract infection.	Positive	B
Echinacea	Preventing or treating viral colds.	Mixed	B
Garlic	Lowering blood cholesterol.	Positive	C
Ginkgo biloba extract	Preventing or treating dementia.	Mixed	B
Ginseng	Improving energy and immunity against infection.	Mixed	C
Glucosamine	Relieving osteoarthritis.	Positive	A
Hawthorn	Improving cardiac function.	Mixed	B
Milk thistle	Improving liver function.	Positive	C
St. John's wort	Treating moderate to severe depression.	Negative	A
	Treating mild depression.	Positive	B
Saw palmetto	Relieving symptoms of benign prostatic hypertrophy.	Positive	B
Acupuncture	Relieving arthritis pain.	Positive	B
	Relieving the pain of tooth extraction.	Positive	B
	Treating hypertension.	Mixed	C
	Relieving nausea from chemotherapy.	Positive	A
	Relieving addiction withdrawal.	Mixed	B
	Treating asthma.	Negative	B
Meditation	Decreasing anxiety.	Positive	B
	Decreasing blood pressure.	Mixed	B
Biofeedback	Preventing migraine.	Positive	B
Homeopathy	Treating asthma.	Mixed	B
	Treating gastroenteritis.	Positive	C
Magnet therapy	Treating plantar fasciitis.	Negative	B
Chiropractic	Treating lower back pain.	Positive	B

Here, A = multiple high-quality, randomized, controlled trials; B = single high-quality trials or smaller, less rigorous trials; C = weaker clinical trials; Mixed = conflicting results among studies of similar quality.

Another common misconception is that the poor are more likely to use TM. At least one study shows that this may not be true. In Zimbabwe, the mean monthly income of households visiting an herbalist, Z$877, was greater than the mean monthly income of households using government clinics, Z$718. Although some traditional healers charge more than conventional practitioners, their fees may be negotiable, the method of payment may be flexible (often on credit or in exchange for labor), and payment may be contingent on outcome. The availability of an outcome-contingent contract favors TM over Western medicine when the disease condition requires providers to both exert effort in curing patients and induce patients to comply with their recommendations. Nonetheless, this strategy may be difficult to apply to the larger health care system.

Furthermore, patients tend to seek care from traditional healers for conditions such as mental illness, impotence, and chronic disorders, which they perceive as requiring greater involvement by the extended family and kinship group. Accordingly, the availability of financial support for seeking treatments for these disorders is greater than it is for illnesses such as malaria or diarrhea, for which patients more often seek conventional treatment.

Rise of CAM in U.S.

In 1992 the U.S. Congress established the Office of Unconventional Therapies, later changed to the Office of Alternative Medicine (OAM), to explore "unconventional medical practices." Two million dollars was appropriated, and OAM began to develop a baseline of information on CAM use in the United States. Alternative Medicine: Expanding Medical Horizons was released in 1995 and summarized the results of two workshops on CAM convened by OAM. The report (often referred to as the "Chantilly Report") examined six fields of alternative medicine and addressed issues such as research infrastructure, research databases, and research methodologies. Many of the recommendations made addressed research needs and opportunities. The report was significant because it was the result of the first NIH-sanctioned meetings held to discuss the field of CAM as a whole.

Responding to public and industry input, Congress passed the Dietary Supplement Health and Education Act (DSHEA) in 1994. DSHEA legally established the term "dietary supplement" and decreed that supplements were to be regulated similar to foods. This distinction exempted manufacturers from conducting premarketing safety and efficacy testing and eliminated the Food and Drug Administrations's (FDA's) premarketing regulatory authority. In 1995, NIH funded the Research Centers Program to provide a nationwide focus for interdisciplinary CAM research in academic institutions. Also in 1995, following a 1994 NIH and FDA workshop on acupuncture, FDA declassified acupuncture needles as an experimental product. In 1996 the Public Information Clearinghouse on CAM was established and NIH sponsored the Consensus Conference on Acupuncture, which provided evidence of the effectiveness of acupuncture for some conditions (e.g., dental pain and nausea). The first large, multicenter trial of a CAM therapy was cofunded in 1997 by OAM, the National Institute on Mental Health, and the NIH Office of Dietary Supplements. The trial tested the effect of Hypericum (St. John›s wort) for depression.

By 1998 the use of CAM was widely discussed and hotly debated. A New England Journal of Medicine editorial argued that "It's time for the scientific community to stop giving CAM a free ride. There cannot be two kinds of medicine—conventional and alternative. There is only medicine that has been adequately tested and medicine that has not, medicine that works and medicine that may or may not work." An editorial in the Journal of the American Medical Association contended that "There is no Alternative Medicine. There is only scientifically proven, evidence-based medicine supported by solid data or unproven medicine, for which scientific evidence is lacking". The American Medical Association devoted space to the topic of CAM in its theme journals and published a total of 80 articles and the results of 18 randomized trials. Included were editorials, descriptive articles, systematic reviews, and results of randomized controlled trials. For the first time, CAM was addressed as a complex issue and journal editors were willing to subject these articles to the same criteria and editorial review as articles addressing topics in conventional medicine.

Meanwhile, Congress, having increased the OAM budget from the original $2 million to $19.5 million, elevated OAM to the level of a national center named NCCAM in 1998, awarded it $48.9 million for fiscal year (FY) 1999, and required that NCCAM appoint CAM practitioners as members of its Advisory Council. In 1999, the Cancer Advisory Panel for CAM was established for the purpose of assessing clinical data related to CAM treatment of cancer and the first Dietary Supplements Research Center was funded jointly by NCCAM and the NIH Office of Dietary Supplements. NIH funded nine Centers for Research of Complementary and Alternative Medicine to conduct interdisciplinary research and training. Three multicenter research studies were funded: one on Ginkgo biloba for the treatment of dementia (cofunded by NCCAM and the National Institute on Aging), one on glucosamine and chondroitin sulfate for the treatment of knee osteoarthritis (cofunded by NCCAM and the National Institute of Arthritis and Musculoskeletal and Skin Diseases), and one on acupuncture for osteoarthritis of the knee (funded by NCCAM). Also in 1999 large pharmaceutical companies entered the CAM market with herbal product lines and other dietary supplements.

Several major events occurred in 2000 and 2001. In March 2000, President Clinton created the White House Commission on Complementary and Alternative Medicine Policy. The purpose of the commission was to "study and report on public policy issues in the rapidly expanding field of complementary and alternative medicine." Furthermore, the commission was asked to report on "legislative and administrative recommendations to assure that public policy maximizes the benefits to Americans of appropriate use of complementary and alternative medicine". The commission's report provided recommendations about research on CAM, education and training in CAM, CAM information dissemination, delivery of CAM practices, coverage and reimbursement for CAM services, the potential role of CAM in wellness and health promotion, and the need for coordination of CAM-related efforts.

The Federation of State Medical Boards began work on CAM guidelines for physicians in 2000. The initiative was focused on "encouraging the medical community to adopt consistent standards, ensuring the public health and safety by facilitating the proper and effective use of both conventional and CAM treatments, while educating physicians on the adequate safeguards needed to assure these services are provided within the bounds of acceptable professional practice". The federation's House of Delegates approved the guidelines in April 2002. The Consortium of Academic Health Centers for Integrative Medicine was launched in 2000 and by 2003 it had 22 member medical schools. To become a member, either the dean or chancellor is required to commit to developing programs in research, education, and clinical delivery of CAM and the school must demonstrate an organized and robust program in two of those three areas. The mission of the consortium is "to help transform medicine and healthcare through rigorous scientific studies, new models of clinical care, and innovative educational programs that integrate biomedicine, the complexity of human beings, the intrinsic nature of healing and the rich diversity of therapeutic systems".

Skeptics of CAM had long contended that the only benefit derived from CAM therapies was due to a placebo effect, not "real" effects. In November 2000 NIH hosted a workshop, The Science of the Placebo: Toward an Interdisciplinary Research Agenda, thereby helping to place placebo in the category of a "real" effect. The August 2001 issue of Science published an article on basic science mechanisms of placebo. These two events triggered expanded interest among the neuroscience community in the study of the impact of nonspecific effects (e.g., expectation, context, belief) on clinical outcomes. Placebo was no longer something to be discarded or dismissed but, rather, something to be studied. Also in 2001, NCCAM and the National Library of Medicine developed CAM. At present, almost 40,000 citations on CAM can be found on the PubMed website. Additionally, clinically significant adverse drug-herb interactions were documented in case studies, and St. John's wort was shown to reduce the level of indinavir, a protease inhibitor taken by AIDS patients, in plasma.

In 2002, NCCAM launched its Intramural Program to explore CAM treatment strategies for patients at the NIH Clinical Center, the world's largest facility dedicated to patient-oriented research. Also in that year, the U.S. Department of Veterans Affairs agreed to provide reimbursement for chiropractic care, the Annals of Internal Medicine began a special series on CAM (17 publications), and Science Xpress published an article on positron emission spectrometry, imaging of the placebo response versus the response to opiod analgesics, thereby signaling continued interest in the application of modern technology to the mechanistic study of placebo-related phenomena. NCCAM, whose budget had grown to $104.6 million in 2002, funded 10 international planning grants, and across NIH more than 200 research projects on CAM were ongoing. Also in that year, IOM established the Committee on the Use of Complementary and Alternative Medicine by the American Public. In 2003, the first two Centers of Excellence for Research on CAM were funded to increase scientific rigor in research on CAM. By 2004 the NCCAM budget was $117.8 million.

Causes of Rise of CAM

The causes of the rise in demand for CAM are largely unknown and little researched. Our somewhat speculative explanations for this social phenomenon include the ageing population, and a growing emphasis on chronic illness and lifestyle-related morbidity rather than acute illness. In such instances, where conventional medicine may be perceived to be less successful, CAM may appear to have much more to offer (e.g., the use of acupuncture for chronic pain).

In this substantively new stage of human history known as the postmodern era, a second explanation might be the so-called postmodern thesis. This suggests that as social change (also involving globalisation) has accelerated, faith in the ability of science and technology (including medicine) to solve the problems of living has declined. Social "green" movements with a preference for organic and non-chemical solutions to problems have arisen. Societal trends toward individualism seem to us to have influenced healthcare trends, with individuals being less prepared to accept traditional authority, such as doctors, and seeking greater levels of control and empowerment over their lives (a trend fuelled by the Internet). The postmodern thesis is an interesting one, but the difficulty lies in translating the broad concept to concrete empirical evidence. While cross-sectional survey data can show that those using CAM hold postmodernist beliefs or opinions, drawing causal inferences from such data is more difficult.

Moreover, any explanation for why more patients are choosing CAM must also account for why patients are increasingly able to exercise this choice, have it met by more CAM providers and, in some instances, paid for by the state and insurance plans. Two broad social changes are implicated. The first is the impact of the consumer movement on healthcare. While postmodernist values can be predictors of use of alternative healthcare, other factors that affect the individual, such as higher education, poorer health, a transformational experience that changed the person's worldview, a commitment to the environment, feminism, spirituality and personal growth have also been predictive. Another important reason for growth in CAM use in the last 20 years is increased migration and the transmission of established medicines from other lands (e.g., Ayurvedic medicine, traditional Chinese medicine).

Allied with this has been the politicisation of health. The clearest example here has been feminism, but it can also be seen in the gay movement (particularly around HIV) and in the green movement. Politicisation of health returns control of health to the individual and control of the healthcare system to the community. It is significant that the growth of CAM has coincided, both in the United States and elsewhere, with a lessening of medical dominance. For much of its history, medicine has contained CAM by ensuring that it was not taught in medical schools or universities; did not have access to research funding; did not get access to hospitals, laboratories and services that might have enhanced their services to their patients; was not covered by government and private insurance; did not obtain state licensure or registration; and that the private educational institutions created by CAM providers did not receive funding. All of these significantly impeded the legitimacy of CAM. Much of it was made possible by medicine claiming to be acting in the public interest. As the consumer movement gained strength and healthcare became politicised, this defence lost its legitimacy and legality. Consumers demanded to act in their own interest and legislation made restraint of trade illegal, even for medicine.

Other specific causes may have contributed to the growth of CAM, and will probably do so in the future. One is the declining competitive advantage of conventional doctors as bulk billing is abandoned, which means patients may be more willing to try alternatives, even though CAM services have never been cheap. Further, as Internet use grows, patients may find more and more useful information about CAM treatments, whatever the problems with some of that information might be.

References

- Historical-and-Cultural-Perspectives-on-Integrative-Medicine: liebertpub.com, Retrieved 21, April 2020
- Rise-and-rise-complementary-and-alternative-medicine-sociological-perspective: mja.com.au, Retrieved 28, January 2020

Chapter 2

Traditional Medicine Practices

Traditional medicine practices include the utilization of skills, practices and knowledge based on theories and experiences of different cultures to prevent, diagnose and treat physical and mental illness. There are different forms of traditional medicine such as traditional Mongolian medicine, traditional Chinese medicine, Iranian traditional medicine, etc. This chapter has been carefully written to provide an easy understanding of the varied facets of these traditional medicine practices.

Traditional Mongolian Medicine

The Mongols materialized the will of their ancestors including Chinggis Khaan to establish the independent country in the Central Asian plateau and aiming to build democracy and civil society, should refine the unquestionable truth through authentic historical facts from the mixture of actualities and illusions. New facts, new materials to enrich history of medical development have continuously been found. More materials are being written and more focus is being paid on the history of medical development covering the period before Indian ayurvedic medicine which was introduced to Mongolia with the third revival of Buddhism from Tibet.

Bone Art

The Mongolian art of bone setting, called 'bone art' in Mongolia, is a fascinating subject. It developed mainly during the Chin dynasty. The eminent practitioners were Tsorj-Mergen, NaraAbai and Heru-Ishinga and various others. Bonesetters (Bariachi) used many interesting methods, such as applying cupping glasses (made of horn) to treat broken bones, or a herbal compress, or, if necessary, used surgery with the aid of ice as a local anesthetic. The Aduuchiin Minister called together 30 professionals in the field and established a special Bone Art Hospital at this time.

Bone Art is a completely independent branch of Mongolian medicine. Bariachi were local people who still believed in Shamanism for they were not educated and therefore untouched by Buddhism. For an accidental bone fracture or dislocation, the Mongols would automatically approach the Bariachi, who had no medicines or surgical instruments. The Bariachi would simply hold the fractured or dislocated limb in their hands and massage it or give it a twist or two. The patient would feel no pain, but was usually advised to rest afterwards. These born healers were just lay people without schooling, but neither spelled charms nor performed rituals. They cured bone disorders perfectly without complaint from the patient or pain afterwards, however serious the injury. The bones would heal quite soon afterwards. These healers had no special training except what was handed down to them, but they needed to have the ability born in them. Their hands were the healing instruments, and setting was done by very sensitive touch. Such healers usually came from a family of traditional bonesetters. Sons or daughters would become bonesetters, having learned from their parents. However, some had a following of disciples who were taught to treat skillfully and professionally.

Balneotherapy

Mongolia has a large land area with many pure rivers, lakes and springs, particularly hot springs. In view of this, balneotherapy has always been widespread in both Outer, and Inner, Mongolia. There are over 30 springs which can be used for treatment. Scholars have written books on the subject and about what kinds of diseases can be treated by it.

Dom Therapy

Mongolia has another kind of therapy called “Dom”, which again, like bone setting, has nothing to do with medical science or religious beliefs, nor was it based on superstition. It falls into the category of folklore and ancient custom. It may be ‘old wives’ tales’ but people still believe in it. It might be termed ‘comfort therapy’. For example, if a person has trouble in their left eye, they are supposed to touch the affected eye with their right knee seven times, early in the morning, before breakfast. That should cure it! If a child can’t sleep comfortably and wakes suddenly or cries in the night for no apparent reason, the parent has only to draw a picture of a fox and hang it over the child’s bed and the child will sleep soundly. If someone has a headache, they should drink a cup of hot tea. If they have stomach trouble they should keep off food for a while. For mental unrest, just count your breath. This probably has more to do with psychology, but gives a person some control over minor ailments.

At the end of the 16th century Buddhism emerged in Mongolia and the Tibetan medicine which was originated from Indian Ayurvedic medicine, was adopted. The change in the medicine was initiated as a result of fights among Mongol nobles for the throne, Manchurian intrusion and religious influence. In such circumstances Mongols adopted Tibetan medical school. After that, Mongols gradually gained much success to plant the Tibetan medicine in the Mongolian soil through renewal of the Tibetan medical theory, substitution of some medical herbs with ones grown in Mongolia, supplementing some treatments with magic treatment elements. These efforts were strengthened by the intellectual scope and capability of Mongols and became the basis to establish a new paradigm of the Mongolian medicine with a blend of Tibetan medicine. Another stimulus to establish the new paradigm was the whole set of differences of Mongols including physiological features, their food consumption, harsh changeable climate, lifestyle, and mindset etc. They faced the necessity to establish theory and practice to heal the diseases occurred due to above mentioned circumstances. For example, Tibetan medicine lacked certain understanding about different types of massage therapy such as gentle rubbing, pressure giving and assembling etc. that were useful to heal fractures, injuries and collision which were common occurrences in daily lives of Mongols. Such deficits were, as shown by some historical facts, completed by Mongol doctors and scholars. As a result, Mongols managed to establish the complete Mongolian medical system based on their original magic treatment with adoption of the Indian Ayurveda, absorption of Chinese acupuncture and theory and methodology of the Tibetan medicine.

Sensitive Period for Traditional Medicine

On March 13th, 1921, the newly formed Communist Party of Mongolia’s Central Committee put together a Mongolian People’s Provisional government, and, after Sukhbaatar’s Mongolian Partisan Army (assembled in February 1921) had defeated the Chinese aggressive forces and regained the Mongolian city of Khiagt (across the border from Kyakhta), a new capital, Ulaanbaatar, was proclaimed. An army of defense, made up of Mongolian and Soviet military forces had been created meanwhile, and by early July it had driven von Ungern-Sternberg's forces out of Niislel Khuree, had occupied the city. On July 11th, the date now recognized as Mongolia's National Day, the rule of the Bogd Khan, a limited monarchy nominally headed by the Jebtsundamba Khutukhtu under the title of Khan, was replaced by the new People's Government of Mongolia.

On September 14th, 1921, the independence of Mongolia was proclaimed, and on October 26th, a legislative assembly, the National Provisional Little Hural, was inaugurated. The formalization of Soviet-Mongolian relations was then accelerated, and, on November 5th, 1921, a Bilateral Agreement of Mutual Recognition and Friendly Relations was signed in Moscow. This officially recognized the authority of the People's Government and facilitated the exchange of diplomatic representatives.

Health beliefs and practices had earlier been based solely on Mongolian Traditional Medicine, with emchi (doctors) and lamas. Nevertheless, health workers mainly those fleeing Czarist Russia, had been developing private health practices using western methods from 1906 onwards. In 1921, the first hospital to combine Traditional and Western medicine practices with outpatients' department and pharmacy was established in Mongolia. There were many doctors on the staff, including a Hungarian and at least 10 Mongolian Traditional practitioners. In addition to this, on August 15th 1021, General Sukhbaatar signed a resolution to establish a military hospital at Niislel Khuree now renamed Ulaanbaatar, and the new Mongolian government invited Dr. P.N Shastin, an eminent Soviet doctor to head it. Several other Mongolian traditional doctors worked alongside Dr. Shastin in the new hospital. However, on March 13th 1937, the government decided to close the traditional medical clinics and pharmacies because of conflicts of ideology. From this time on, the practice of traditional medicine was officially suppressed and eventually forgotten in Mongolia until the end of the 1980's. After the collapse of socialism, the democratic government realised the importance of traditional medicine to satisfy the needs of a population whose health system had broken down, and made efforts to revive it.

Traditional Mongolian Practices

Social health elements were initially developed among the sedentary societies, yet the Mongolians created preventive health measures that suited their nomadic lifestyle, and they have been converted to daily routines and traditions over the years. To keep drinking water clear, Mongolians did not prohibit animals from grazing around the source of any river, nor did they throw any garbage, food, or drink into water. Their ancestors treated water with great respect calling it chindamani (wishing jewel) and taught their children not to pollute any water areas. There was a tradition of not spoiling north-side areas with excretions. This was a result of observing wind directions, which usually blow from the north to the south. By never polluting on the north sides of land, the people avoided spreading viruses carried by the winds. Generally, they treated human waste very carefully. Women usually relieved themselves on the southeast side of their ger (traditional Mongolian dwelling) while men relieve on the southwest side. They use euphemisms instead of direct expressions to relieve themselves. For example, men say "to watch their horse", but women say, "to watch a mare or cow". In addition, ash and other dry wastes were thrown to the west side. Before moving to other places; wastes had to be buried; any holes of stakes were filled with soil; and the surrounding areas were cleared up.

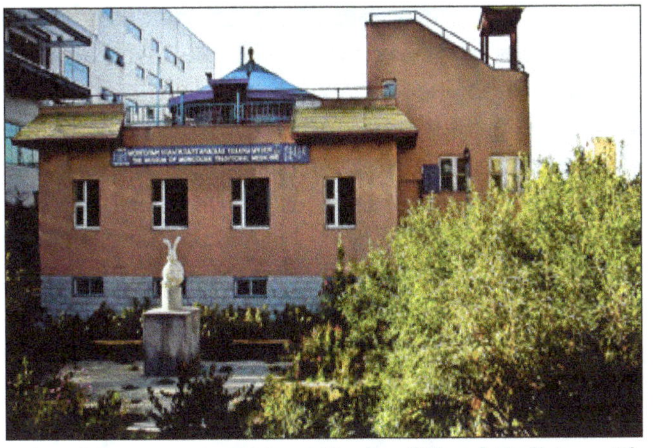

Figure: Exterior of the Museum of Mongolian Traditional Medicine, with a statue of a rabbit, the symbol of traditional Mongolian medicine.

Furthermore, their ancestors developed many traditions to form healthy lifestyles by preventing infections. Traditional Mongolian dress was created for four seasons and suited their daily activities well, such as riding horses, dealing with horses and livestock, and hunting.

A short deel (clothing), loose pants and boots worn by Mongolian soldiers were one factor in defeating Jao soldiers who wore clothes with long sleeves and skirts. The Mongolian deel has many important uses. It can be used as a blanket when someone needs to sleep outside, it can be used as a shield when they relieve themselves, and it can protect the upper and lower parts of the body from heat and cold equally. Mongolian boots have a turned-up nose to prevent the nose from digging into the ground and soil.

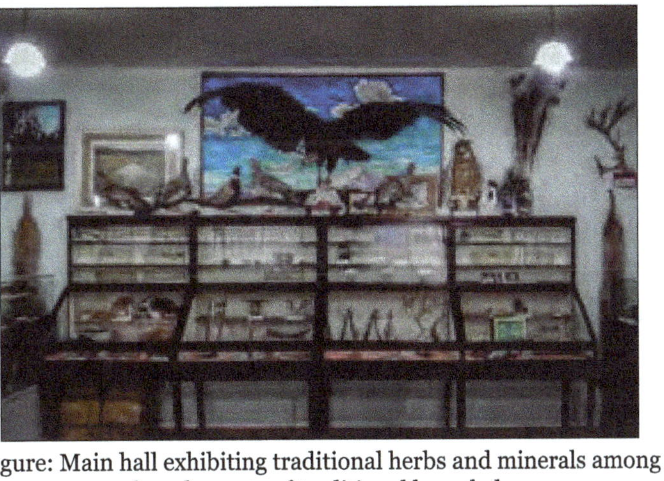

Figure: Main hall exhibiting traditional herbs and minerals among other elements of traditional knowledge.

All Mongolians had their own special cups. When they visited families, men sat on the right side and women sat on the left side in accordance with their age. Hostesses took their cups from them and filled them with tea. The cups were carried in small bags. In the beginning, wooden and gradually copper, silver and golden cups were used. Having their own cups helped prevent infections. Another thing is the Mongolians carried their own handkerchiefs and they never exchanged them. Wealthier ones carried woollen cloth, and after eating they wiped their mouth and hands with the cloth.

Belts have special significance in Mongolia. Belt, belly or back bands were important for health, especially to protect people's backs from cold winds. The belt was thought to keep a man's spirit, so the belt was always treated with respect. In early times, both men and women wore belts. However, when the distinction between men's and women's work later appeared, women eventually stopped wearing them after marriage. During the wedding ceremony, the groom cut his bride's under-belt. Thus, women got the name busgui, (literally, "without belt") after their wedding.

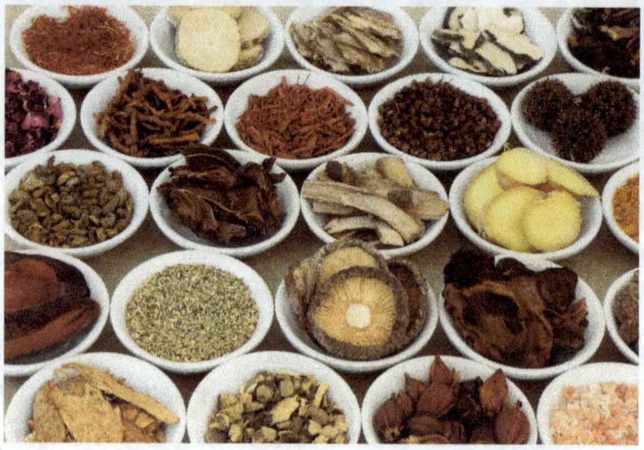

Figure: Collection of dried berries and minerals used in making traditional medicine.

Mongolians had unique child-rearing traditions, especially in relation to infants. The adults made nappies by latticing wood pieces or using sheep fur. From the 13th century, nappies were made of metal and Mongolians also used nappies made of animal wool and ash. The woollen nappy was placed in the crotch to absorb the liquid, keeping the infant's skin dry, and ash nappies were placed under the infant's bottom. A piece of a tail of a sheep has been given to infants to suckle to make them healthier. Sheep's tail has been identified to include unsaturated fatty acids. It is amazing that early Mongolians discovered the benefits of this and put it into practice.

When boys turned three, the parents tied the boys to a saddle on a horse and led them on a gallop. After the boys reached four or five, their parents prepared a small bow and arrow and gave them introductory tips on how to hunt. Mongolian children grew up strong, lively and skilful. Mongolians also paid special attention to their children's diet. For instance, children were not allowed to eat bone marrow to prevent early sexual development. Also, they were not allowed to drink tea with certain ingredients until marriage to avoid increasing body heat, which could hurt the liver and bladder. Instead, they drank boiled water with milk. There were many taboos concerning health and hygiene among Mongolians. It was forbidden to visit the mother and the baby within a month after the birth. If a boy was born, a sign was hung on the right. On the contrary, if a girl was born, a sign was hung on the left.

Mongolians have been producing dairy products since they domesticated animals. Over 2,000 years ago the Hunnu fermented horse milk and started to make curds. Because milk products were considered a healthy food, and a basis for a long healthy life, milk products have been a main part of the diet. Mongolians have gained much knowledge in preparing and using milk products. For instance, raw milk is rarely drunk. Instead they drink boiled milk or milk tea. A wide range of products such as tarag (like yogurt), curds, and cheese can be made from milk.

People in the olden days used to live longer as they followed correct lifestyle in comparison with modern people who crave sweets, ignore good advice, and refuse to follow a healthy life plan.

People, who understand the need for a right lifestyle, do not excessively consume meat and fat. They restrict desires and emotions and keep a good physique thus saving strength. They tolerate sadness and depression, ignore unnecessary desires, avoid inappropriate appetites and concentrate on solidifying internal strengths, thus keeping their composure. People who take care of themselves usually do not eat until hungry. They do not eat when they're full. They drink when they are thirsty. They usually do not eat and drink in large quantities. Overfeeding damages the lungs but hunger hurts your strength.

- Do not lie down when you're full. It causes various diseases.
- Do not be exposed to wind or coldness after having hot food and drink when you are sweating. This is to prevent headaches, exhaustion etc.
- Do not eat too much late in the afternoon. Avoid sleeping in areas where it is cold and possibly there is a draught.
- Do not relieve yourself in a north-westerly direction.
- Go to the toilet at regular intervals.
- Do not relieve yourself in the direction of the sun, moon, stars, temples, monasteries or springs.
- Do not hum or make loud noises during the night.
- Do not eat 12 parts of meat relating to birthday organs on you or your parents' birthday.
- Sit straight and try to concentrate.
- Do not stand for long hours. It will harm your bones.
- Do not sit for long hours. It will damage your blood.
- Do not walk for long hours. It will damage your sinews.
- Do not lie for long hours. It will kill your strength.
- Do not wash your head after eating.
- Restrict love affairs if your eyes are hurt. Otherwise this could lead to albugo.
- Do not be exposed to coldness or any wind after washing your body as the skin pores are open.
- Do not go in and out during strong winds, heavy rain, cold or hot temperatures.
- Do not blow out candles. It will weaken your strength.
- Do not stare or glance straight at the sun when it is bright as it will hurt the eyes.
- Do not attempt to see long distances with great intensity as this will affect eye strength.
- Do not sit or lie on the wet ground.

- Do not sleep in candle light.
- Close your door and burn incense when lightning strikes during heavy rain. The gods may pass by.
- Do not spit in your immediate environment.
- Do not have tea on an empty stomach.
- Do not eat rice soup after the hour of the monkey.
- Our ancestors taught us to boil down glass noodles, meat and to have less vodka.
- People in olden times took times of themselves all throughout their life while people in the modern era neglect their own personal welfare until their bodies start to complain.
- If you press your eyes with your palm after rubbing them before sleeping, it will prevent eye diseases.
- If you massage gently your face with your palm after rubbing them before sleep, it will prevent the appearance of 'chancre'.

Herbs in Mongolian Medicine

About 3160 species (included 133 subspecies and 33 varieties), 684 genera, and 108 families of vascular plants exist in Mongolia. Among them, herbal plants rich in vitamins, essential oils, tannins, dyes, flavonoids, alkaloids and coumarins were distinguished.

Table: The classification of the Mongolian plant species.

No.	Plant Specie	Content
1	Herbal medicine	~1100
2	Ornamental plants	480
3	Alkaloid bearing plants	280
4	Tannins bearing plants	250
5	Flavonoid bearing plants	231
6	Essential oil producing plants	200
7	Dye-stuff plants	200
8	Industry-use plants	200
9	High vitamin content plants	150
10	Soil protecting plants	68
11	Coumarin bearing plants	65

About 32% of the total vascular plants found in Mongolia are registered as medicinal plants, and among them more than 200 plants species could be used for manufacturing modern western medicines. Fabaceae, Asteraceae, Rosaceae, Ranunculaceae and Papaveraceae are the most dominant families in the Mongolian herbal plant species.

Table: The plant species of families of the vascular flora.

No.	Family Name	Genera Name	Genera Number	Species Number	Percent of Total Flora
1	Fabaceae	Faba	6	40	1.3
2	Asteraceae	Aster	12	23	0.7
3	Rosaceae	Potentilla	3	16	0.5
4	Ranunculaceae	Ranunculus	6	9	0.3
5	Papaveraceae	Papaver	2	6	0.2
6	Brassicaceae	Draba	4	5	0.2
7	Lamiaceae	Lamium L	3	3	0.1
8	Plumbaginaceae	Limonium	1	3	0.1
9	Juncaceae	Juncus L	2	2	0.1
10	Plantaginaceae	Plantago L	1	1	0.1

The main life form of the plant species with orthodox seeds is a perennial followed by annual and biannual grasses.

Table: Distribution of different plant life forms.

No.	Plant Life Form	Content, %
1	Perennial grasses	72.2
2	Annual/biannual grasses	13.5
3	Semi-shrubs/shrubby	3.7
4	Shrub	6.0
5	Shrubby	2.0
6	Low trees	1.6
7	Large trees	0.7
8	Vines	0.3

Useful Medicinal Herbs

In 2013, member states of WHO's Western Pacific Region introduced details the nature and application of the most useful medicinal herbs found in Mongolia. Most of the Mongolians apply the medicinal herbs in their everyday life. There are some samples of the most popular medicinal herbs:

1. Mongolian Name: Ikh Shuudergene

Tibetan Name: Donroiselva

English Name: Greater Celandine

Traditional Uses: It is bitter in taste with cooling potential and is used for treating typhoid fever, bile disorder burn wounds alleviating fever, soothing pain dermatitis and papillomas.

Chemical Constituents: 1.4-4.3% organic acids, 0.01% essential oil, saponins, flavonoids, phenol carboxylic acid, alkaloids: chelerythrine, sanguinarine chelidonine, berberine, coptisine, chelidimerine, chelirubine. The main alkaloids are chelidonine, chelerythrine, sanguinarine and berberine.

Bioactivities: Sedative, anesthetic, spasmolytic, antifungal, antiviral antibacterial, hypotensive, analgesic, cytostatic, cytotoxic, antitumor antimicrobial, stimulation of the dopaminergic system and inhibition of the serotonergic system.

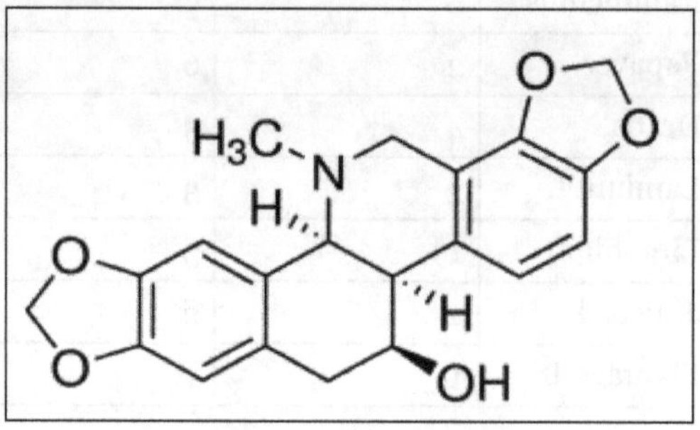

Figure: Chelidonine.

2. Mongolian Name: Ikh Tavansalaa i Ukher-Uurgene, Khongolon

Tibetan Name: Taram

English Name: Rippleseed Plantain

Traditional Uses: It is sweet in taste with warming potential and is used for treating diarrhoea, hematuria and as diuretic drug.

Chemical Constituents: The leaves contain sugars: 20% polysaccharide, pectic acid, mannitol, sorbitol, iridoids: 1% aucubin, catalpol, phenolcarboxylic acids and their derivatives: vanillic, n-hydroxybenzoic, chlorogenic and neochlorogenic acids, flavonoids: baicalein, baicalin, scutellerein, luteolin and others, alkaloids, and terpenoids.

Bioactivities: Sedative, antihypertensive, anti-inflammatory activity, ulcerogenic, antimicrobial activity, mucolytic.

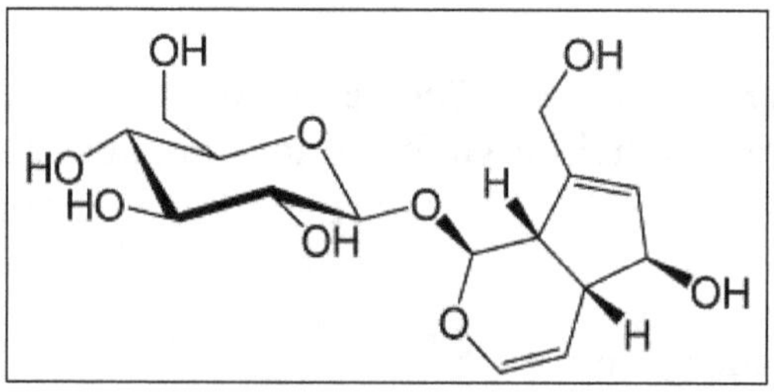

Figure: Aucubin.

3. Mongolian Name: Yagaan Mugez (Altangagnuur)

Tibetan Name: Tsanser

English Name: Rose boot

Traditional Uses: It is bitter in taste and has astringent and cooling properties, and is used for treatment of inflammation of the lung fever and to strengthen the body. In addition, it is used to tap the mouth to refresh the breath.

Chemical Constituents:

Sugars: glucose, galactose, arabinose, rhamnose, organicacids, 15.9-20.3% tannins, 0.8-0.9% essential oil: n-decanol, geraniol, geranyl formate, geranyl acetate, benzyl alcohol, phenylethyl alcohol, linalool, nonanal, decanal, nerol and cinnamyl alcohol, phenylpropanoid: rosavin, rosin, rosarin; phenylethanol derivatives: salidroside, tyrosol; flavonoids: rodiolin, kaempferol, astragalin, rodionin, rodiosin, acetylrodalgin, trycin, kaempferol-7-rahmnoside, trycin-7-glucoside, 8-methylgerbacetin, rhodioflavonoside and others; terpenoids: rosiridol, rosiridin, rhodiolosides A-E; steroids: b-sitosterol, daucosterol; phenol carboxylic acids: chlorogenic, 4-hydroxycinnamic, gallic, isochlorogenic, neochlorogenic acids and lotaustralin.

Bioactivities: Cytotoxic, antibacterial, central nervous system effects.

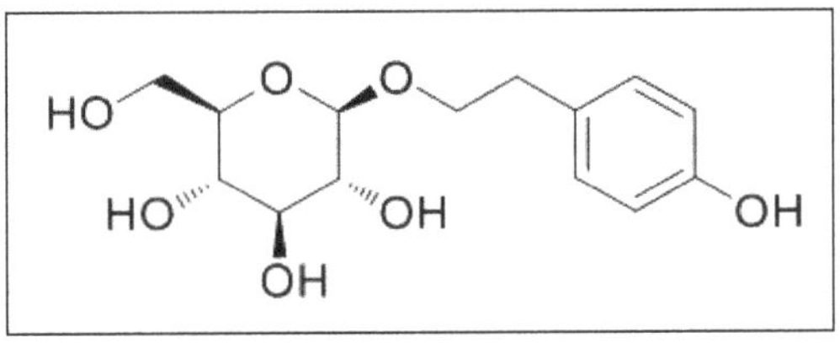

Figure: Salidroside.

4. Mongolian Name: Yulden Taravganshiir

Tibetan Name: Saradgar

English Name: Lanceolata Thermopsis

Traditional Uses: It is bitter in taste with cooling properties and is used for treating wounds and fever, and to fortify the body.

Chemical Constituents:

Alkaloids: cytisine, anagrinepachycarpine, rhombifoline, N-methylcytisine, N-formylcytisinethermopsine, thermopsidin, lupaninspartein, 5, 6-dihydro-lupanin, baptifoline, epibaptifoline, 17-oxosparteine 11,12-dehydroanagyrineammodendrine, isoammodendrine.

Bioactivity: Mucolytic.

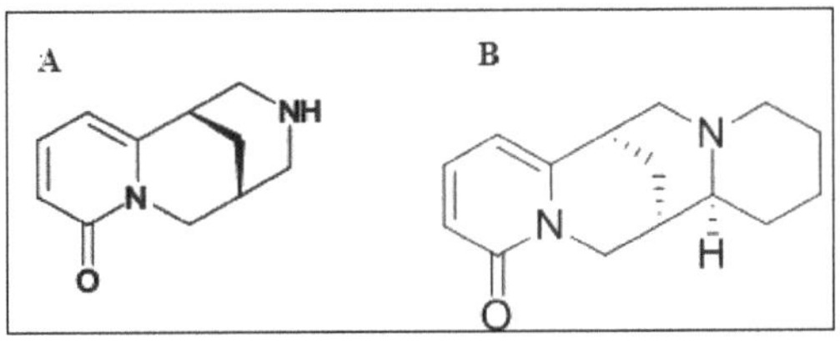

Figure: A-Cytisine, B-Thermopsine.

Risk of Extinction of Valuable Species

Due to the progressive degradation of the natural environment, drastic climate changes, and especially illegal, mass acquisition of rare medicinal plants, many species of Mongolian herbs are in danger of extinction. About 40% of natural habitats of rare, endangered plant species have been included in areas with special protection.

Table: The classification of threatened of the plant species.

Plant Species	Content of Plant Species	Percent of the Extremely Threatened, %
Medicinal	75	26.6
Natural food	11	54.5
Industrial	16	25.0
Ornamental	55	18.2
Soil protecting	15	33.3

Traditional Chinese Medicine

TCM is a healing system that was developed in China about 3000 years ago. Compared to many other alternative or complementary medicines TCM has many unique features. Firstly, even TCM has abstract ideas like ying, yang and the five elements, It is a complete and rational system consisting of diagnosis, treatment, prognosis and prevention. It seeks to treat all kind of illness people could encounter. Secondly, even though most of the knowledge was transferred verbally at the beginning of TCM history, the knowledge has systematically been handed down since the first textbook (The Yellow Emperor's Internal Medicine) dated back to 800 BC – 200 BC, a textbook that is still in use. Lastly, TCM has been continuously developing since its dawn. It is still an important health system for the Chinese people of today.

At 2200 BC early Chinese inhabitants empirically found different ways of healing. For instance, while using hot stones to warm themselves, inhabitants realized that pressing them against certain parts of the body could give relief for certain sicknesses. They also found that pricking themselves with bone needles in particular spots could relieve pain in other areas of the body. This is the acupuncture at its very beginning. At this stage, however, the medicine was much intermixed with magic and other rituals. The classic books of The Yellow Emperor (The Yellow Emperor's Internal Medicine) and Fire Emperor (Classic of Herbal Medicine) lay the fundament for the theory and philosophy of TCM as well as principles of herbal and acupuncture treatment. The books have a huge impact on later TCM development. Both books are dated to 2nd and 1st century BC. Although the books are attributed to the Yellow Emperor and the Fire Emperor, they were in fact written by several authors over a long period of time. In ancient time it was common for the Chinese authors to assign authorship of books to the great teachers or important persons who influenced them.

At Han-dynasty 200 BC–200 AD, Zhang ZhongJing wrote a book called Shanghan Zabinglun (Discourse on Fevers and Miscellaneous Illnesses), about the treatment of febrile conditions. At this stage there was no distinction between febrile illness caused by infection or non-infection. However, it is still significant as it discusses diagnosis and treatment methods based on an assessment of the symptoms of different pathological conditions. Hua Tuo (145-208AD) is famous for his skill as a surgeon and his use of anesthesia. The anesthesia was called mafeisan and was taken by the patient before surgery. Mafeisan combines ma ("cannabis, hemp, numbed or tingling"), fei ("boiling or bubbling"), and san ("to break up or scatter", or "medicine in powder form"). Therefore, the word mafeisan probably means something like "cannabis boil powder". Unfortunately, many of Hua Tuo's works have been lost. Additionally, surgery became unpopular because religious and cultural belief. To some extent surgery in TCM died with Hua Tuo. Besides performing surgeries, Hua Tuo also recommended physical exercises to his patients. He devised movements that were similar to the movements of five different animals: tiger, deer, bear, monkey and bird.

From 200 AD – 580 AD the concept of blood and circulation was fully developed in the practice of TCM. Two separate systems of circulation within the body was defined, each with a specific substance flowing through it. Blood goes from the heart and into vessels throughout the body. Qi was thought to be an abstract form of energy that circulated throughout the body in invisible tracts called meridians or channels. Wang Shuhe (265 317 AD) wrote the Maijing (Pulse Classic or Manual on the Pulses), which was a summary of the available knowledge on pulse diagnosis up to this point in history. In TCM diagnostics, examination of the pulse is central as different pulse is thought to indicate different diseases. All together 24 different kind of pulses were identified in this book. Lei Xiao's Liu Juanzi Guifang around 500 AD provides information of the treatment of wounds caused by metal instruments and disease affecting the skin such as anthrax and abscesses. Mercury is also mentioned for curing some skin conditions.

In the Tang Dynasty 618-907 AD, due to China's expansion and improvement in communication and transportation systems, medical knowledge was exchanged between different countries. TCM concepts were brought to foreign cultures. In return, these foreign cultures added new ideas to TCM. TCM doctors travelled to countries which is today's Korea, Japan, India and Vietnam. Many of the previously mentioned Chinese medical texts were translated into these countries' languages. From Korea, herbs such as ginseng, giant Typhomium tuber (bai fuzi), Korean pine and others were introduced to China. From Vietnam came vanilla grass, sappan wood, and cloves. Ophthalmology was quite undiscovered in TCM before Tang dynasty. It was developed by Buddhist monks who were popular both in China and India. Herbs such as ephedra, ginseng, and angelica were also brought from China to India.

In the Jin-Yuan period 1115-1368 AD, several schools of thought evolved, each with their own concept of factors that contribute disease and with contrasting approaches to treatment. Mongolian physicians additionally have their own set of thoughts that was distinctly different. Liu Wansu (1120-1200) emphasized the importance on the elements of fire and heat. He frequently prescribed herbs with cold properties to treat disease arising from these influences. His school is later called "School of cooling". Herbs that were frequently used are cassia twig, rehmannia root, ephedra and mint.

Zhang Congzheng (1150-1228) had an innovative approach to medical treatment and advocated that the treatment should follow the progress of the illness: "the medicines of yesterday could not use to treat present-day illnesses". He is best known for his theory of the "six doors and three methods." The six doors refer to the six influences (wind, summer heat, dampness, fire, dryness and cold) that Liu Wansu observed and thought was the etiology of different illness. The three methods are the therapeutic regimens Zhang used to induce sweating, vomiting and purging for cure. Li Gao (1180-1251) is famous for his work about how social factor could affect the body's functions. He believed that a person's emotions, including anger, joy, sadness and grief, could influence the qi, and that illness was caused by a society plagued by poverty, war and oppression. He might be classified as the first doctor in community medicine in TCM history.

Nomadic Mongols were known to be furious warrior and was constantly involved military activity. This stimulated the development of external medicine. Wei Yilin wrote Shiyi Dexiaofang (Efficacious Remedies of the Physicians), a textbook about treatment of fractures and dislocations of shoulder, hips and knee. It was the start of orthopedics in TCM. Around the time of Ming dynasty, Wu Youxing discovered that some diseases were caused by a transmissible type of Qi, which called liqi (pestilential Qi). Liqi had the following characteristics:

- It could be cured by herbs.
- The site of entrance to the body was the mouth and nose.
- The severity of the disease depended on the amount and intensity of the excessive influence, and the body resistance.
- Each pestilence was associated with its own particular liqi.

Wu's thinking has some resemblance to microbiology and is the first in TCM history to propose germs as a cause of epidemic diseases.

Concepts of TCM

TCM is built upon philosophical concepts drawn from the human body and the external environment. In contrast to Western medicine, TCM is more of a philosophy than science. Inside the human body, TCM will tell you that there are internal organs (Zhongs–Fus) but they are not synonymous with the human organs as described by distinguished Renaissance anatomists such as Leonardo da Vinci or Vesalius. The definitions of acupoints and meridians are equally conceptual and they do not correlate with known anatomical landmarks or conduits, such as the lymphatic systems as understood by Western medicine. Due to Chinese beliefs of Taoism and Buddhism, it is a forbidden to dissect a human body and hence TCM is not based on internal human anatomy. The meaning of health in TCM is synonymous with the functional interactions between entities inside the body in response to the natural forces of the environment. It is the overall dynamic equilibrium between the Yin–Yang, Qi–Xue and Zhongs–Fus that a TCM practitioner wants to achieve in order to re-establish health, not a treatment of any entity in isolation.

Yin–Yang

Yin and Yang are probably the two key principles that underlie TCM. In the broadest sense, Yin and Yang are two opposing entities that coexist in a dynamic equilibrium within the universe. In any system or space, there is Yin and Yang. Yang represents light, uprising, heat, mobility, the sun and the male gender. Yin represents the opposite: darkness, down-going, cold, rest, the moon and the female gender. Due to their opposing nature, Yin and Yang cancel each other out in any system when either entity exceeds a certain level. In extremis, they can interconvert, i.e. Yin becomes Yang and Yang becomes Yin. Yang cannot exit on its own and has to be rooted with Yin and vice versa. Inside a living body, any functioning organ or tissue, there is, by definition, a coexistence of Yin and Yang in dynamic equilibrium. Their dynamic interactions define life and their degree of interplay reflects the state of health. When there is imbalance, health deteriorates; when Yin–Yang decouples, death ensues.

Qi–Xue

Both are conceptual materials circulating inside the meridians and the main internal organs (Zhongs and Fus). Qi refers to the intangible energy inside the human body and constitutes the essence of life. Qi is contained inside the 12 meridians that are sequentially connected in a grand circle ramifying through different parts of the body including the Zhongs and Fus. Qi is also compartmentalized in each organ for its normal functions. Qi cycles through our body 50 times a day. Qi is categorized as a Yang entity and best kept in incessant flow. When Qi is deficient, the meridian or organ will be weakened and malfunction or increase susceptibility of the body to attacks by the six pathogens. Symptomatically, Qi deficiency is recognized by fatigue, malaise, shortness of breath, low voice, pale complexion, pale tongue and a thread-like pulse. When the level of Qi is normal but its flow is sluggish, it results in a stagnation syndrome where internal organs maybe bloated or pain will develop at sites where Qi cannot flow through the meridians. In these situations, acupuncture achieves its therapeutic effect by activating the flow of Qi in the affected meridians and unblocking the acupuncture points.

Xue is a Yin entity that coexists with Qi and is driven through the meridians by Qi. While Qi energizes an organ or bodily part for normal functioning, Xue provides the building blocks that form the organs or bodily parts. As a word, Xue is translated as 'blood' but is not synonymous with the anatomical entity as in Western medicine. Deficiency syndrome of Xue leads to multiple diffuse aches, pale complexion, irregular or scanty periods in females, pale tongue and a narrow pulse. Like Qi, when flow of Xue is blocked or sluggish, it results in a stagnation syndrome, which is recognized by sharp nocturnal pain at fixed areas of the body, a dark-purple tongue and an irregular pulse.

Zhong–Fu

Zhong and Fu are conceptual correlates of the major internal organs inside the body. There are five Zhongs (heart, liver, spleen, lungs and kidneys) and six Fus (bladder, gall bladder, stomach, small intestine, large intestine and pericardium). The Zhongs are considered solid entities and hence correlate with the Yin, while the Fus are considered hollow entities and correlated with the Yang. For a Zhong to be in its optimal state, it has to be filled with Qi or Xue, failure to do so results in a Deficiency Syndrome. On the contrary, a Fu needs to be emptied and drained constantly to maintain its hollow state, failure to do so will lead to a blockage or stagnation syndrome. The best example is constipation where the larger intestine, a Fu, is not emptied properly and hence the blockage presents with pain and bloatedness. Moreover, each Zhong or Fu is associated with a meridian ramifying a different part of the body. A Zhong and a Fu pair up as a functional dual. The five Zhongs correlate with the five elements of nature and promote/suppress each other to achieve equilibrium.

Five Elements

The concept of the Five Elements originates from the earliest archives of Chinese philosophy, Yi-Jing, or 'Book of Changes' in 300 BC In our nature and environment, it is believed that there are five main elements that interact and constitute everything as we know it: Earth, Wood, Water, Fire and Metal. Between them there exists a mutual promotion–suppression relationship that keeps them in equilibrium. The five elements promote each other in the following way: Earth → Metal → Water → Wood → Fire → Earth. Conversely, they suppress each other also in this particular manner: Earth → Water → Fire → Metal → Wood → Earth. So in a way, there exist an intricate pull–push dynamics among all five elements that form the basis of clinical diagnosis and therapy in TCM.

Table: The Zhong–Fu pairing and their designation with the Five Elements.

Zhong	Fu	Member of Five Elements
Liver	Gall bladder	Wood
Heart	Small intestine	Fire
Spleen	Stomach	Earth
Lung	Large intestine	Metal
Kidney	Bladder	Water

Human beings are part of nature and in the theory of TCM, the internal organs are believed to correlate with the Five Elements according to their behaviours and functions in the body: Earth–spleen (spleen digest all crops harvested from earth); Wood–liver (liver likes to spread and extend the Qi like branches of the tree); Fire–heart (heart governs the blood which is red like fire); Water–kidneys (kidneys governs the waterworks); Metal–lungs (lungs maintains the cleanliness like pure metal). So translating to Zhongs (the solid organs in TCM), the same promoting relationships exists: spleen → lungs → kidneys → liver → heart → spleen and the suppressive relationships are seen: spleen → kidneys → heart → lungs → liver → spleen. A schematic diagram showing the promotion–suppression relationships of the Five Elements is given in figure. These inter relationships help to understand the aetiology of disease and the formulation of treatment. For example, in Excess Syndrome of the liver, the spleen will be weakened as Earth is suppressed by Wood under the Five-Elements rule, and hence the treatment strategy is to abate the Wood (liver) and support the Earth (spleen), possibly via strengthening of the Fire (heart) as Fire promotes Earth.

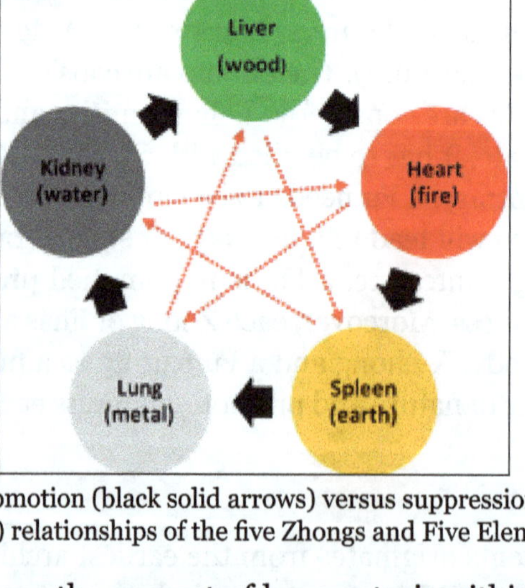

Figure: The promotion (black solid arrows) versus suppression (red broken arrows) relationships of the five Zhongs and Five Elements.

In Western medicine, we do have the concept of homeostasis within organ systems but we often emphasize the 'single disease–single organ–single treatment' dictum wherever possible. We do not need to consider cross-systems homeostasis unless in dire situations of multi-organ systems failure. This illustrates how TCM differs from Western medicine where multiple interacting factors and organ systems have to be conside red in every diagnosis for achieving an overall balance of health for that particular individual. This TCM paradigm maybe valuable especially at times of deadly epidemics that baffle Western medicine.

Causes of Diseases

1. Six Agents: Just as nature is susceptible to seasonal change, TCM believes that the human body is equally susceptible. Six agents are identified: Wind, Cold, Heat, Dampness, Dryness and Fire, which are predominant in different seasons of the year Per se, they are natural stages of the four seasons that all humans are subject to, and they only cause diseases when they appear too soon, last too long or come in far excess. Equally, if there is already an imbalance (of the Yin–Yang, Qi–Xue or Zhong–Fus) inside the body, there is increased susceptibility to these external agents. These six agents can affect the human body in isolation or in combination as the seasons go round. In addition, pandemics and plagues were explained in the ancient TCM archives as unexpected excess of these natural agents—this maybe the very first reference to abrupt changes in seasons leading to spread of air-borne pathogens.

Table: Six agents and their properties.

Agent	Predominant Season of the Year	Nature
Wind	Spring, autumn, winter	Yang
Cold	Winter	Yin
Heat	Summer	Yang
Dampness	Spring, summer	Yin
Dryness	Autumn	Yang
Fire	Mid-summer	Yang

2. Seven Emotions: According to the theory of TCM, there are seven emotions recognized in the humans and when in excess can cause diseases and illness. They are Joy, Anger, Worry, Contemplation, Sorrow, Fear and Shock. In brief, they affect the movement of Qi and Xue in different ways. One must avoid getting into extreme swings of emotions, nor should one dwell in any particular type for too long, otherwise our health will be jeopardized. Crude as it seems, these references may well count as the earliest descriptions of psychosomatic symptoms and illnesses in humans as described in present day Western medicine.

Table: Seven emotions and their effects on Qi and Xue.

Emotions	Effect on Qi and Xue
Joy	Slows
Anger	Upsurges
Worry	Blockade
Contemplation	Interruption
Sorrow	Stagnation
Fear	Sinking
Shock	Disarray

Four Pillars of TCM Diagnosis

Observation

Like Western medicine, TCM diagnosis starts with general observation of the patient. TCM stresses on the assessment of 'spirit' of the patient that is exhibited by the general demeanour, physical agility, facial complexion, skin hues, speech clarity and rate of breathing. In brief, good spirit means a robust flow of Qi and Xue with dynamic equilibria among their Zhongs and Fus as seen in good health. Disease of any Zhong or Fu often manifest as a particular facial skin hue of the corresponding member of the Five Elements. For example, a heart problem often shows up with a red hue (Heart → Fire = Red), lung problem with a white pale hue (Lung → Metal = White), kidney problem with a dark hue (Kidney → Water = Black), spleen problem with a sallow hue (Spleen → Earth = Yellow) and liver problem with a green hue (Liver → Wood = Green). The other main observation is of the tongue. TCM places a lot of emphasis on tongue diagnosis and in the diagnostic indicators that are listed in table. A few examples of tongue diagnoses are given as below:

1. Listening and smell: TCM practitioners will listen to the intensity and the tone/pitch of a patient's voice. They also assess the patient's way of breathing and cough as an assessment of Qi/Xue and the state of the Zhong/Fus. Furthermore, any particular smell or odour, from the patient's body or excrement, is a diagnostic indicator for syndromes relating to an imbalance of the Zhong/Fus. For example, foul-smelling diarrhoea often indicates stagnation of the large bowel with excess of heat, whilst odourless diarrhoea means excess of dampness and cold in the stomach.

2. Taking a history: TCM emphasizes a good history taken from the patient based on the 'Song of Ten Questions' regarding:

- Head and body.
- Degree and timing of sweating.
- Feeling of hot or cold.
- Urination and bowel movement.
- Appetite and diet.
- Breathing cough and chest (breast).
- Hearing.
- Thirst.
- Previous illness and their causes.
- Gynaecological, obstetrical and paediatric infections.

TCM archives have records of ancient practitioners specializing in women's health, paediatrics and infectious diseases, hence the coverage of these areas in the history taking. Arguably, this could be interpreted as the earliest model of history taking as taught today in Western medicine.

Table: Some common tongue signs and their diagnoses.

Tongue Sign	Diagnosis
Pale tongue	Xue deficiency.
Red tongue	Normal variant; heat excess.
Purple tongue	Blood stagnation.
Purple tongue with dark spots on underside	Extreme blood stagnation with 'clots'.
Thin and narrow tongue body	Yin deficiency.
Thick tongue body	Qi deficiency.
Thick tongue body with teeth marks along border	Deficiency of spleen.
Thin white tongue coating	Normal health.
Thick white tongue coating	Excess of cold.
Thick yellow tongue coating	Excess of moisture and heat.
Thick black tongue coating (moist)	Excess of dampness and cold.
Thick black tongue coating (dry)	Excess of heat.
No tongue coating, glossy tongue	Stomach Yin deficiency.
Patchy coating	Stomach Qi deficiency.

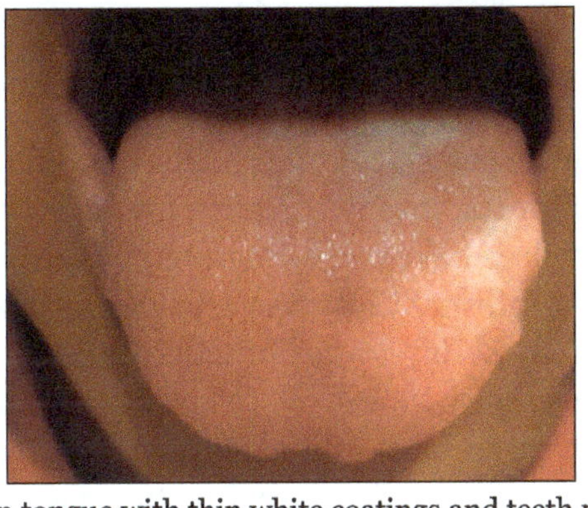

Figure: Fat swollen tongue with thin white coatings and teeth marks on the side, signifying weakness of spleen with excess of water and moisture.

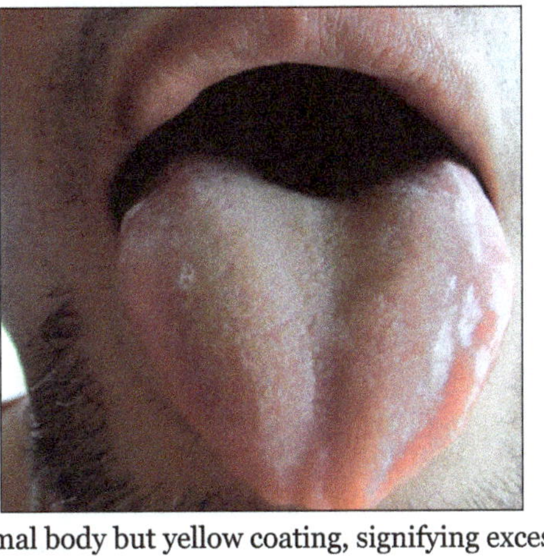

Figure: Tongue with normal body but yellow coating, signifying excess of moisture and heat.

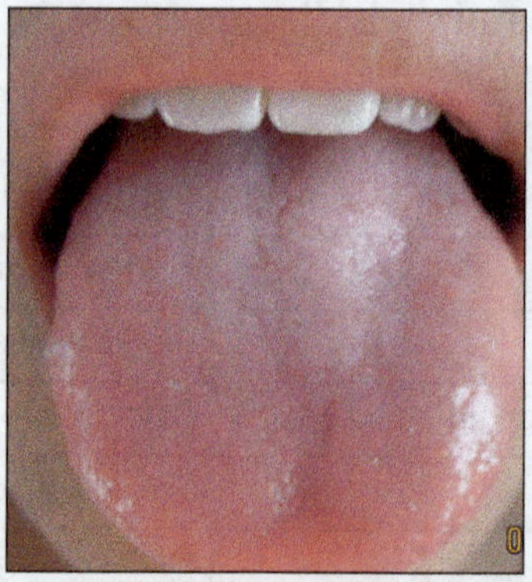

Figure: Tongue from a 13-year-old male with redness at tips and prominent taste buds, signifying heat of the heart meridian (this child has mild insomnia).

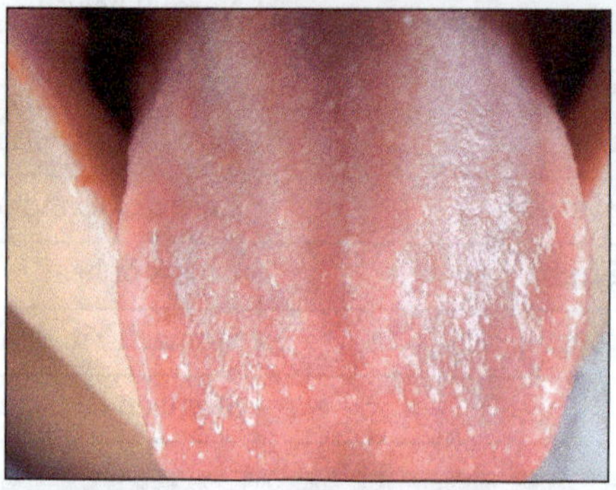

Figure: Tongue of an 8-year-old male with normal looking body but lack of tongue coating, signifying weakness of stomach. He has low appetite for food.

3. Taking the pulse: TCM practitioners place three fingers (index, middle and ring) along the radial artery of the patient to feel for the intensity, rate, rhythm, wave characteristic and resilience of the pulse. Up to 28 types of pulses have been described in the ancient archives of TCM like the Su Wen of the Yellow Emperor's Internal Classic in 260 BC and the Mai Jing in 280 AD. Despite fewer pulses being recognized in most day-to-day practice, taking the patient's pulse is considered a mandatory diagnostic step, together with tongue inspection. There have been attempts to scientifically analyse the dynamic behind the various pulses but so far they have not been successful. An editorial regarding the evaluation of conduit artery function mentions some similarities with the TCM pulse diagnosis but they are hardly comparable. Pulse taking remains a diagnostic skill that has to be acquired through good apprenticeship and is refined during years of clinical practice.

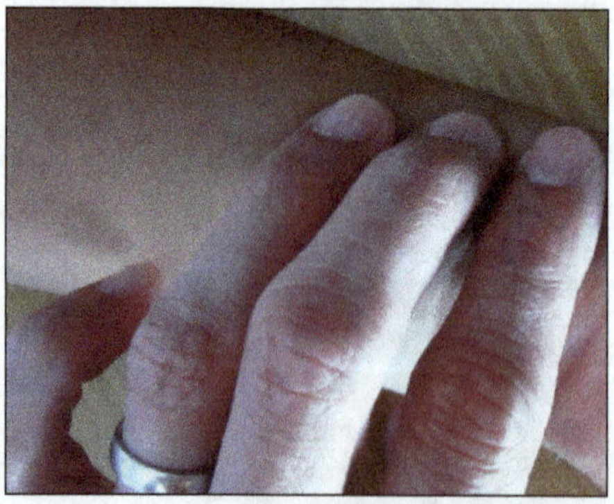

Figure: Taking the pulse in the TCM manner. Note the standard positioning of the index, middle and ring fingers of the TCM practitioner over the radial artery of the patient in that order.

Categorization into Eight Syndromes

In the language of TCM, health is based upon a dynamic balance between opposing (e.g. Yin–Yang) and interacting entities (Zhong–Fus and Qi–Xue) that coexist inside the human body. Any disease state can be categorized by one or a combination of the Eight Syndromes, each of which carry specific signs and symptoms:

- Yang Syndrome: Yang symbolizes activity, motion, uplift and intensity. Patient presents with fever, excessive movements, nervousness, excessive speech/thoughts, rapid bouncy pulse, insatiable appetite, increased libido, red complexion, red tongue with dry and thick coating.
- Yin Syndrome: Yin symbolizes quiescence, inactivity, downturning and weakness. Patient looks pale, easily fatigued, hypothermic, feeble speech, paucity of thoughts, slow thread-like pulse, loss of appetite, decreased libido, and pale narrow tongue with thin wet coating.
- Superficial Syndrome: Usually refers to the early stage of diseases due to invasion from the six external agents when they are still contained at the superficial domains of the bodies (surface meridians and the skin). Prognosis for superficial syndrome is good and full recovery is expected with or without treatment.
- Deep Syndrome: Refers to diseases that affect the Zhong–Fus or deeper meridians of the body, either due to deterioration of the Zhong–Fus or progression of the superficial syndrome due to delayed or inappropriate treatment. Prognosis is generally worse compared to superficial syndrome and if the patient escapes death chronic ill health is expected.
- Cold Syndrome: Occurs when Yin is in excess or the body is afflicted by external agents like the Cold and the Dampness. Patient presents with hypothermia, fatigue, pallor, nocturnal pains, fear of cold, watery stool, clear urine, pale tongue with thick moist coating and a slow thread-like pulse.
- Heat Syndrome: Occurs when Yang is in excess or body is afflicted by external agents like Fire or Summer Heat. Patient often has a fever, craving for cold drinks, red face, constipation, dark/yellow urine, red tongue with yellow/black greasy coating.
- Deficiency Syndrome: Often used to specify the deficiency of a particular category (e.g. Yin/Yang) or of a particular Zhong. (Fu is never deficient as Fu is hollow in its natural state.) Symptoms and signs are analogous to those of Yin or Cold Syndrome where the patient looks pale, lethargic, shortness of breath with pale tongue and slow pulse.
- Excess Syndrome: The reverse of Deficiency Syndrome and refers to excess of a particular category or of a particular Fu (when it is congested or with stagnation of Qi/Xue). Symptoms and signs are similar to that described for Yang or Hot Syndrome: fever, thirst, hyperactivity, abdominal fullness, constipation, rapid bouncy pulse and a red coated tongue.

This system of categorization forms the essential algorithm upon which a TCM practitioner reaches a diagnosis and initiates treatment for the patient at a particular time. Such categorization often changes over time as the illness progresses.

Herbs in TCM

Traditional Chinese Medicine (TCM) is an incredibly complex system used to balance health. Focused on consuming foods that keep the body's humors in check, it uses ingredients including herbs, fruits, and pulses that have some great health benefits.

Ginseng

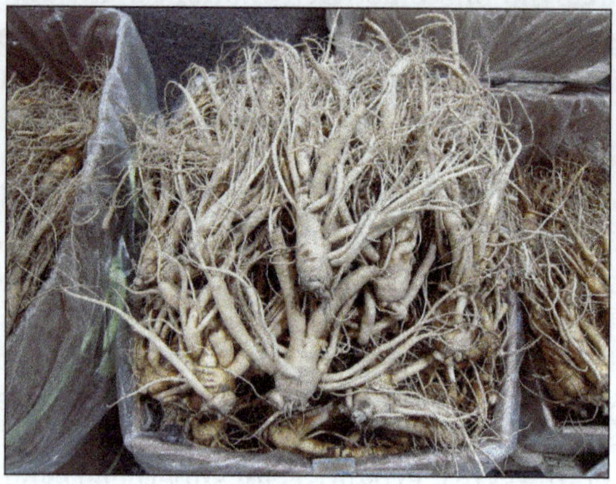

This gnarled rhizome is perhaps one of the best known of the Chinese herbs. The name literally translates to "human root" because the shape of it vaguely resembles a human body – in TCM, it's thought that the shape symbolizes ginseng's potent ability to cure human ills, replenish qi (vital energy), and warm the body. Aside from that, ginseng is an antioxidant, which helps rid the body of free radicals. There is also some evidence that ginseng boosts the immune system, which can help the body fight off infection and disease.

Walnuts

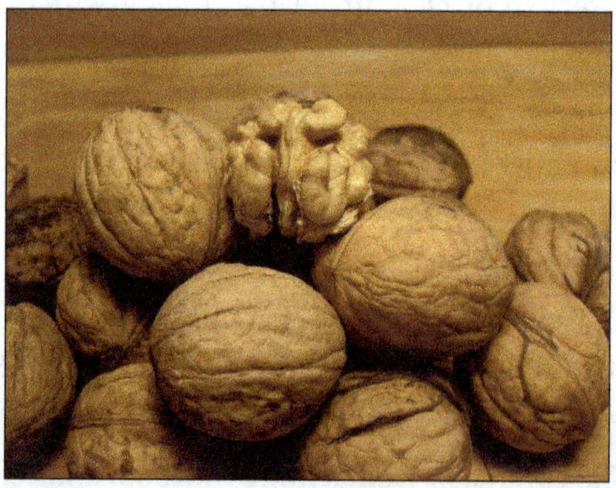

The Chinese have long believed that eating walnuts can sharpen the mind and boost concentration and memory. This stems from the fact that the crinkled appearance of a walnut resembles the folds of a human brain – and according to TCM principles, like replenishes like. TCM also considers walnuts as a warming food, which means they're a great winter time snack. Walnuts are also chock full of goodness as well, including omega-3 fatty acids, vitamin E and folates – all of which aid the heart and brain.

Cinnamon

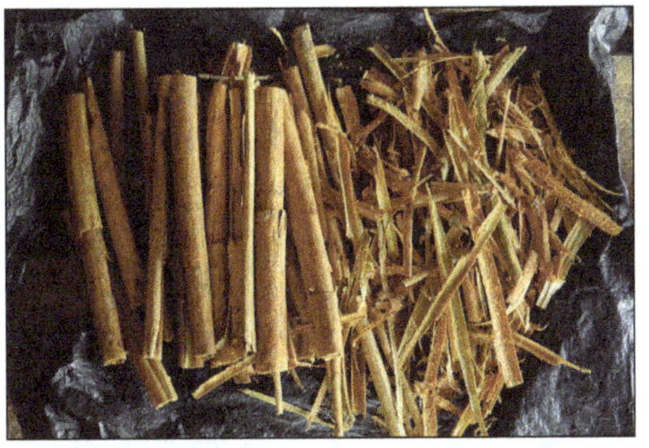

TCM says the branches and bark of this large tropical tree warm the body, invigorate the circulation, and harmonize the energy of the upper and lower body. Modern studies demonstrate that cinnamon helps to reduce allergic reactions and increases circulation. You'll most often find it combined with other TCM ingredients mixed into a tea, or bobbing around in a hot pot.

Ginger

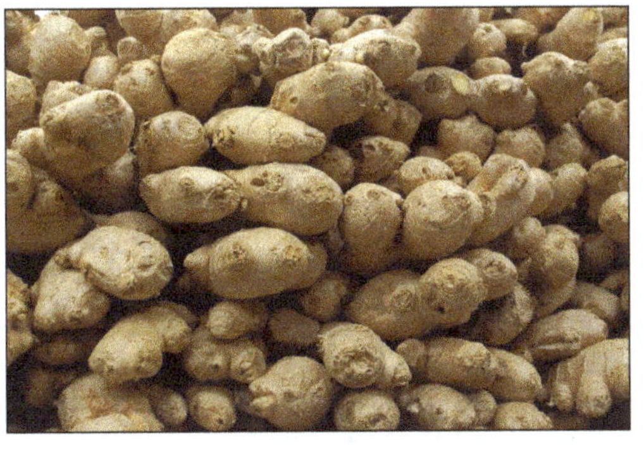

This spicy rhizome is said to benefit digestion, neutralize poisons in food, ventilate the lungs and warm circulation to the limbs. Today, ginger is commonly used in cooking, as well as in teas and candies and has been shown to help counteract nausea and aid digestion. It is also simply delicious in the winter time when steeped with red sugar and jujubes.

Lotus Seed

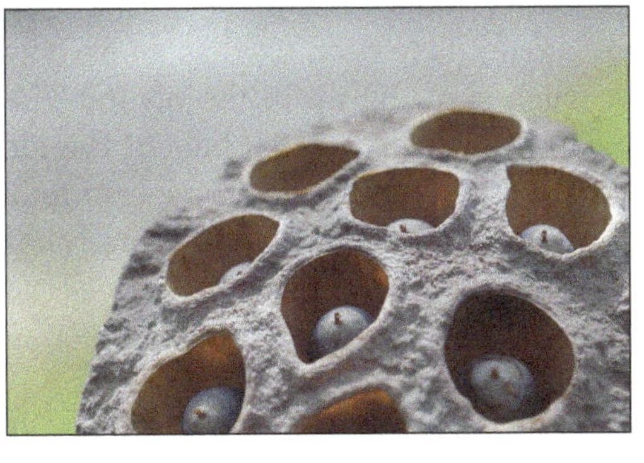

Lotus seed may not be as famous as ginseng, but it is ubiquitous in China, found in soups, teas and even fresh in stir fries. In TCM, it is thought to improve the functions of the spleen and kidneys, as well as helping regulate diarrhea. Lotus seeds are also rich in calcium, phosphorus and potassium, which are great for nourishment – and the fiber improves digestion as well.

Hawthorn Berries

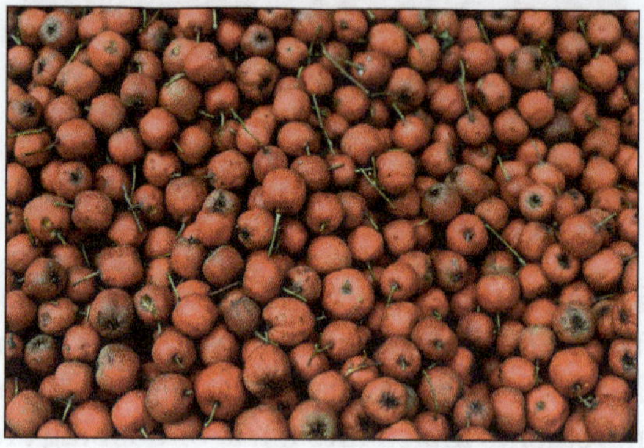

Though best known as the primary ingredient of the much beloved haw flake candies, hawthorne is actually a common ingredient used in traditional Chinese medicine. The berry itself is incredibly sour, like a crab apple, and traditionally used as a digestive aid and to reduce indigestion and heartburn. There is some evidence in modern research that it also might help treat cardiac weakness. But best off, it's just a delicious addition to candies, teas and baked sweets.

Goji Berries

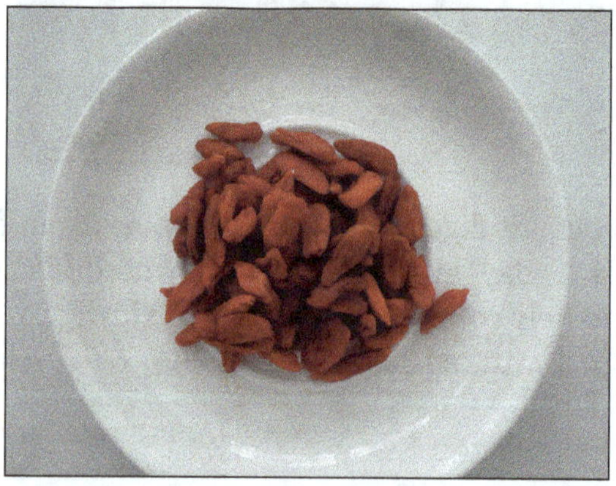

Also known as wolfberries, goji berries have been used as an herbal remedy for over 3,000 years, with their first recorded use as such showing up in the pivotal The Classic of Herbal Medicine. They are thought to be anti-ageing because they can benefit the kidneys and to nourish jing, or kidney essence, which underpins human vitality. These vibrant and lightly floral berries are also rich in vitamin C, antioxidants, fiber and vitamin A, and generally come in dried form, used in teas and several dishes to improve nutrition and eyesight.

Jujube

Deeply red jujube dates have been used in TCM recipes for centuries, the sweet, spongy fruits often steeped in teas or cooked in congee (rice porridge) to aid circulation and to bolster qi. These fruits are thought to promote blood flow, calm the mind, and soothe the nerves, and are often used to treat insomnia. They are also high in vitamins B and C, and can help lift mood and soothe anxiety.

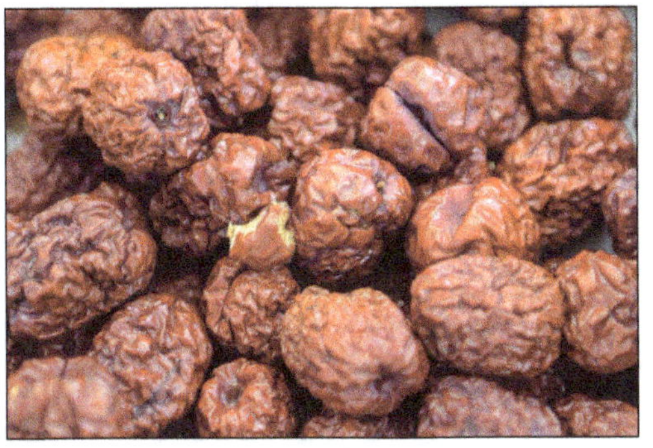

Licorice Root

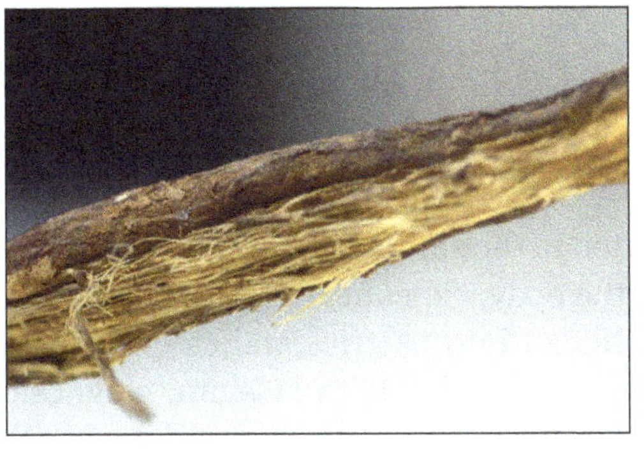

Licorice root is thought to replenish vital energies, help stomach functions, clear out heat and control coughing. Due to its sweetness, it's also often used in TCM herb tonics to ease bitterness and to help 'harmonize' the harshness of their flavors – basically to help the medicine go down! It has also been depression, cold, flu, cough, heartburn and many more. It is used in Chinese medicine to harmonize all the other medicinal herbs that goes into a formula. In addition, there is some evidence that licorice can help with swelling, itching and redness that goes along with skin rashes.

Aged Mandarin Peel

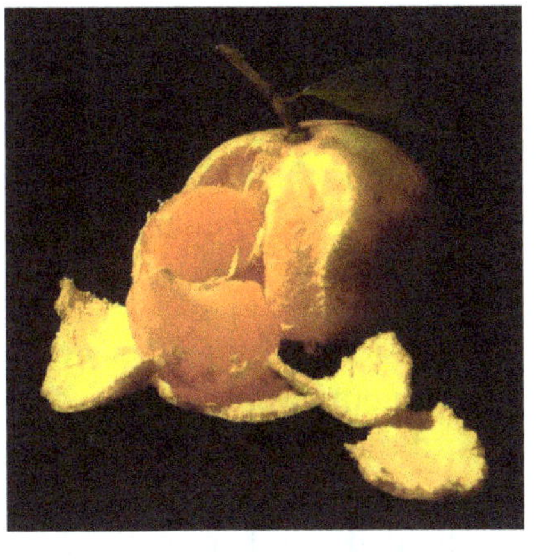

Mandarin tangerine peels, after being sundried, are often used as a warming agent to help the functions of the spleen and stomach, and balancing qi. Like the citrus fruit itself, mandarin peel is also rich in vitamin C, and antioxidants are also found in higher concentrations in the peel, which means more fighting off of free radicals. You'll most often find mandarin peels used in teas, as well as a flavoring in stir fries with meat.

Mung Beans

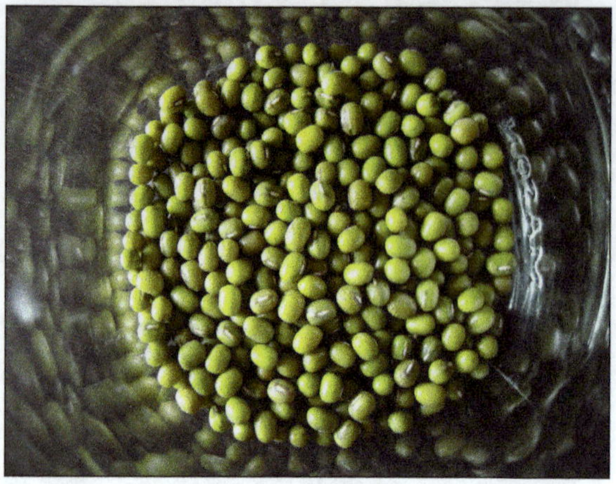

These little pulses are often eaten in the summertime as they are an essential yin food that, according to TCM, helps to detoxify the body, expel heat and add moisture. You'll find sweet mung bean soups, as well as mung bean added into pastries and eaten for breakfast in congee. These little nutritional powerhouses are also packed with potassium, magnesium, folate, fiber, and vitamin B6, which can help smooth over mood swings and control stress. The fiber also helps to regulate digestion and keep things moving.

Traditional Iranian Medicine

The Traditional Iranian Medicine (TIM) is a school that views the world as a good and seeking discipline created by the wise and omniscient Almighty. TIM consists of the sum total of all the knowledge and practices used in diagnosis, prevention and elimination in Persia from ancient times to present. It is based entirely on practical experience and observations passed down from generation to generation. TIM roots back to over 8000 yr B.C. and it is a branch if not the root of the so called Arabic-Unani medicine as quoted by Cyril Elgood, the English medical historian, was more advanced than that of Assyria and it is not too bold to go even further and claim that the Persians taught the Greeks the elements of that system of medicine, which has been known ever since as Greek medicine.

According to Ibn Khaldoon, Among Persians, rational sciences had a high status. Such sciences had a vast scope since Persians' governments were majestic and long-lasting. Words have it that after Darius' murder by Alexander and the occupation of Kelikiyeh, and access to the countless Persian books and sciences, such sciences were passed to the Greeks. Considering the definitions given by the WHO, the TIM can be divided into two sections: A Written Traditional Medicine & B-Verbal Traditional Medicine.

Structure of Tim

The Traditional Iranian Medicine has two main branches, namely a theoretical branch and a practical branch which each also branch into sub-branches as follows:

- The theoretical branch of TIM: This branch is a science which discusses the status and changes of the human body and the causes and signs of health and disease.
- The practical branch of TIM: This branch is also a science, although it may remind us of practical procedures but it is really the science of how to keep health and how to bring it back after the occurrence of diseases.

Seven Natural Affairs

In the TIM, physiological functions of the human body are considered to be based on seven factors, known as "Umoor-e-Tabee-e-ya". These are as follows:

- Elements [Arkan].
- Temperament [Mizaj].
- Humors [Akhlat].
- Organs [Azaa].
- Spirits [Arwah].
- Faculties or Forces [Quwa].
- Functions [Af'al].

Prevention, Diagnosis and Treatment

TIM has given more attention and importance to the prevention of disease rather than its cure. Maintaining health was so important that the main duty of the physicians were to keep people healthy and to treat them if they became sick. There are six factors, which are essential for the maintenance of good health, which is referred to as: Setteh-e-Zarurieah. These essential factors are as follows:

- Air.
- Food and Drink.
- Sleep and Wakefulness.
- Evacuation and Retention.
- Body movement and Repose.
- Mental movement and Repose.

Modes and Strategies of Treatment in Tim

The imbalance in body temperament and humors leads to the onset of disease condition. Therefore, treatment is based on the correction of temperament and humors to achieve a balanced state. Every humor has a specific temperament as described earlier. So, the drug used for the treatment should possess the opposite temperament than that of the diseased humor, resulting in normalization of the temperament. A disease, which is cold in nature, can be cured by a drug, which has hot temperament and so on. It should be noted that not all the diseases in the TIM are treated based on the temperaments, because there are three forms of disease according to TIM:

- Distemperaments (distortion of the temperament of a single organ up to the whole body).
- Disfigurements (distortion of the anatomy or the structure of an organ).
- Disconnections (distortion of the correlation and connection between organs).

The Distemperaments are the ones mostly treated by correction of temperament and the two latter are mostly treated by special drugs or manipulation especially including surgery. TIM physicians have mentioned four modes of treatment:

- Correction of the six essentials (Tadbir ba Sitteh-e-Zarurieah).
- Diet-o-therapy (Tadbir ba Ghaza).
- Pharmacotherapy (Tadbir ba Dawa).
- Manipulation or physical therapy (Aamale yadaavi).

These modes might also be considered as levels of treatment, where if a level fails or is inadequate the next level is considered.

Some of the earliest practices of ancient Iranian medicine have been documented in the Avesta and other Zoroastrian religious texts. During the Achaemenid era (559-330 BCE), the 21 books of Avesta encompassing 815 chapters were an encyclopedia of science consisting of medicine, astronomy, law, social science, philosophy, general knowledge, logic and biology. It can be inferred from these books that Zoroastrians placed great importance on personal hygiene, public health and the prevention of contagious diseases. The best teachers of medicine and astrology were Iranian Magi and Mobeds (Zoroastrian priests) who passed their knowledge on to their pupils from one generation to the next. According to Avestan texts, King Jamshid was the physician who initiated the custom of bathing with hot and cold water. Iranians refrained from polluting the four elements. They would not bathe or wash dirty objects in flowing water, and urinating or spitting into water was considered a great sin. Odorous materials were never thrown into the fire. Wild rue and frankincense were always burned inside houses to kill insects and bacteria, a custom which continues to this today.

The Persians, who lived in an empire stretching from the Indus valley in the east to the Aegean Sea in the west with considerable variation in climate and vegetation, became familiar with a vast range of medicinal plants. The Avesta mentions several medicinal herbs including basil, chicory, sweet violet, and peppermint, while Bundahishn cites the names of thirty sacred medicinal plants. Avestan texts list not only the various parts of plants such as roots, stems, scales, leaves, fruit and seeds used for treatment but also indicate which plant is the remedy for each disease. According to the Zâdspram, a Pahlavi text of the ninth century AD, there are thousands of species of medicinal plants created by Ahura Mazda for the prevention of thousands of sicknesses created by Ahriman and that the best of these plants is haoma (Vedic soma). Haoma (Ephedra Vulgaris) is indigenous to the Iranian plateau and contains a large quantity of Ephedrine which is effective in the treatment of cardiovascular and respiratory diseases. Garlic was used to reduce blood pressure, combat heart disease and treat infections. Rue was once a popular remedy for earache, easing shaking fits and joint pain; it was also used to disinfect the house. Bangha, extracted from Cannabis Indica seeds, has hallucinatory effects and was used as an anesthetic.

Frankincense was used for inhalation therapy. Aloeswood was used in the treatment of cardiac disease and irregular heartbeat. Many modern-day Iranian herbalists prescribe plants such as Borage, Sweet Marjoram, Fenugreek and Chicory as treatment. Ancient Persian physicians believed that good health is the result of the 'right' measure of the elements of humor, and that sickness is the product of their excess or deficiency.

Therefore, the medicine of the body consists of keeping the body in good health and re-establishing balance and the medicine of the soul involves curing the body and preserving it from sin. The Vendidad tells of three kinds of medicine practiced; medicine by the knife (surgery), medicine by herbs, and medicine by divine words, which according to the sacred text, is the best form of the three. A Mazdean physician-in-training was required to treat and cure three non-Mazdean patients before receiving permission to treat Mazdeans. In this way physicians were taught to treat any and all patients, whether friend or foe. Avestan scriptures did not restrict giving treatment to Mazdeans alone. The Ordibehesht Yasht classifies physicians under five categories:

- Health Physician (Ashoo Pezeshk): This physician was in charge of the well-being of the city, preventing the spread of contagious diseases by quarantining, keeping the four sacred elements of water, wind, earth and fire free from contamination, and making sure the sanitation of houses was maintained.
- Medical Examiner (Dâd Pezeshk): Similar to modern-day pathologist/coroners, their duties included examining the dead, performing autopsies when required, the issuance of burial licenses and ascertaining the cause of death with an eye toward finding cures for future cases.
- Surgeon (Kard Pezeshk): Archeological excavations in the Burnt City in Sistan have yielded skulls that show signs of surgery. Surgical procedures, difficult and dangerous even in the present time, were much more so in the past when it was not possible to properly anaesthetize patients and medical instruments were rudimentary.
- Herbalist (Gyâh Pezeshk): The origin of herbal medicine predates the development of agriculture and cultivation in Iran, yet some believe that the ancient Persians were the first to document the properties of herbs and to use plants to cure diseases.
- Psychiatrists (Mantreh Pezeshk): This physician used holy words and prayers to cure patients suffering from a sickness of body and soul which could not be cured with herbs. Treatment consisted of verbal communication, the reading of poetry, listening to music and the recitation of prayers, including ones from the holy books of other nations, which were designed to console and heal the patient. Avestan texts tell of consultation among the surgeons, herbalists and psychiatrists which indicates a form of medical association at the time.

Essential Foods in Iranian Medicine

Oral Food

Oral food includes all edibles and drinks which usually are consumed by a person. According to ITM, oral food must have some properties to ensure fitness. It, at first, should be Halal; hence, it would be obtained through loyal legitimate way and its eating would be allowed by religion. ITM scholars believe that Lord has not put the human health in unlawful and ill-gotten food. Second, oral food should be compatible with individual temper to reach the best physical and mental fitness. Otherwise, it can lead to mal-temperament, a condition that makes the people susceptible to illness. According to ITM, every edible has a specific temper, and it is better to consume with its corrector (Mosleh). For example, fish and yogurt have a cold temper and should be used with hot spices such as pepper, cinnamon, ginger, and mint. Meanwhile, simultaneous consumption of two or more food with similar temper is forbidden in ITM; so, for example, fish and yogurt should not be eaten with each other. The food's temper should be also compatible with the season. Because, according to ITM, every season has a specific temper. For example, winter has a cold-wet temper, so consumption of hot-dry foods in this season is more compatible with fitness. In addition, different geographic conditions of the habitat influence on the human temper. For example, if cold-dry foods are consumed in regions with hot and wet weather, the human health would be more insurable. Third, the food, if possible, should be gentle (Latif) righteous chime (Saleh chime), and nutritious (Kasirol-ghaza). This means that it is easy to digest and absorb, its digestion creates normal blood and humor, and it has sufficient nutrients to meet the body needs.

Fourth, ITM scholars emphasize on the quantity of oral food. According, the best program for the main meals is consumption up twice a day, a full meal in the morning, and the second one in the evening. Fruits and other proper edibles can be eaten for lunch and other snack times. Fifth, some healthy behaviors toward oral food have been recommended by ITM scholars to keep us healthy which include well chewing and mastication, hand washing before and after the meal, start the eating with the name of god, beginning the meal with a bit of salt, and finishing it with a little of sweets.

Imaginary Food

According to ITM, individual thought content, either positive or negative, is considered as imaginary food. It influences directly on mental and physical fitness and could disturb the balanced temperament. Positive thoughts and feeling like self-confidence, reliance to God, trust to others, kindness and love, etc., all have a positive effect on the human health and well-being. Reversely, negative thoughts and feeling such as frustration and disappointment, pessimism and distrust to others, diffidence, etc., are considered as a pest against health and reasons for mal-temperament. Today, many studies have explored the significant role of meditation interventions to heal the chronic diseases, either physical or psychological. Meditation is a practice to train the mind or to induce a consciousness state, either to appreciate some advantage or for the mind to simply admit its content without becoming recognized with that content or as an end in itself. It refers to a wide range of drills including techniques planned to promote relaxation, make internal energy or life force (qi, ki, prana, etc.) and develop compassion, love, patience, generosity, and forgiveness.

Auditory Food

All sounds surrounding us are considered as the auditory food, according to ITM. Some of these sounds are sedative and lead to the balanced temperament, for example, natural sounds such as sounds river falls, sounds of rain, and song birds; spiritual and beautiful words such as song Qari Quran, sounds of worship, names of God; and eastern music such as song straw and song def. Vice versa, inharmonic industrial sounds, such as traffic sound, train horn, and factory siren; ugly and unworthy words, such as cuss and curse words; and nearly all western music, such as jazz lead to an imbalanced temperament. Lord says in Holy Quran: "Verily in the remembrance of Allah do hearts find rest". Accordingly, every word, sentence, sound, etc., by which we remember Lord could calm down us, an example for auditory food. Today the role of music therapy has been determined to reduce pain and other physical and psychological problems in several conditions, according to many studies.

Visual Food

According to ITM scholars, everything that is in the range of human vision can be considered as visual food. What a person sees affects his/her mind and thought. Natural beautiful scenes such as mountains, forest, sea, river, etc., have almost a warm temper and help to balance human temperament. Reversely, all ugly and nasty scenes such as the view of accumulated waste could disturb the human temperament and have negative effects on fitness.

Natural views improve attentional performance in them. Natural view through a window could accelerate recovery from surgery in patients. Natural view has also showed a positive effect on psychological well-being and reduction of stress in persons. Seeing violence views, however, has induced negative effects on well-being. Moreover, every color is actually a visible light which affect persons in different ways, so different persons show variable reactions to each color. Color therapy or chromo therapy is an ancient branch of alternative medicine with more than several 1000 years oldness rooted in ancient Egypt. Recent studies have determined that every color could affect human emotions to different amounts.

Olfactory Food

Olfactory food includes all scents and odors around us which could stimulate the smell. Natural fragrant odors such as the scent of fresh flowers have often a warm temper and help to improve humor and moderate the temperament. For example, breathing of a gentle fragrance of flowers in cold seasons which have cold temper could moderate the temper and help to reinforce of central nervous system. On the other hand, unnatural chemical odors like cologne have almost a cold temper leading to brain coldness disorders such as depression and dementia.

Aromatherapy is one of the ancient medical sciences according which many of human diseases are treated through essential oils obtained from natural herbs. Today, these natural oils are widely used in developed countries. Moreover, the WHO has approved the aromatherapy as a complementary medicine technique since 1992. For example, many studies have run after 2000 which have determined the significant efficacy of the aromatherapy in treatment of sleep disorders. In addition, the effectiveness of aromatherapy for stress management has been shown in recent several randomized clinical trials. Aromatherapy has also presented a significant efficacy to treat the hypertensive patients, according to some recent studies.

Touch Food

Touch food includes all objects and materials that are in direct contact with body skin, such as textiles and clothes, which have a determinant role in temper moderation in case of being natural. According to ITM resources, the material of clothes has a determinant role to the human well-being. For example, wearing of cotton or linen clothes has been recommended by ITM scholars, and adversely, wool, hair, and chemical clothes have been forbidden for wearing.

According to many studies, it has been determined that chemical textiles such as polyester have negative effects on human health. There are also some research evidences toward negative effects of wooly and hairy clothes on human fitness. For example, studies have shown a higher severity of microbial burden in polyester textiles compared to cotton ones. Moreover, the prevalence of contact dermatitis in polyester and other chemical clothing has been reported more than natural clothing, particularly cotton. In addition, the sexual activity of men with polyester underclothing has been less than men with cotton underclothing.

Sexual Food

According to ITM, every person naturally needs sexual food; hence, a healthy human should be able to express his/her love to others and/or also be loved by them. It is beyond the sexual activity alone and includes all romantic behaviors in a person. Accordingly, sexual fulfillment could insure human fitness and prevent mal-temperament.

Studies have determined that sexual satisfaction has a significant effect to keep human health. Meanwhile, romantic relationships are considered as natural psychological behaviors; so without it, mental and psychological well-being would not be prepared. Loving and the sense of belongingness have a determinant role on emotional aspects of human personality and on cognitive processes. Without love and belongingness, health, adjustment, and well-being are in danger.

Familiarity Food

Familiarity food can be provided by companion with friends, relatives, and family members; so according to Islamic resources and psychological studies it has a significant role to prevent of diseases and increase human life time. Based on Islamic doctrine, the human is naturally social and the path of his/her evolution passes through community. Mental fitness and relaxation, and friendship have been mentioned as the main goal of marriage in Holy Quran. A well-structured family has an important role to keep and promote personal and social human fitness. Divorce and other familial disrupting events have significant deleterious effect on human health, according to many recent studies. Social isolation and staying away from the community and family could lead to harmful effects on the human fitness, particularly within mental health; the fact that many studies have approved it. Today, the role of friendship and social advocacy in health, particularly in later life, has been determined; so, friendship is considered as an important health factor in health-related studies.

Herbs and Plants in Iranian Medicine

Although plants have been used for millennia as medications, it was not until the 19th century when analytical chemistry became available and scientists began to extract and modify the active ingredients from plants in a pure form and later chemists learned to synthesize those ingredients in the laboratory. Almost one-fourth of modern pharmaceutical drugs are derived from plant extracts and pharmacists are searching mountains, forests and oceans in search of new medicinally effective plants.

Papaver somniferum, from which opium is extracted and has been known for millennia, contains many alkaloids with various properties including morphine, heroin and codeine which are the most potent analgesics known to man. History of Aspirin, originally extracted from the leaves of the Willow tree as Sodium salicylate to treat pain, fever and inflammation has been known for several thousand years until it was synthesized as Acetylsalicylic acid in the 19th century by the chemist Charles Frederic Gerhardt. Other well-known herbal remedies include Quinine, extracted from the bark of the Cinchona tree to treat malaria and Digitalis, extracted from the common Foxglove plant or Digitalis purpurea to control cardiac arrhythmias. More recently, the production of Paclitaxel (brand name Taxol) from the needles of the European Yew tree has been used extensively in the treatment of certain types of cancers.

The Solanacea family of plants includes tomatoes, potatoes and aubergine as well as belladonna or the 'deadly nightshade', the foliage and berries of which are extremely toxic, contain tropane alkaloids which can cause delirium, hallucinations and death. The Atropa genus, to which the Belladonna species belong, has a long history of use as a medicine, cosmetic and poison. Modern pharmaceutical preparations from the nightshade species include atropine, Hyoscine and scopolamine. Its name, 'belladonna', meaning 'beautiful woman' derived from Italian, is due to its use by ancient Egyptian women as eye drops to cause pupillary dilatation which has a subconscious attractive effect on men. All of these plants and many other herbal medications have many side effects and are poisonous unless the proper dose, methods of preparation and administration are carefully controlled.

Iranian Medicinal Plants

Of course, the most popular herbal remedies in Iran are different from those in Europe and North America. In the western world, the most popular remedies include Echinacea, Ephedra, Kava, St. John's wort, Ginkgo, Ginseng, Valerian, Chamomile, Ginger and several others. A group of researchers conducted a study to evaluate the efficacy and safety of alternative therapies and found significant hazards in the use of some herbal remedies including Ephedra, Kava and St. John's wort as well as the fact that many Ayurvedic medicinal products contained significant levels of lead, mercury and arsenic. St. John's Wort plant because of its interference with performance of oral contraceptives (OCP), ginkgo and ginseng due to interactions with the action of warfarin, and keratome drugs due to being agonistic with opioid receptors can be referred.

In some countries, such as the Germany, all forms of herbal compounds are not OTC and are not available for use without prescription. In Iran, herbal medicines are traditionally different from those in the west. Since the Islamic revolution, governmental, university and religious leaders have encouraged the resurgence of traditional 'Iranian' and 'Islamic' medical practices most of which are neither Iranian nor Islamic and are an amalgam of ancient Greek and other retrogressive medical practices.

Of the 8100 plant species in Iran, approximately 2300 species are aromatic and medicinal and about 450 species are sold by herbal apothecaries without any controls as to their purity. The consumers of these herbal medications have no knowledge of their toxicity, side effects or their interactions with other herbal or pharmaceutical medications nor are they instructed as to their dosage and specificity of their actions. Development of herb shops in recent years and the lack of proper monitoring, as well as the misuse of some profiteers through the extensive and exaggerated propaganda of medicinal plant compounds such as weight loss and obesity, etc. which is often non-scientific and commercial in nature, make it more necessary to monitor these kinds of activities.

The most common herbal medicines sold in Iran, according to a survey carried out by Tehran University of Medical Sciences are, Borage (golgavezaban), Valerian (sonboletip), Rocket seeds (khakeshir), Violet (banafsheh), Chicory (kasni), Thyme (avishan), Marshmallow (khatmi), as well as Foxglove (gole angoshtooneh), Castor (karchak), Liquorice (shirin bian), Stramonium (taatooreh), Cordya (sepestan) as well as a host of other plants.

Most of these plants are quite harmless and have a long history as ancient medicinal plants, but the multiple medicinal properties claimed for each have not been scientifically proven in evidence based clinical trials but merely extracted from ancient pharmacopeias. Some, however, can be toxic if consumed in excess, such as Borage (golgavezaban) which contains pyrrolizidine alkaloids that are hepatotoxic and Stramonium (taatooreh) belonging to the Solanacea family can cause confusion, hallucination, delirium and coma. Some may interfere with blood clotting and blood pressure medications or anesthetics and therefore care must be exercised under such circumstances.

Unani Medicine

Unani medicine originated in Greece and is primarily based on the principles propounded by the ancient Greek practitioners Hippocrates and Galen. Over the subsequent centuries, a number of Arab and Persian scholars enriched the system, among them Ibn Sina, who is also known as Avicenna. He was an Arab philosopher and physicist, who wrote Kitab-al-shifa (Book of Healing) and the Canon of Medicine. This system, earlier known as "Galenics", later became known as Unani Tibb, (Unani being the Arabic word for "Greek" and Tibb an Arabic word for "medicine").

Unani medicine states that disease is a natural process and that symptoms are the reactions of the body to disease. It employs the humoral theory which presupposes the presence of four akhlaat (humours) in the body – dam (blood), balgham (phlegm), safra (yellow bile) and sauda (black bile). Each humour has its own temperament: blood is hot and moist; phlegm is cold and moist; yellow bile is hot and dry; and black bile is cold and dry. According to Unani, if the four main humours and the four primary temperaments (hot, cold, dry, moist) are all in a state of mutual equilibrium, the person is considered healthy. In Unani medicine, six key factors are evaluated in relation to health. These six factors are called "al-umoor al-tabiyah". Each has a close relation to, and a direct bearing on, the state of health of an individual. Therefore, it is necessary for a Unani medicine practitioner to take all these factors into consideration in order to arrive at a correct diagnosis and decide how to treat the ailment.

Concepts of the Stages of Digestion

According to the Unani system of medicine, there are four stages of digestion:

- Gastric digestion followed by intestinal digestion, when food is turned into chyme and chyle and carried to the liver.

- Hepatic digestion, when chyle is converted into the four humours in varying quantities, blood being the largest. Thus, the blood that leaves the liver is intermixed with the other three humours; phlegm, yellow bile and black bile.
- Vessel digestion, in which every tissue absorbs nutrition by its attractive power and retains it by its retentive power.
- Tissue digestion is the digestive power that, in conjunction with the power of assimilation, converts the nutritive elements into tissue.

The waste material remaining in the humours at this stage is excreted by the expulsive power. Unani practitioners maintain that when any disturbance occurs in the equilibrium of the humours, it causes disease. Therefore the Unani mode of treatment aims to restore the equilibrium of the humours.

States of the Human Body (Haalaat al-jism)

According to Unani medicine practitioners, the states of the body are grouped under three headings:

- Health, in which all the functions of the body operate normally.
- Disease, the opposite of health, in which one or more forms or functions of the bodily organs are at fault.
- Neither health nor disease, where there is neither complete health nor actual disease, such as in the case of elderly individuals or those who are convalescing.

Diseases are of two types, namely simple or complex. A simple disease is one that completes its course without complications. A simple disease may manifest itself in three forms:

- Imbalance of the humours (dyscrasia).
- Structural diseases.
- Diseases of disharmony.

Physical Temperament (Mizaj)

The interaction of the elements produces various states, which in turn determine the temperament of an individual. It is of paramount importance to keep that temperament in mind while prescribing a course of treatment. Each individual has a unique temperament, which may potentially be real equitable, equitable or inequitable. The state of real equitable never occurs in reality, rather it is a theoretical situation in which the temperaments of the four elements used are equal. An equitable temperament denotes an appropriate and required amount of compatible temperaments. An inequitable temperament results from an inappropriate distribution of temperaments for the requirements of the individual's condition.

Prevention of Disease

Unani medicine has long recognized the influence of surroundings and ecological conditions on the state of health of human beings. It has a theory on the six essential prerequisites for the prevention of disease and it places great emphasis on the maintenance of a proper ecological balance and on keeping water, food and air free from all pollution. These prerequisites, known as al-asbab al-sitta al-dharuriya (six essentials) may be briefly explained as follows:

- Al-hawaa (air): Good, clean air is necessary for health and many diseases are said to occur owing to changes in the air. Abu Sina, the famous Unani medicine practitioner, said that a change of environment can relieve patients of many diseases. Abu Sina also emphasized the need for open, airy houses with proper ventilation and for playgrounds and gardens in the cities so that everyone could get plenty of fresh air to allow for maintenance of a proper ecological cycle.
- Al-maakool wa al-mashroob (food and drink): Food should be fresh and free from putrefaction and pathogens. Drinking water should also be pure.
- Harakat wa sukoon al-baden (physical exercise and repose): To maintain positive health and fitness, the body requires both exercise and rest. Inflammation and fractures require total rest for an optimum healing. On the other hand, afflictions such as paralysis demand specific types of movement. Several exercises help muscles to grow and ensure increased blood supply and proper functioning of the excretory system. Exercise also keeps the heart and liver in good condition.
- Mental exertion and repose: Psychological factors such as happiness, sorrow, and anger are believed to have considerable bearing on the health of the human being. Unani medicine practitioners maintain that certain diseases and disorders are caused by emotional strain and maladjustment. Therefore, when dealing with such cases, the practitioner should try to take all these factors into account. There is a branch of Unani medicine known as "psychological treatment" that deals with the abovementioned factors, and many diseases are treated by psychological methods. Sometimes this type of treatment is used alone, while at other times it is used in conjunction with various medicines. Unani medicine practitioners have also recognized the effects of music, pleasant company and beautiful scenery.
- Sleep and wakefulness: Normal sleep and wakefulness are essential for health. Sleep is an ideal form of rest; physical as well as mental. Lack of sleep causes dissipation of energies, mental weakness and digestive disturbances.
- Evacuation and retention: Waste products of the body, if not completely and properly excreted, produce disease. The natural means of excretion are diuresis, diaphoresis, vomiting, defecation, excretion through the uterus in the form of menses, excretion through the eyes, ears and nose and respiration. Proper and normal functioning of the excretory processes must be ensured in order to maintain what, in Unani medicine, is considered perfect health. Any disturbance in the normal excretory balances, whether it is excess, diminution or blockage, may lead to disease.

Faculties/Powers (Quwa)

According to Unani medicine there are three kinds of powers: psychic (natural) power, power of metabolism and power of reproduction.

- Psychic and nervous power is present in the brain and is made up of two other powers: perceptive power, which conveys impressions or sensations, and motive power, which brings about movements as a response to the sensation.

Perceptive power may be external or internal. The external perceptive power recognizes objects outside the body and is served by the five senses. The internal perceptive power operates when perceptions do not come from the outside, but are inferences drawn from external impressions and realizations. Internal perceptive power uses five other powers:

- Composite sense, which collects together all external realizations.
- Imagination, which stores all the materials collected by the composite sense.
- Conceptualization, which correlates all external realizations and draws conclusions from them.
- Memory, which stores the conclusions drawn by conceptualization.
- The modifying faculty, which gives the capacity to explain the same thing in different ways and interprets all internal and external realizations.

- The seat of the power of metabolism is the liver, but the process is active in every tissue of the body. The process of metabolism is conducted by two powers:
    - Nutritive power is developed in the liver from the food eaten and is conveyed to all parts of the body. It is served by four other powers: attractive, retentive, digestive and expulsive.
    - Growing power is responsible for the development and growth of the human organism and is served by three other powers – receptive power, power to retain nutrition and assimilative power.
- Reproduction is accomplished by two powers: generative power and formative power.

Therapeutics

This system, the entire personality of a patient is taken into account. Each individual has got its own basic structure, physique, make-up, self-defence mechanism, reaction to environmental factors, likes and dislikes.

Main Types of Treatment in Unani Medicine

1. Regimental therapy (Ilaj-bil-Tadbir): Regimental therapy is special technique/physical methods of treatment to improve the constitution of body by removing waste materials and improving the defence mechanism of the body and protect health. In other words these are the best known “detoxification methods”. Important techniques in regimental therapy along with the ailments for which they are considered effective are briefly described below:

- Venesectio (Fasd): This method of treatment has been found very effective for:
    - Correction of blood related problems and relieve high blood pressure.
    - Prevention of toxicity and accumulation of waste matter in the blood.
    - Excretion of waste matters from various parts of the body.

- Stimulation of metabolic processes.
- Cure of ailments due to certain menstrual disorders.
- Correction of hot material in temperament.

- Cupping (Al-hijama): This method of treatment is used for:
  - Cleaning the skin of waste matters.
  - To stop excessive menses or epistaxis.
  - To correct liver diseases.
  - To treat malaria and spleen disorders.
  - To treat piles, inflammation of testes and uterus, scabies, boils etc.
- Sweating (Tareeq): Waste matter from skin, blood and from other parts of the body is excreted through the normal process of sweating. It helps in reducing excessive heat. Dry or wet fomentation, bath with warm water, massage and keeping the patient in a room having hot air are some of the methods of diaphoresis.
- Diuresis (Idrar-e-baul): Poisonous matters, waste products and the excess of humours are excreted through urine. It is applied as a cure for diseases of the heart, liver and lungs. Sometimes diuresis is affected by keeping the patient in a cold room and applying cold water.
- Turkish bath (Hamam): This is recommended for:
  - Resolving the waste matter and increasing sweating.
  - Providing light heat.
  - Increasing nutrition.
  - Decreasing fat.
  - Increasing fat.

  Cold bath is preferable in normal health. Hot bath is generally applied for the cure of diseases like paralysis and muscular wasting etc. after massage.
- Massage (Dalk, Malish): Soft massage is sedative and relaxant; dry and hard massage is deobstruent and increases the blood supply while the massage with oil relaxes the muscles and softens the skin.
- Counter irritation: This technique provides relief in pain, burning sensation and irritation. It helps to reduce inflammation and heals tumours.
- Cauterization (Amal-e-Kae): It prevents the poison malignancy of one organ from transferring it to other organs. In case of pain of hip joint, this technique is found very useful. By

this technique the pathogenic matters, which are attached to some structures, are removed or resolved.

- Purging (Ishal): Unani medicine widely uses purgatives for intestinal evacuation. There are written rules for using this method. This method influences normal metabolic process.
- Vomiting (Qai): Emetics are used to cure headache, migraine, tonsillitis, bronchopneumonia and also bronchial asthma. This also cures mental diseases like mania and melancholia.
- Exercise (Riyazat): Physical exercise has great importance for maintenance of good health and for treating certain diseases. It is said to be good for stomach and for strengthening digestion. There are laid down rules, timings and conditions for various types of exercises.
- Leeching (Taleeq-e-Alaq): This method is used for removing bad matter from the blood. This is useful in skin diseases and ringworms etc. The system describes specific conditions for applying it.

2. Dieto therapy (Ilaj-bil-Ghiza): In Unani treatment, food plays a key role. By regulating the quality and quantity of food several ailments are treated successfully. There are several published books, which deals with the subject of diet in relation to specific diseases. Certain foods are considered as laxative, diuretic and diaphoretic.

3. Pharmacotherapy (Ilaj-bil-Dawa): This type of treatment involves the use of naturally occurring drugs, mostly herbal. Drugs of animals and mineral origin are also used. Natural drugs only are used because they are locally available and have no or less after effects on the body. Unani medicine presupposes that the drugs also have their own temperament. Since in this system, emphasis is laid on the particular temperament of the individual, the medicines, administered are such as go well with the temperament of the patient, thus accelerating the process of recovery and also eliminating the risk of reaction. Drugs are supposed to act by their temperament of being hot, cold, moist and dry. As a matter of fact, drugs are classified into four classes according to their temperament and the physicians consider its potency, age and temperament of the patient, nature and severity of diseases. Drugs are used in the form of powders, decoctions, infusion, Jawarish, Majoon, Khamira, Syrup and tablets etc. The system has set rules for prescribing alternative drugs.

4. Surgery (Ilaj-bil-Yad): This therapy is of very limited use, although the Unani system is credited to be pioneer in this field and having developed its own instruments and techniques. At present only minor surgery is in use in the system.

Herbs in Unani Medicine

S.No.	Botanical Name	Indian Name	Unani Name
1.	Abelmoschus moschatus Medic, syn. Hibiscus abelmoschus Linn.	Mushk-dana (H,B,Bo)	Mushkdana
2.	Abies spectabilis (D.Don) Spach, syn.A. webbiana Lindl.	Talishapatri (Tamil, Telgu)	Talipatra
3.	Abutilon indicum (L) Sweet, syn. A. asiaticum (L) Sweet	Kandhi (H), Kankati (S)	Kanghi
4.	Acacia catechu Willd.	Khair(H), Khadira(S)	Katta

5.	Achyranthes aspera Linn	Chirochita (S)	Chirchita
6.	Aconitum ferox Walld. Ex Ser.	Bich (H,B), Visha (S)	Bish
7.	Aconitum heterphyllum Walld. Ex Royle.	Atis (H), Ativisha(S)	Atis
8.	Acorus calamus Linn	Vacha (S), Bach (H)	Wuz
9.	Adhatoda vasica Nees	Bakas (B), Vasaka (S)	Banga
10.	Aegle marmelos Correa ex Roxb.	Bel (B,Bo), Bilva (S)	Belgiri
11.	Aleurites triloba Forst.	Jangli akhrot (H)	Chahar-maghz-e-hindi
12.	Alpinia galangal Willd.	Bara kulanga (Bo,H)	Kulanjan
13.	Althaea officinalis Linn	Gul-khairo (H,Bo,D)	Gul-Khairo
14.	Amorphophallus campanulatus Blum ex Decne.	Zaminkand (H) Kanda (H)	Zaminkand
15.	Ananas comosus Merr, syn. A.sativus Schult f.	Anannas (H), Ananasa (H)	Ananas
16.	Andropagon miliaceus Retz.	Usira or Virana (S)	Usir
17.	Annona squamosa Linn	Sharifah, Sitafal (G.M.D)	Sharifah
18	Aquilaria agallocha Roxb.	Agar (H)	Agare-hindi or Aude-hindi
19.	Areca catechu Linn.	Supari (H,B), Sopari (Bo, G)	Supari
20.	Aristolochia indica Linn.	Saapasan (H) Isharmul (H,B)	Zaravande-hindi
21.	Artemisia absinthium Linn.	Afsantin (H, D)	Afsanthin
22.	Artemisia vulgaris Linn.	Majtari or Mastaru (H)	Afsantine-hindi
23.	Artocarpus heterophyllus Lamk, syn. A. integrifolia Linn, f., A. integra (Thunb.) Merril.	Kathal (H), Panasa (S)	Kathal
24.	Asparagus ascendens Roxb.	Safed Musli (H, G)	Shaqa-qule-hindi
25.	Asparagus racemosus Willd.	Satwar (H), Satvari (G)	Shaqaqul
26.	Asteracantha longifolia T. Nees, syn. Hydrophila spinosa T. Anders.	Tal-makhana (H, M)	Talmakhana

Chumash Medicine

In 1542, the Spanish explorer Juan Rodriguez de Cabrillo sailed along the coast of California. While he really didn't discover anything, he did encounter the Chumash Indians who occupied the three northern large islands of the Santa Barbara archipelago and the shoreline from Malibu Canyon to Estero Bay. The Chumash were a coastal people with a maritime lifestyle. Cabrillo described the Chumash this way: "They were dressed in skins and wore their hair very long and tied up with long strings interwoven with the hair, there being attached to the strings many gewgaws of flint, bone, and wood." Regarding Chumash on Santa Cruz Island he reported: "They are fisherman; they eat nothing but fish; they sleep on the ground; their sole business and employment is to fish."

The Spanish noted that there were 10 rancherias (small Indian settlements) on Santa Cruz Island. In addition, the Spanish mention the names of more than 20 villages on the mainland coast. It is generally estimated that at the time of contact with the Spanish, there were 75-100 Chumash communities with a total population of 20-30,000. The villages usually contained between 15 and 50 houses roughly aligned along a street. Chumash houses were bowl shaped structures made of poles and covered with thatched tules. "The structure was hemispherical, made by planting willows or other poles in a circle and bending and tying them together at the top."

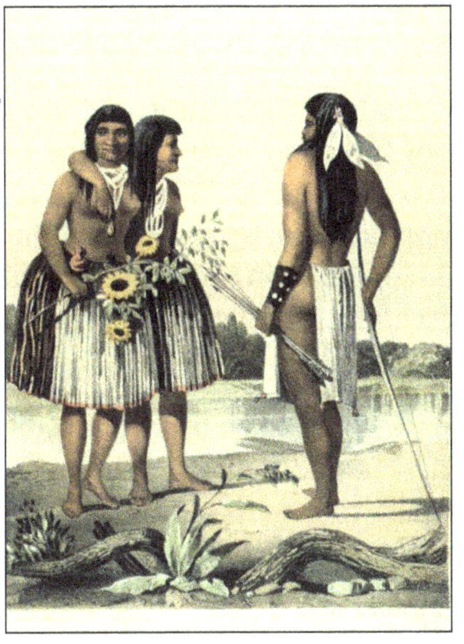

The house diameters ranged from four to seven meters. Next to many of the houses were temascal, smaller dome-shaped structures covered with mud which were used as sweat houses. One of the substances gathered and used by the Chumash was bitumen, a naturally occurring type of tar from the Channel Islands. The Chumash used this as a kind of all-purpose glue. "The Chumash gathered naturally occurring bitumen from numerous seeps throughout the islands. They used the gooey substance to waterproof canoes, line baskets used as water bottles, and to plug holes in shells that they used as food containers. They even chewed it."

On the negative side, the polycyclic aromatic hydrocarbon toxins in the bitumen may have led to major health problems, such as cancer, damage to internal organs, and reproductive impairment. This may have also lead to an overall decrease in Chumash stature of about four inches. According to the oral history of the Chumash, all of the people originally lived on Santa Cruz Island. One day Xoy split the people into two groups. One group, the ka'ikiku, went over a rainbow bridge to Mount Pinos. The other group, the molmolokiku stayed with Xoy and learned how to make plants and animals for the ka'ikiku to use. Thus the ka'ikiku asks the molmolokiku for guidance in using plants and animals. Many of the plants were used medicinally and spiritually.

For the Chumash, as for many of the Indian peoples of California, one of the most important spiritual plants was jimsonweed (Datura) which was used to help produce visions. In many of the tribes, it was felt that jimsonweed was so powerful that it should be used only once. However, among the Chumash, "Individuals were allowed to use the plant as often as they saw fit, and they could take it right in their own village." Use of jimsonweed was seen as important to a person's life, and higher status Chumash individuals tended to use it more than once in order to gain spiritual power.

Among the Chumash, both men and women used jimsonweed. The first infusion of Datura was usually administered by a paid specialist who was skilled at preparing the plant. In some villages, the initial experience was supervised by five elders. Boys were always initiated alone, but girls were sometimes initiated as a group. After ingesting an infusion of the root of the plant, the initiate would become dizzy and start to tremble. The specialist would then tell the initiate to sleep and to dream. The initiate would generally sleep for 18-24 hours. As the initiate began to revive, the specialist would sing and the elders would ask about the dream and then interpret it.

There were a number of reasons why the Chumash would use jimsonweed after initiation. This would include the strengthening of the bond with the spirit helper, acquiring additional spirit helpers, and acquiring spiritual power in general. Women would use the plant to become immune to danger and to attain courage. John Baker notes that among the Chumash: "A person who ingested Datura for visionary purposes might do so in order to communicate with the spirit of a beloved person who had died, or to obtain a glimpse of his or her own future. Datura could also be used to locate lost objects."

In addition to spiritual uses, jimsonweed was also used medically. Jimsonweed (Datura) was used as an anesthesia when setting bones. In addition, it might be ingested when treating bruises and wounds. "Datura was taken internally to 'freshen the blood' and to treat alcohol-induced hangovers (a post-contact innovation) and applied externally to treat hemorrhoids. "It is clear that the Chumash use of Datura was based upon a thorough empirical knowledge of the effects of the plant." Specialists understood both the dosages needed to achieve different ends as well as the preparation and environmental factors which can influence outcomes.

Among the Chumash, a tea made from the root and rhizomes of Anemopsis californica (commonly called yerba mansa, swamp root or lizard tail) was used as a drink for colds, asthma, and urinary tract disorders. It was also used to wash cuts and sores and for bathing arthritic joints. "This plant has been used for a long time in California and should be investigated by scientists interested in new drugs for the treatment of venereal diseases and asthma." For headaches, stomach problems, and arthritis, the Chumash ate the root of hog fennel (Lomatium californicum). In addition, hog fennel seeds were eaten to treat colds and sore throats. Hog fennel root was worn on a necklace or on a belt as a means of repelling rattlesnakes.

Red shank (Adenostoma sparsifolium, also called greasewood or ribbonwood) had a number of medicinal uses among the Chumash. Sore throats, stomach problems, respiratory problems, and colds were treated with a tea made from red shank bark. A tea made from small branches was used for treating toothaches and for washing wounds. Ephedra californica (commonly called joint fir, Indian tea, and desert tea) was used by the Chumash for purifying the blood and for treating urinary tract infections and venereal diseases. Other California tribes used this plant for stomach problems and backaches. Since one of the active ingredients found in the plant is psuedoephedrine, it was also used as a nasal decongestant and as a stimulant.

The Chumash and the Kumeyaay used an elderberry (Sambucus mexicana) flower tea for treating colds, flu, and fevers. This tea was also used to relieve premenstrual syndrome and dysmenorrhea. The inner bark of the elderberry was used as an emetic and its berries were used as a laxative.

Techniques used in Chumash Medicine

Traditional Chumash healing starts with God. The Healer may use prayer and fasting to invite

God to help with the healing. Fasting is a self-denial that enhances the spirituality of the Healer, facilitating communication with God. In fact, all healing must involve God. The spirit is always involved in the healing process. The reason for this is that many diseases start with the spirit. The spirit forgets to be well. Another way of thinking of this is that the spirit may be overstressed with work or concerns, depressed, overburdened with addictions or neglected from not enough prayer. When the spirit forgets to be well, the body becomes ill. The spirit may neglect the sick body and prevent healing. Treating the body alone leaves the spirit still sick. This may result in more illness.

The Healer is not alone in this spiritual healing process. The sick person's family, friends and other community members may aid in prayer, fasting, dancing and generally reassuring the person that he or she is loved. This reassurance is comforting and helps the spirit to feel well again. When the spirit is well, the body can recover from disease. Dancing, like singing, can be used as prayer.

This spiritual healing is very dissimilar to standard health care, where doctors, nurses, pharmacists and other health care workers may not pray with the patient, despite the fact that prayer has been shown to be beneficial to the majority of patients. Prayer comforts patients. At the very least, prayer does no harm and costs nothing. While in hospital, the patient may feel isolated from family and friends. The spirit may not become well quickly. The approach with standard health care is that the body is treated and made well. The spirit should then follow and recover as well. However, many patients complain of uncertainty with their healing even after their bodies are supposed to be well again.

Prevention of disease was a major concern of Healers in the old days. People were encouraged to work hard every day for the village. This helped keep them physically fit and helped them feel needed. Everyone had a job that was necessary for the village. Being physically fit and thin tends to lower the chances of having high blood pressure, high blood cholesterol, diabetes, heart disease and other conditions. These problems can be caused by visceral fat that secretes cortisol and induces the metabolic syndrome. Obesity was uncommon in the old days, because each person was physically fit. The Healer worked hard at keeping everyone working. Healers of the past used humor in the healing process. Helping patients laugh at a joke can help relieve their anxiety. Sometimes when people become sick, it is almost as if they are taking on the misery of the world. They need attention and love, from their family, friends and Healer. They also need to have a different perspective on their situation. Humor can help take them away from their despair for a while and give them a new perspective. Then they can allow the healing process to begin.

White Sage

The Healer frequently starts treatment with white sage (Salvia apiana), which purifies the central nervous system to help a person maintain integrity. White sage is wey'wey in Chumash (pronounced waykway). White sage can help a patient become calm enough to be rational. White sage may be the foundation of treatment since it can help set the spirit back to normal. White sage tickles the spirit and sets it right again. White sage is our protection. Ideally, we should all take white sage every day to help maintain spiritual health, when used with prayer. This can be done by planting and maintaining white sage plants in gardens. Seeds or plants can be obtained from some nurseries and botanical gardens. The Tongva and other people used to plant and tend white sage near their village sites. White sage bushes grow in full sun, in sandy soil and are drought resistant. They have long, thin leaves about 3 inches long with a silver, green color and a pleasant sage smell. The flowers are small, white, sometimes with purple, and have long anthers that emerge out of the flowers. The shiny, black or brown seeds have a pleasant sage flavor.

White sage, like any plant, should be collected with prayer. Only the amount needed should be collected. A small branch or a single leaf can be broken off for each use. Each leaf contains vital medicine for the health of the spirit. The leaves can be dried for later use, if necessary. The best way to use white sage is to put it in the water a patient drinks. Simply put an entire leaf in the water bottle the patient drinks from. Water bottles typically contain ~1 L of water. Allow the leaf to flavor the water over 30 min or so before allowing the patient to drink the water. The leaf can be re-used in four bottles of water. The water may develop a very slight sage flavor and smell. Only use the leaf for 1 day. After 1 day, the leaf will start to degrade. Another way to use white sage is to put half of a leaf in the mouth and suck on it. The leaf will fill the mouth with sage flavor and soothe the throat. White sage contains cineole, also called eucalyptol, which is soothing. Salvia plants contain many active compounds including many active diterpenoids that can be antibiotic or anti-allergic. Also present are anti-inflammatory compounds, antibiotic compounds and anti-anxiety compounds. White sage can also be drunk as a tea. Start the water at room temperature. Add a white sage leaf and heat the water until it just starts to boil. It must be tended so the water does not boil, or it will lose its effect.

Of course, white sage is also used when blessing people. The traditional Chumash way to do this is to use small branches, about 6 inches long, of dried white sage. The white sage should not be bound with yarn or string. This can cause the white sage to mold. Gently suck on the end of the branch and gently touch each leaf after harvesting. Remember that white sage is spirit medicine and should not be wasted by simply burning it like incense. When white sage is smudged, everyone should be praying. The smoke brings the prayers to God. The smoke also invites God to participate in the healing process. Certain people in each group are recognized for their ability to bless others with white sage, and are invited by the group to administer the blessings. A Healer may also smudge white sage to help with a healing process.

Mugwort

Dreams are an essential part of health. Dreams help the spirit remember to be normal, to be happy. Dreams help heal the spirit. Many patients have trouble dreaming because they are under too much stress. They cannot relax their minds at night and simply dream. Many patients use drugs to help them sleep. These drugs usually prevent dreaming and may cause patients to wake up with some lingering depression, hung over. Patients who are addicted to drugs or alcohol may have trouble dreaming. Patients with heart disease may also find it hard to dream and sleep.

Dream sage is used by Healers to promote good dreams. Dream sage is also called mugwort, Artemisia douglasiana. It is called molush in Chumash. To use dream sage, collect the stalks, leaves and seeds, dry them and sew them into a small pillow ~15 cm × 15 cm × 7 cm. Place the small pillow under the normal pillow to promote dreaming. Dream sage contains camphor, linalool, cineole and other pleasant-smelling compounds. The pleasant, sage smell of the dream sage induces aromatherapy that will help promote dreaming. This helps heal the spirit. When the spirit remembers to be normal, the body can heal. Various sesquiterpene lactones such as absinthin and a hallucinogenic compound thujone are also present in Artemisia plants. These are the principle ingredients in absinthe.

One of the most romantic things a young man can do for his girlfriend is to make her a small pillow of dream sage. This shows her that he cares about her and her dreams. Hopefully, she will dream pleasant dreams about him. Dream sage is a common plant that grows in deep canyons near water. It is best to collect some of the seeds from this plant in the autumn, plant them in a garden and tend the plant for later use. It may also be possible to find a nursery or botanical garden that may sell the plant. The plant grows in partial or full shade and requires watering.

Californian Sagebrush

Sometimes, when the spirit is sick, just remembering pleasant thoughts can be helpful in healing. A Healer may use Californian sagebrush, Artemisia californica, to help promote pleasant memories. The smell of Californian sagebrush reminds many Californians of the smell of grandmother's house. A pleasant smell, like Californian sagebrush, can help the patient remember long-lost memories. Aromatherapy is a very powerful way of bringing back pleasant memories.

Californian sagebrush is a common plant. It can be purchased from some nurseries or botanical gardens to grow at home. It grows in full sun and is drought resistant. The leaves are thread-like and have a strong sage smell when crushed. There have been few scientific examinations of the active compounds in Californian sagebrush. However, the active compounds are probably similar to those found in mugwort, such as the sesquiterpene lactone, artecalin. Anyone can benefit from this aromatherapy each time they walk past Californian sagebrush.

Californian Bay

In the old days, the Chumash people bathed frequently in hot springs. The pool was prepared with prayer. Red maids, Calandrinia ciliata, called khutash in Chumash, were sprinkled onto the water. The water was treated with a few Californian bay leaves, Umbellularia californica, psha'n in Chumash (pronounced pshokn). People bathed in the water to soothe themselves, comfort their arthritic joints and to feel normal again. Of course, warm water is soothing to arthritic joints and can help relieve pain and swelling, at least temporarily. Patients can benefit from this therapy in their own tubs at home.

Californian bay used to be eaten as a flavoring for food and as a way of strengthening the immune system. It was eaten during the first 2 weeks or so of a new season. This means it was eaten four times each year. It was used to help people adjust to the changing seasons and to the changes of life. It can be used by Healers to help the spirit adjust to the changes needed in healing. Usually Californian bay leaves are crushed and smelled. This aromatherapy helps open the breathing passages and can relieve headaches, even migraine headaches. Since Californian bay helps people adjust to the changing seasons, it also helps enhance immunity to colds and flus.

Californian bay is a large tree that can grow to nearly 150 feet tall. The long, thin leaves are ~4 inches long and smell of bay. The fruit is a soft, green drupe about three-quarters of an inch in diameter. Californian bay trees grow in shady, moist canyons and slopes. In Oregon, this tree is called Oregon myrtle. This tree can be purchased from some nurseries. The leaves and fruit contain many fragrant compounds. Sabinene smells like pine. Cineole smells like eucalyptus. Thujene smells like grass and soy sauce. There are probably many other compounds in Californian bay yet to be identified. Aromatherapy with Californian bay is comforting and recommended. However, there are some people who complain of headache from excessive aromatherapy with this plant. The leaves make a very pleasant spice in soups and stews. They are more flavorful than commercial bay leaves and have a similar flavor.

Californian Rose

When a baby cries from teething, Californian rose (Rosa californica) can help. It is called watiqoniqon in Chumash and can be pronounced wotteekwoneekwone. Chumash people used to mash the petals in water and rub the fluid on their baby's gums to relieve the pain of teething. Rose petals have a pleasant, sweet flavor. While chewing the petals, the nose fills with the smell of rose. Adults can chew the petals or drink a rose petal tea. Californian rose helps relieve anxiety. This helps the spirit become more receptive to healing.

Californian rose, probably like most rose species, contains many fragrances, called monoterpenes. Geraniol, nerol, citronellol and other monoterpenes are found in the petals and are used in the perfume industry. These wonderful fragrances have strong effects on people. Some people become happy, others soothed, when smelling rose fragrance.

Momoy

Momoy, Datura wrightii or Californian jimson weed, was used by sucking on part of a leaf to protect the spirit. However, it can be used in other ways to help with spiritual healing. Momoy is the Chumash name for the plant. Some patients, who do not listen well, need to breathe the aroma of the crushed stems. This opens up their breathing passages and their ears. When patients live with too much stress from jobs and relationships, they may find it difficult to take a moment to rest and breathe. Momoy helps them breathe and in general opens them to listening to God and healing.

Some patients need to soak their feet in solutions made from momoy. This is especially true of domineering people, who may be very decent, but are basically mean. The roots or stems of momoy, ~0.25 kg, are fermented in the sun in ~1 L of water for 3 days. The fluid is then heated on the stove to body temperature, or slightly warmer. The patient may then soak their feet for ~15 min. Some patients may need to soak their feet every night for a week before bed. This may help them relax and become receptive to God.

Momoy contains atropine, scopolamine and other compounds. This plant has been used as a way of inducing sacred dreams in order to talk to God. The dose that causes a sacred dream, hallucination, is very close to the dose that inhibits breathing. This makes the plant very dangerous. In addition, scopolamine crosses the blood–brain barrier slowly and may not penetrate adequately until up to 13 h. This makes using momoy for induction of sacred dreams very dangerous. The seeds contain ~0.1 mg of atropine and 0.05 mg of scopolamine each. As few as seven seeds have resulted in poisoning leading to hospitalization. Death may occur with blood levels of 47 ng/ml of atropine and 21 ng/ml of scopolamine, or urine levels of 200 ng/ml of atropine and 95 ng/ml of scopolamine. However, it is safe to use momoy for aromatherapy or as a foot soak. Momoy should also be used as part of Chumash religious practices, as protected by religious freedom laws, provided that its dangers are well understood.

Fire

Fire is a very important part of Chumash religion and healing. The Chumash religion centers around the fire. Fire is the symbol of purity. Fire purifies everything it consumes. Fire is also a symbol of joy for most people. Just looking at a fire makes most people feel happy. Since fire purifies, it can help calm patients and help them stop fretting. Since fire brings joy, it can help patients laugh and give them a new perspective. Fire can help patients accept healing.

In the old days, it was common for the patient to lie beside a fire during a healing ceremony. Singers stood on one side of the patient. Dancers danced on the other side of the fire. Friends formed a circle around the patient, dancers, singers and the fire. The friends were there to let the patient know that he was loved. The singers sang prayers of healing. The dancers danced prayers of healing. The fire purified and brought a new perspective for the patient. All this was directed by the Healer who also administered medicines to the patient.

The Chumash saw fire as a good force in nature. Whenever a brush fire came, the next year the plants and animals would be stronger and more plentiful than before. People would be less hungry in the next winter time. The Chumash were good farmers and grew chia sage, Californian tobacco, red maids, fire poppies and possibly other plants. Every year, they burned their fields in order to have a good harvest the next year. Today, forest fires and fire storms fill us with the dread of people losing their houses or lives. Unfortunately, the chaparral is overgrown and is a fire hazard in many areas during dry seasons. However, when carefully controlled and tended in a proper camp fire or ceremonial fire, fire still purifies us and brings us joy.

Siddha System of Medicine

Siddha is one of the oldest systems of medicine discovered in the South India as a part of the trio, the other two being the Ayurveda and Unani. It is based on the principles similar to Ayurveda. According to the ancient Siddha texts, a human body is made up of several elements. It is a microscopic component of the universe. The elements that form a human body are the earth (munn), fire (thee), water (neer), air (vayu) and space (akasam). Additionally, there are three humors or the DOSHAS called the Vata, Pitta, and Kapha. Siddha medicine believes that diseases occur when there is a disequilibrium or imbalance in these humors or if their individual harmony is disturbed. The balance can be restored by correcting the underlying dosha by the application of the Siddha medicine system.

These three Doshas co-exist in all the cells of the body. They function in a harmonious manner to create a balance. Vata is formed by Vayu and Akasam. It controls the sensory and motor functions of the nervous system such as sensation and movement. Pitta is formed by Thee (fire). It controls the metabolic processes in the body such as digestion, and assimilation, and helps to maintain the warmth of the body. Kapha is formed by Neer (water) and Munn (earth) and controls stability. The three doshas are considered the three pillars of health and support the structure and functions of the body. These Tridoshas are involved in regulating all the functions of the body, and maintain the balance in the physical, emotional and mental spheres.

Origin of Siddha

Siddha system that originated in the South India derives its name from the term 'Siddha' which means an achievement. The practitioners of this medicine system are called the Siddhars. They need to attain the physical and spiritual excellence to be able to treat people. Eighteen Siddhars have been believed to have contributed towards the development of this system. The Siddha texts are in Tamil language and the system is practiced mainly in the Tamil-speaking parts of the world.

History of Siddha

It is believed that the place for the beginning of the human civilization as allotted to the mankind by the Creator was in the temperate zone and the fertile regions of the East, which includes India. Human race evolved in this region. Hence, India is considered the first country from which the human civilization began and spread. According to the Indian history, the Dravidians were the first inhabitants of India among whom the Tamilians were quite prominent. The Tamilians were also the earliest civilized humans. They made considerable progress in the civilization than the other ancient people.

During those times, the languages of India were grouped largely into two classes: Sanskrit in the northern regions and Dravidian language in the southern regions. So, the Siddha science of medicine, which is of fundamental importance for the well-being and survival of humans and has its literature in the Dravidian Tamil language, is believed to have originated in the South India during the period the mankind evolved and developed as the civilization spread.

The Siddha system was prevalent in the south India and the Ayurveda, which was largely in the Sanskrit language, developed in the north. However, instead of giving the name of any human as the founders of these medicine systems, our ancestors attributed the creator for their origin and development. Hence, Siddha medicine is considered to have been created by Lord Shiva, who unfolded the knowledge of medicine to his concert Parvati, who later handed it down to the Nandi Deva and the Siddhars. The Siddhars were considered scientists in ancient times. Though it is difficult to determine the exact point of time when this system originated, it is considered eternal. It began with the mankind and is expected to end with it.

Basic Concepts and Principles of Siddha

The fundamental and applied principles of Siddha system of medicine have a close similarity to the principles of Ayurveda. According to the Siddha system, a human body, as well as the plants and other living species, are the replica of the elements of the universe irrespective of their origin. This system believes that all the objects in the universe are made of five basic elements which are:

- Earth
- Water

- Air
- Fire
- Sky

The food we consume and the medicines we take are also composed of these five elements. The amount and proportion of these elements in the medicines vary. It is their preponderance that is responsible for the medicinal actions and therapeutic results they produce. Siddha system considers a human body as a conglomeration of 3 doshas, 5 elements, and 7 basic tissues together with waste products such as sweat, feces, and urine.

The food, which is the basic building material for the human body, gets processed into these body tissues, humors, and waste products to determine the balance of the doshas in the body. The equilibrium of humors ensures optimum health while any disturbance in these results in diseases. Siddha system also deals with the concept of salvation in life. Siddhars propose that the state of salvation can be achieved through the use of natural Siddha medicines and meditation.

Mode of Action of Siddha Medicines

Siddha Medicine works by revitalizing and rejuvenating the organs. This helps to correct the dysfunctions responsible for causing the diseases. It restores the normal functioning of the organs and maintains the ratio of the three doshas – Vata, Pitta, and Kapha, thereby providing a healthy state of equilibrium in the body. No artificial chemicals are involved in Siddha medicine. Siddha medicine also believes that the universe consists of two entities.

- Matter
- Energy

The Siddhars call these energies, the Siva (male) and Shakti (female, creation). It proposes that matter cannot exist without the energy inherent in it and vice versa. Thus, the two co-exist and are inseparable.

Materia Medica of Siddha Medicine

The Siddha system has developed a rich treasure of medicinal knowledge that includes the use of herbs, metals, and minerals. Depending on the nature and duration of the illness, the results with these medicines may take a variable time to be noticeable. Siddha Medicine can provide an instant relief in some cases, whereas in other cases, the results may take a longer time. Once the disorder is completely cured, the patient can stop taking the medication. Here are the basic forms of medicines in this system:

- Siddha medicine has 25 varieties of inorganic and water-soluble compounds like alkalis and salts that are called 'UPPU.'
- It has 64 varieties of drugs prepared from minerals. These medicines are not soluble in water and are vaporized when put in the fire. Out of these, thirty-two are natural and the rest are artificial.

- Some medicines exhibit properties like sublimation on heating. These medicines contain mercury and its different forms such as mercuric chloride, red sulfide of mercury, and red oxide of mercury.
- The system has a separately classified group of medicines prepared from metals and their alloys, which liquefy when heated and solidify upon cooling. These medicines are prepared from metals like gold, silver, lead, copper, tin, and iron that are incinerated by special processes.
- Sulfur, which is insoluble in water, is also used for treating several ailments owing to its therapeutics properties.

Efficacy and Limitation of Siddha Medicine

The Siddha system can help in treating several diseases although its use in the emergency cases is limited. This system is effective in treating most skin problems including psoriasis as well as urinary tract infections, hepatic diseases, general debility, digestive disorders, arthritis, allergic disorders, postpartum anemia, and fever. It is also effective in the management of viral infections, chronic inflammation, endocrine disorders, and functional disorders.

Diagnosis in Siddha Medicine

Siddha medicine relies on the examination of pulse, eyes, urine, tongue, voice, skin color, and the status of the digestive system to diagnose diseases. This system provides a detailed procedure for the examination of urine including the study of its color, density, smell, oil drop spreading pattern and quantity to determine the cause of illness. The system advocates a holistic approach and the diagnosis is based on the study of the person as a whole and not just the examination of the affected parts of the body.

Siddha Medicine Treatment

The Siddha System emphasizes that the treatment of a patient should be based not just on the disease but also his physical, mental and spiritual state. It also takes into account the environment, age, gender, habits, habitat, mental frame, and the meteorological considerations while recommending the treatment. It also considers the appetite, diet, and physiological constitution of the patient. This means the treatment is individualistic and aimed at removing the root cause of the illness.

Benefits of Siddha Medicine

- Traditional Siddha medicine upholds maintaining the equilibrium of elements in the body and eliminating pathogens for treating diseases and boosting the health.
- It stresses on the importance of prevention of diseases rather than treating them.
- According to the Siddha medicine, diet and lifestyle play an important role in maintaining health and curing diseases.
- The medications are aimed at restoring balance in the body.

- Siddha medicines do not react adversely with the modern medications. Hence, patients who are using allopathic medicines can continue using the same while taking Siddha medicines, but keeping at least 3 hours gap between both.
- All Siddha medicines are natural and do not produce any side effects.

References

- Traditional-Chinese-Medicine-A-Beginner's-Guide-229432202: researchgate.net, Retrieved 08, March 2020
- Chinese-tcm-ingredients-scientifically-proven-to-improve-your-health: theculturetrip.com, Retrieved 12, July 2020
- The-Traditional-Iranian-Medicine-Point-of-View-on-Health-and-Disease-228675430: researchgate.net, Retrieved 26, February 2020
- Iranian-medicine: multiscreensite.com, Retrieved 17, May 2020
- BenchmarksforTraininginUnaniMedicine: who.int, Retrieved 08, August 2020
- Ayurvedic-drugs-in-unani-material-medical-224898925: researchgate.net, Retrieved 15, June 2020

Chapter 3

Ayurveda: An Integrated Study

Ayurveda is a form of alternative medicine having roots in the Indian subcontinent. Various topics studied under Ayurveda are history and eight branches of Ayurveda, Dosha in Ayurveda, Ayurvedic herbs, Ayurvedic acupressure, Dincharyah and Rasa Shastra. All these topics have been carefully analyzed in this chapter.

History of Ayurveda

Ayurvedic medicine has a rich history. Originally shared as an oral tradition, Ayurveda was recorded more than 5,000 years ago in Sanskrit, in the four sacred texts called the Vedas: the Rig Veda (3000-2500 BCE), Yajur Veda, Sam Ved aand Atharva Veda (1200-1000 BCE). Ayurvedic theory states that all areas of life impact one's health, so it follows that the Vedas cover a wide variety of topics, including health and healthcare techniques, astrology, spirituality, government and politics, art and human behavior.

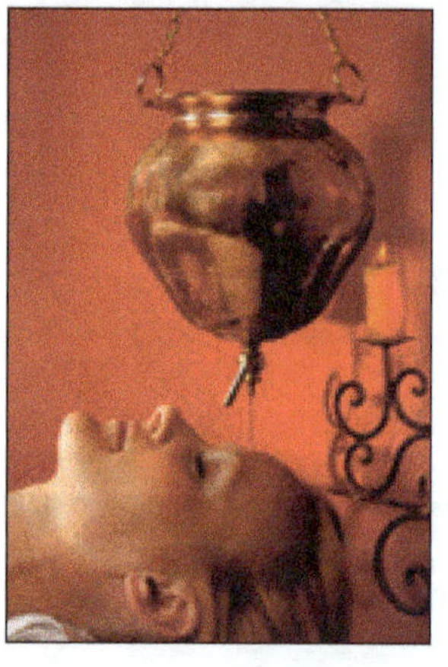

Ayurvedic medical books, available by the eighth century BCE, provide not only procedural instructions but also a history of how Ayurvedic medicine evolved over time. Current knowledge about Ayurveda is primarily based on "the great triad" of texts called Brhattrayi, which consists of the Charak Samhita, Sushurta Samhita and Ashtanga Hridaya. These books describe the basic principles and theories from which modern Ayurveda has evolved.

Major Ayurvedic Classics

Brhattrayi

- Charak Samhita by Charaka: Charak Samhita, which dates back to approximately 800

BCE, is a major compendium of Ayurvedic medical theory and practice that Charaka, an internist at the University of Taxila, compiled in Sanskrit. Presented as poetry, Samhita contains more than 8,400 verses in its 120 chapters. Modern Ayurvedic physicians still use Samhita in their medical training and the text has been widely translated.

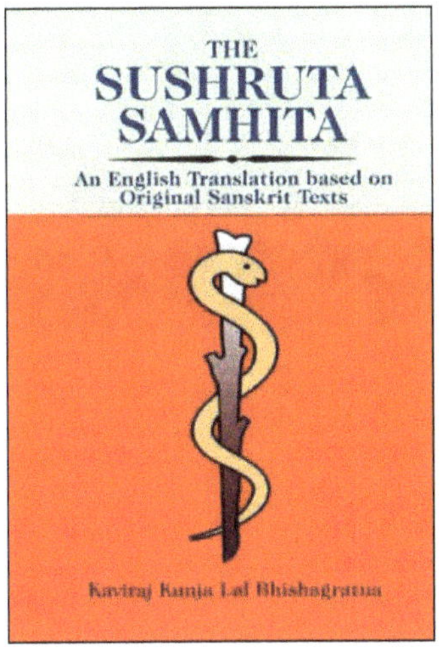

- Sushruta Samhita by Sushruta: This surgical text, which dates back to approximately 700 BCE, contains seminal content such as the Ayurvedic definition of health, information on blood and the description of five subdoshas of Pitta and the marma points. This volume also includes pioneering techniques in skin grafting and reconstructive surgery.

- Ashtanga Sangraha and Ashtanga Hridaya by Vagbhata: Ashtanga Sangraha and Ashtanga Hridayam, dating back to approximately 400 CE, were written by an Ayurvedic physician from the Sindh region of India. The Sangraha is primarily written in poetry, while The Hridayam is presented as prose. These texts define the five subdoshas of Kapha and emphasize the material value of life. The Hridaya is still highly regarded as a primary Ayurvedic medical textbook.

Minor Ayurvedic Classics

The Lghutrayi

- Sarangadhar Samhita by Sharngadhara: This text was written in the 13th century CE and is valued for its explanation of the Ayurvedic concept of materia medica, as well as for its pharmacological formulations. It is also considered the foremost text on pulse diagnosis.

- Bhav Prakash Nighantu by Bhavamisra: This 16th century text contains approximately 10,278 verses of varying meters and focuses on herbal descriptions, food, the therapeutic use of trace metals and rejuvenation therapies. Information on sexually transmitted diseases, particularly syphilis, is also included.

- Madhava Nidan by Madhava Kara: This text was written between 700 CE and 1100 CE and is valued for its precise classification of diseases and disease etiology, particularly in the fields of bala (pediatrics) and toxicology.Madhava Nidan is considered the Bible for Ayurvedic clinical diagnosis.

Eight Branches of Ayurveda

The major eight disciples of Ayurveda are:

- Kaya Chikitsa.
- Kaumar Bhritya.
- Graha Chikitsa (Bhoot Vidya).
- Shalakya Tantra.
- Shalya Tantra.
- Agad Tantra.
- Rasayana.
- Vajikarana (Vrishya Chikitsa).

Kaya Chikitsa

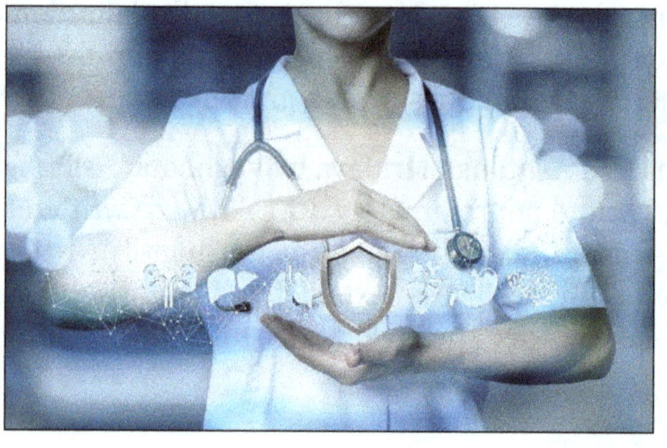

Kaya Chikitsa refers to internal medicine or general medicine in Ayurveda. It is a major branch of ayurvedic medicine deals with prognosis, diagnosis and treatment. Sanskrit word Kaya denotes to the body or metabolism in the body and Chikitsa words indicates towards the diagnosis and treatment. It is a main discipline of Ayurveda. It includes diagnosis techniques, bio-cleansing or detoxification (Panchakarma), herbs and ayurvedic medicines, so it is a complete health science.

Kaumar Bhritya

Kaumar Bhritya deals with health and diseases of children and obstetrics diseases. It can be divided into two parts as per modern sciences. One is Pediatrics and another is Obstetrics. In ancient times, Ayurveda had put these two branches of medical science in a single discipline because both concerned with children. According to Ayurveda, Kaumar means child of age 0 to 16 and Bhritya refers to care and hygiene. Kaumarbhritya is the science that provides preventive and curative measures from the fertilization of eggs to the development and growth of children up to the age of

16. It is the backbone of Ayurveda and human sciences. Ayurvedic scholars believe that care during this period is the backbone of the whole life of an individual.

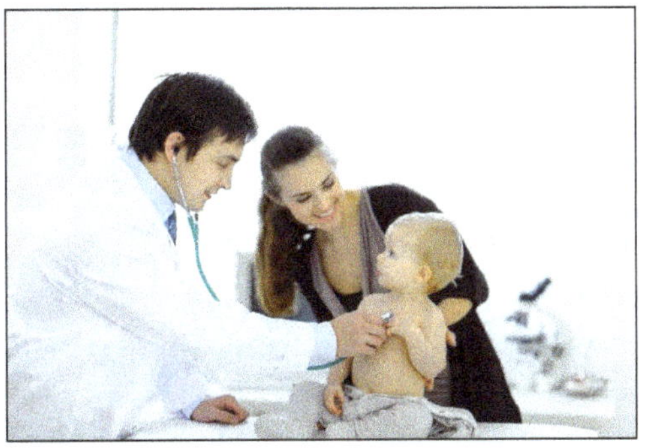

Graha Chikitsa (Bhoot Vidya)

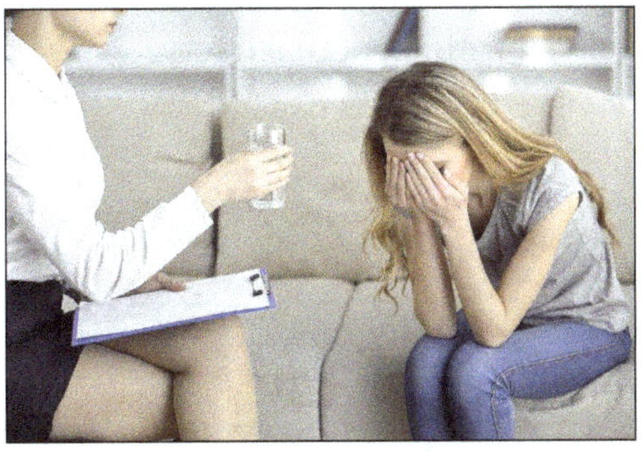

Graha Chikitsa (Bhoot Vidya) is the science of mental life, mind and its characteristics. It is the branch of ayurvedic sciences dealing with the prevention, diagnosis and treatment of mental disorders. The methods used in Bhoot Vidya are related to correcting emotions, mental beliefs, eradicating illusions and providing calmness to the mind through herbal smokes. In modern, it can be correlated with:

- Psychiatry
- Psychology
- Psychotherapy

Shalakya Tantra

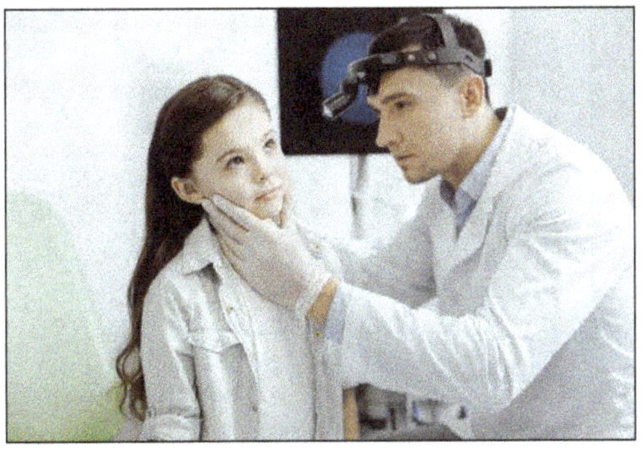

Shalakya Tantra deals with the ear, nose, throat and eye. Therefore, it belongs to Otorhinolaryngology (ENT) and Ophthalmology (Eye), as per modern medical science.

Shalya Tantra

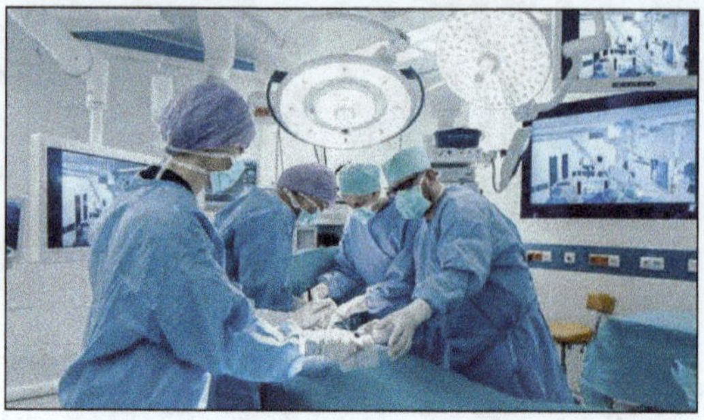

Shalya tantra is the branch of ayurvedic science that treats and manages injuries and diseases by operative procedures. It is correlated with modern surgery.

Agad Tantra

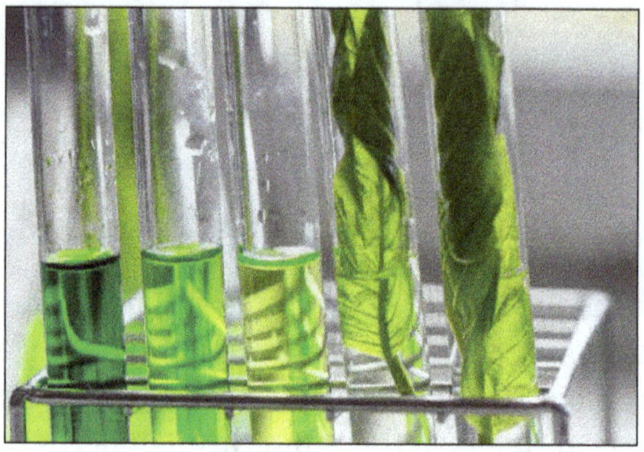

Agad Tantra is the branch of ayurvedic pharmacology that deals with the effects and nature and treatment of poisons. It also deals with the laws and principles of medical practice and laws of medical sciences that lead courts to make appropriate decisions. It also includes forensic techniques and scientific tests used in the investigation of crimes. In modern sciences, Agad tantra relates to the Toxicology, medical jurisprudence and forensic sciences.

Rasayana

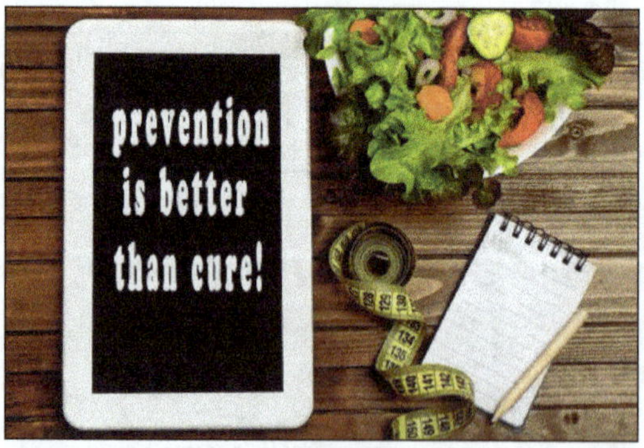

Rasayana is the branch of ayurvedic sciences deals with the rejuvenation of the body, prevention of the diseases and ways for long and healthy life. It includes ayurvedic nutrition, ayurvedic supplements, ayurvedic medicines used in old age for prevention from diseases, detoxification and immunology. In modern, it can be correlated with dietetics, immunology, geriatrics and preventive and social medicine.

Vajikarana (Vrishya Chikitsa)

Vajikarana (Vrishya Chikitsa) is the science of aphrodisiacs. It includes aphrodisiacs herbal and ayurvedic medicines for improving physical strength.

Dosha in Ayurveda

The three primordial forces (sattva, rajas & tamas) interweave to create the five elements (panchmahabhutas) which birth the entire creation. According to Ayurveda everything in life is composed of the Panchamahabhutas – Akash (Space), Vayu (Air), Jal (Water), Agni (Fire) and Prithvi (Earth). Omnipresent, they are mixed in an infinite variety of relative proportions such that each form of matter is distinctly unique. Constantly changing and interacting with each other, they create a situation of dynamic flux that keeps the world going.

This is a small example: Within a simple, single living cell for example the earth element predominates by giving structure to the cell. The water element is present in the cytoplasm or the liquid within the cell membrane. The fire element regulates the metabolic processes regulating the cell. While the air element predominates the gases therein. The space occupied by the cell denoting the last of the elements. In the case of a complex, multi-cellular organism as a human being for instance, Akash (space) corresponds to spaces within the body (mouth, nostrils, abdomen etc.); Vayu (air) denotes the movement (essentially muscular); Agni (fire) controls the functioning of enzymes (intelligence, digestive system, metabolism); Jal (water) is in all body fluids (as plasma, saliva, digestive juices); and Prithvi (earth) manifests itself in the solid structure of the body (bones, teeth, flesh, hair et al).

The Panchmahabhutas therefore serve as the foundation of all diagnosis treatment modalities in Ayurveda and has served as a most valuable theory for physicians to detect and treat illness of the body and mind successfully. For example if a person has more of the fire element in the body he may suffer from more acid secretion (gastric/digestive), which if causing harm in the form of hyperacidity etc., can be controlled by giving him food which contains more of jala (water) mahabhuta in it like sugarcane juice etc.

Panch Mahabhutas	Sense Organs	Sensory Faculty	Properties	Actions
Space	Ears	Hearing	• Creates natural space in the body. • No distinct taste.	Produces softness, lightness and porosity.

Air	Skin	Touch	• Light, clear and dry. • Governs breathing, movement of eyelids, joints and other motor functions. • Slightly bitter taste.	Creates dryness, lightness and wasting.
Fire	Eyes	Sight	• Rough & bright. • Controls temperature and luster of body color. • Pungent taste.	Helps in digestion, improves eye sight.
Earth	Nose	Smell	• Heavy, immobile, compact & rough. • Controls organs as teeth, nails, flesh, skin, tendons & muscles. • Sweet taste.	• Increases firmness & strength of the body. • Acts as a nutrient and purgative.
Water	Tongue	Taste	• Cold, heavy fluid. • Slimy, fat and sweat by nature. • Sweet & astringent, sour & saline taste.	• Imparts glossiness. • Enhances fluid content & purgative. • Acts as nutrient, purgative.

Language of the Doshas

The Physical, psychic and cosmic language of the body is created from the circadian rhythm of the universe set in motion some billions of years ago when the five great elements were born. Space, air, fire, water and earth, the first material for life, are the basis of the Vedic sciences. In Ayurveda human physiology and anatomy is rooted in bodily humors (doshas) tissues (dhatus) and wastes (malas). These three principles support all of life and are more than the physical substance of our anatomy.

Doshas are three in number called Tridoshas (tri meaning three and doshas being the basic physical energies/humors). They are the primary and essential factors of the human body that govern our entire physical structure and function. Derived from the Panchmahabhutas (five elements), each dosha – which like the elements cannot be detected with our senses but their qualities can be. They are the combination of any two of the five bhutas (five elements) with the predominance of one. Called Vata, Pitta and Kapha in Sanskrit, these three are responsible for all the physiological and psychological processes within the body and mind – dynamic forces that determine growth and decay. Every physical characteristic, mental capacity and the emotional tendency of a human being can therefore be explained in terms of the tridoshas. When existing in the body of all living organisms, the five elements congregate in a certain pattern and are known in Sanskrit as doshas, the literal meaning of which is, "that which is quick to go out of balance." Doshas imply that the human system maintains a delicate balance, its dynamic elemental composition always being on the verge of disorder.

The doshas are a classic example of energy and matter in dynamic accord. All matter born from energy remains intricately woven within its core nature of energy. In a state of balance or equilibrium, doshas are considered an energy force in that we cannot visibly detect them as they move through and support bodily function. For example most of the physical phenomena ascribed to the nervous system by modern physiology for example, can be identified with Vata. Just as the entire chemical process operating in the human body can be attributed to Pitta, including enzymes, hormones and the complete nutritional system. And the activities of the skeletal and the anabolic system, actually the entire physical volume of an organism, can be considered as Kapha.

In a state of imbalance or disequilibrium the doshas become visible as excessive mucus, bile, flatus and physical matter. When these early signs of disorder are ignored, imbalances can quickly become full-blown diseases. In this unique system of explaining health, air and space—both ethereal elements form one of the three doshas called Vata. Here air exercises its power of mobility only when space is available.

The elements fire and water form a second dosha called Pitta. Here the bodily water protects the heat of the body from burning through. An example of bodily fire is the acid in our stomachs, which, if leaked from the stomach, is capable of burning the organism with the force of a raging fire. Water is the buffering force that contains the body's fires.

The elements water and earth combine to form the third dosha called Kapha. Because of their mutual density, water gives earth its fluidity. Without water, earth would become stagnated and inert. Thus, the Kapha dosha enables certain fluidity in the body without depriving it of its solid support. Thus the three doshas co-exist in all living organisms. It is important to realize that these three are forces and not substances. Kapha is not mucus; it is the force that causes mucus to arise. Similarly pitta is not bile; but that which causes bile to be produced. And they are called doshas – literally meaning `faults' or `out of whack'-as they indicate the fault lines along which the system can become imbalanced.

It is equally important to understand that the three doshas within any person keep changing constantly due to their doshic qualities (explained in the next chapter), the specific lifestyle and environment of the person, time and the season. Remember that these three are not separate energies but different aspects of the same energy, present together in an infinite variety of combination .The degree to which each dosha exists within a person determines the individual's constitution, commonly referred to as body type. Each dosha thus shares a quality with another (although there remain slight differences in the nature of shared quality). Also, each has an inherent ability to regulate and balance itself, which comes from the opposite qualities that arise from the doshas constituent (basic) elements.

When the doshas are in balance i.e. in a state of equilibrium, we remain healthy. As Charaka, the great ayurvedic sage, explained: "Vata, pitta and kapha maintain the integrity of the living human organism in their normal state and combine so as to make the man a complete being with his indriyas (sense organs) possessed of strength, good complexion and assured of longevity." It is only when that there is imbalance within these three doshas that disease is caused. And since it is the strongest dosha in the constitution that usually has the greatest tendency to increase, one is most susceptible to illnesses associated with an increase of the same.

Three Doshas and their Basic Qualities

Vata (Air and Space)	Pitta (Fire and Water)	Kapha (Water and Earth)
Light	Light	Heavy
Cold	Hot	Cold
Dry	Oily	Oily
Rough	Sharp	Slow
Subtle	Liquid	Slimy
Mobile	Sour	Dense
Clear	Pungent	Soft
Dispersing Erratic Astringent		

Eash dosha also has a primary function in the body. Vata is the moving force, Pitta is the force of assimilation and Kapha is the force of stability.

Vata, the most dominant of the doshas, governs bodily movement, the nervous system and the life force. Without Vata's mobility in the body, Pitta and Kapha would be rendered lame. Pitta governs enzymatic and hormonal activities and is responsible for digestion, pigmentation, body temperature, hunger, thirst and sight. Further, Pitta acts as a balancing force for Vata and Kapha.

Kapha governs the body's structure and stability. It Imbricates joints, provides moisture to the skin, heals wounds and regulates Vata and Pitta. Vata, Pitta and Kapha pervade the entire body, but their primary domains are in the lower, middle and upper body, respectively. Kapha rules the (Upper) head, neck, thorax, chest and upper portion of the stomach, fat tissues and the joints. Pitta pervades the (Middle) chest, umbilical area, stomach, small intestines, sweat and lymph glands and the blood. Vata dominates the (Lower) body, pelvic region, colon, bladder, urinary tract, thighs, legs, arms, bones and nervous system.

Apart from its main site, each dosha has four secondary sites located in different areas of the body. Thus each dosha then has five sites considered to be its centres of operation, which include the various outreach systems because of which the entire body functions. The doshas interact continuously with the external elements to replenish their energy within the body. Each of the three doshas' five sites has a specific responsibility towards the maintenance of the organism.

Physio-Psychological and Pathological Nature of the Doshas

Five Airs of Vata

The five sites or centres of operation and systemic outreach through which Vata casts its influence on the entire organism are called the five airs of Vata, namely: prana, udana, samana, apana and vyana.

- Air of Respiration (Prana): Prana means 'life' is the first air of the universe and of the body. Although located in the body between the diaphragm and throat, it not only pervades the region of the heart and chest, but also up into the face and brain. Prana aids in the chewing and swallowing of food and provides immediate nourishment to all vital tissues of the body. The system is constantly being rejuvenated through the natural rhythm of the breath's inhalation, exhalation and timely retention. The activity of the colon is attuned to the respiration's rhythm; the main function of prana is extracting 'prana' i.e. life from the digested food and diffusing it into all of the tissues in the body. When the colon is disturbed and unable to fulfill its natural ability to extract and diffuse prana, this unused prana becomes waste.

Prana facilitates all movement in and out of the body. It moves in the region of the heart, causing it to beat. It carries food through the oesophagus into the stomach. Prana sustains the heart, arteries, veins, senses and our wisdom faculty, (buddhi). When prana cannot function properly our very life force is threatened. Respiratory ailments such as bronchitis and asthma result. Heart ailments and the impulse to vomit are also related to prana's imbalance.

- Air of the Throat (Udana): Udana, the second air of Vata, which means "rising air," flows upward from the umbilicus through the lung and into the throat and nose. Known as the air of ejection, it provides us with our vocal powers and clarity of sense perceptions. It also preserves our body's natural forces, such as its strength of will and capacity for effort. Udana has the supreme task of keeping track of the number of breaths we expend.

- An equally supreme task is udana's capacity to preserve memory, both experiential (memories gathered within a present lifetime) and cognitive (cumulative memories carried into all lives from the beginning of creation through all time). Impairment of udana can result in loss of memory, impaired speech, giddiness or heaviness in the head, deep-seated fears and a shortened life span).

- Air of the Stomach (Samana): Samana, the third air of Vata, is located between the diaphragm and navel. It aids the movement of food through the stomach and small intestines, fans the fires of digestion by stimulating the production of gastric juices and digestive enzymes and helps in the assimilation of nutrients extracted from our food. Samana is the moving force that transports these nutrients to the various tissue elements and discharges wastes into the colon. When the samana air is disturbed, it can cause mucus accumulation in the stomach called 'ama', indigestion, poor assimilation and diarrhoea.

- Air of the Colon (Apana): The fourth air of Vata, apana, is located in the colon and the organs of the pelvic region. Also known as the air of elimination, apana's primary function is to relieve the body of feces, urine, flatus, semen and menstrual waste. Its down ward pressure maintains position of the foetus and the flow of its eventual birth. Apana is the most dominant of the five airs, situated as it is in Vata's primary location. Apana maintains the delayed nutrition of prana in the organism. When apana is impaired, diseases of the bladder, anus, testicles, uterus, menstrual problems and obstinate urinary diseases, including diabetes, prevail.

- Air of Circulation (Vyana): Vyana is the fifth and final air of the Vata and is located in the heart. It diffuses the energy derived from food and breath throughout the entire organism including the skin. Circulatory in nature, Vyana functions in the body's circulation channels, such as the blood vessels, to transport nutritive juices and blood throughout the body. Vyana also carries sweat from the glands to the skin and is the force behind bodily expressions such as yawning and blinking. When vyana malfunctions, there is dryness of the skin and other body extremities, poor circulation and diseases such as fever.

Doshas	Site	Normal function
Prana	Heart & Head, between diaphragm and throat	Breathing and swallowing of food, life & thinking, heart rhythm.
Udana	From umbilicus to lung, throat and nose	Speech, voice, colour, strength, immunity, energy, memory, capacity for effort.
Samana	Between diaphragm and navel (stomach and intestines)	Helps action of digestive enzymes, assimilation of end products of food and separation into their various tissue elements & waste products.
Apana	Colon & organs of pelvis	Elimination of stool, urine, flatus, semen, fetus and menstrual blood.
Vyana	Heart	Diffusion of energy from food and breath in the whole body helps in the functioning of circulating channels as blood vessels.

Five Fires of Pitta

Pitta, formed from the elements of fire and water, also is said to reside in five sites. These sites are the centers of operation and systemic outreach through which the Pitta dosha influences the entire organism; they are: pachaka, ranjaka, sadhaka, alochaka and bhrajaka.

- Fire of the Stomach (Pachaka): Pachaka is referred to in Ayurveda as the first fire of the body. It exists in the small intestine, duodenum, gall bladder, liver and pancreas and supports the remaining four fires, to be discussed below. Pachaka's main action is to dissolve and digest the food we eat. It also regulates body temperature. Once digestion has taken place, pachaka separates the food's nutritive elements from its waste elements. An imbalance in this first fire, pachaka, causes indigestion as well as revulsion for food.

- Fire of the Blood (Ranjaka): True to its name, ranjaka, the second fire of Pitta, controls the formation and preservation of blood. Located in the liver, spleen and stomach, ranjaka provides the blood with its colour and oxygen. When ranjaka is impaired, bile compounds may appear in the blood and diseases such as anaemia and jaundice may follow.

- Fire of the Heart (Sadhaka): The finest of the fires, sadhaka, the third fire, is central to the activity of Pitta. It reigns along with prana, in the heart. With udana, it governs memory and the retention and wellness of all mental functioning. When sadhaka is impaired, there may be psychic disturbances, mental disorientation, extreme emotional states and craving for extreme foods, drugs and so on.

- Fire of the Eyes (Alochaka): Alochaka, the fourth fire of Pitta, exists in the pupils of the eyes. It gives the eyes their lustre and diffuses light and its spectrum of colours throughout the body. When the fourth fire is vitiated, there is impairment of vision and yellowness may appear in the eyes.

- Fire of the Skin (Bhrajaka): The fifth fire, bhrajaka, is located in the skin, given the skin its lustre and gleam. Bhrajaka protects the body from extreme atmospheric conditions and facilitates the assimilation of light, wind, water and oil through the skin. When this fire is disturbed, skin diseases such as psoriasis, eczema and leukoderma may result.

Doshas	Site	Normal function	Ailments caused by its vitiation
Pachaka	Stomach & small intestines, gall bladder, liver, pancreas	Digesting and dissolving of food, regulating body temperature, separation of nutritive elements from wastes.	Indigestion, Anorexia.
Ranjaka	Liver, spleen and stomach	Blood formation and preservation.	Anemia, Jaundice Hepatitis.
Sadhaka	Heart	Memory and other mental functions.	Psychic disturbances, Cardiac diseases, mental disorientation and extreme emotional states.
Alochaka	Eyes	Vision, lusture of eyes.	Impairment of vision, yellowness of eyes.
Bhrajaka	Skin	Colour and glaze of the skin.	Leucoderma, Other skin diseases e.g. psoriasis, eczema.

Pitta Dosha Imbalance

All the above mentioned functions of pitta and its various subtypes are executed when they are in their balanced state. Due to various reasons *pitta gets imbalanced and causes the following results. If pitta dosha is in excess it results in:

- Ambition
- Anger
- Envy
- Fear of Failure
- Sarcastic speech and actions
- Skepticism
- Excessive thirst
- Loss of sleep
- Frustration

- Hate
- Jealously
- Judgemental or critical tendencies
- Lack of discernment
- Pride
- Burning sensations
- Craving for cold
- Fever

Decreased Pitta results in:

- Indigestion
- Abnormal loss of body heat

- Loss of luster in the skin Irregular bowel movements.

Five Waters of Kapha

Kapha, formed from the elements water and earth, also manifests in five doshic sites, through these centres of operation and systemic outreach it influences the entire organism. The five waters of Kapha are: kledaka, avalambaka, bodhaka, tarpaka and slesaka.

- Water of the Stomach (Kledaka): The first water of Kapha, kledaka, originates in the stomach. It is the cause of mucus formation in the body. Most important of the waters, kledaka's moist foamy liquid aids digestion, liquefies foods and nourishes the remaining waters of Kapha. When the first water is aggravated, the digestion process becomes impaired, heaviness of the abdomen prevails and nausea may also occur.
- Water of the Heart (Avalambaka): The second water of Kapha, avalambaka, resides in the chest and heart. It provides a plasmic (fluid) tissue covering to the heart, thus insulating it from heart & acting as a shock absorber. Avalambaka also provides the limbs with their energy. When this water is disturbed, laziness and lethargy ensure. Heart originating diseases such as rheumatic fever and pains in the pericardium (tissue around the heart) may also occur.
- Water of the Tongue (Bodhaka): Bhodhaka, the third water of Kapha, is the one which joins the five waters of body's river. It sends water to the tongue and palate and gives the perception of taste. It registers each of the six tastes in nature and sends the appropriate impulses to the receiving tissue long before the food is ingested. Bodhaka water also liquefies the food. When this water is disturbed, crimes against the body's natural instincts are committed, due to the impairment of taste. This creates Ama, the foul undigested remnants of food which stick in the tissues and promote diseases such as obesity, bulimia and anorexia. Generally, a thick white coating on the tongue indicates the presence of ama in the body.
- Water of Head (Tarpaka): Tarpaka, Kapha's fourth water, flows in the brain and spinal cord. It soothes the sense organs and, as a result lubricates and protects the nervous system. When this water is out of balance, the sense organs become impaired. Loss of memory and dullness of sensory perceptions are the natural result.
- Water of the Joints (Shlessaka): The fifth water of Kapha, slesaka, is located in the joints. It lubricates the joints and gives them their solidity. Slesaka's unctuous gel protects the joints from heat and gives ease and flexibility of movement. When this water is impaired, the joints may become swollen, painful and dysfunctional.

Doshas	Site	Normal function	Ailments caused by its vitiation
Kledaka	Stomach	Moistens food, which helps in digestion, formation of mucus in body.	Impairment of digestion, heaviness in abdomen, nausea.
Avalambaka	Chest & Heart	Energy in limbs, controls temperature of the heart.	Laziness, Rheumatic heart disease.
Bodhaka	Tongue, palate	Perception of taste.	Impairment of digestion, bulimia, anorexia, obesity.
Tarpaka	Brain, spinal cord	Nourishment of the sense organs, lubrication and protection of nervous system.	Loss of memory, Impairment of function of sense organs.
Shlesshaka	Joints	Lubrication of joints, protection of joints from heat.	Pain in joints, Impairment of function of joints.

Kapha Dosha Imbalance

All the above mentioned functions of kapha and its various subtypes are executed when they are in their balanced state. Due to various reasons *kapha gets imbalanced and causes the following results. If kapha dosha is in excess it results in:

Boredom
Carelessness
Lack of compassion
Greed
Feeling lack of support or love
Obsessive behavior
Unkindness

Lack of interest
Secretions from the mouth
Lethargy
Excessive sleep
Improper digestive function
Obesity
Nausea

And decrease Kapha gives way to:

Thirst
Giddiness
Body aches
Dryness of mouth
Cramps

Agni

Being the biological fire that governs metabolism, agni encompasses all the changes in the body and mind from the dense to the more subtle. Such changes include the digestion and absorption of food, cellular transformations, assimilation of sensory perceptions and mental and emotional experiences. Agni therefore covers all the sequences of chemical interactions and changes in the body and mind. Digestive abilities are directly proportional to the strength of agni.

Agni and pitta are closely connected. While both are hot and light, agni is subtle and dry, while pitta is gross & liquid .The heat energy to help digestion contained by pitta is agni. Pitta is therefore the container and agni the content. Agni is acidic in nature and stimulates digestion. It is subtly related to the movement of vata. In every tissue and cell agni is present and is necessary for maintaining the nutrition and auto-immune mechanism which is performed by destroying micro-organisms, foreign bacteria and toxins in the stomach and the intestines.

A balanced agni therefore is vital for health. The strength of the body to resist disease and also its physical strength are directly related to its heat energy determining the metabolic processes of the body. Disturbances to Agni are usually the chief causes of disease leading to ama in the body.

As per Ayurveda there are thirteen types of Agni in the body and mind according to the conversion and the transformation made. The most important of them is the Jatharagni, the gastric fire; responsible for digesting the food eaten (can be correlated to hydrochloric acid in the stomach and the digestive enzymes and juices secreted into the stomach, duodenum and the small intestines). If digestive agni is low and the its capacity is impaired, one may experience pain, discomfort, feeling of heaviness or gases gurgling, constipation or loose stools.

Ayurvedic Herbs

Owing to fast paced world that we are living in, we are getting far from the nature. While the lifestyle that we live can have adverse effect on us, it is important to know that by introducing small changes in our daily life can go a long way in keeping us healthy and energetic. Therefore, the importance of Ayurveda holds true in today's life as it is based on the principal of bringing us close to nature and relying on its natural powers to cure us and keep us healthy without any side effects. Thanks to the use of natural ingredients and medicinal herbs, Ayurvedic medicines and products today have become a symbol of safety in contrast to synthetic drugs that are considered unsafe and hazardous for overall health.

One way of understanding the basic fundamentals of Indian Ayurveda is to spend more time with nature and observe the plants and herbs. Each plant or herb has a specific quality and can be used to treat multitude of ailments and diseases. Medicinal plants like aloe, turmeric, tulsi, pepper, elachi and ginger are commonly used in a number of Ayurvedic home remedies and are considered to be the best aid among fighting ailments related to throat and skin. As a rich source of nutrients, anti-bacterial and antioxidant properties, ayurvedic herbs are non-toxic in nature and so the products or remedies made using them are often recommended for their high therapeutic value. Treatment with herbal medicinal plants also hold a strong ground because these plants are considered to be safe and have no side effects. Since they are in sync with nature, they hold greater advantage over chemically treated products and synthetic medicines. As opposed to other drugs and medicines, Ayurvedic herbs are known to treat the disease from the root and thus aid in keeping you healthy and fit in the long run.

Apart from medicinal use, these herbs can also be used for purposes like pest control, natural dyes and formulation of food items, teas and perfumes among others. If we look at various researches from across the world, a sudden spurt in cases of people turning to natural herbs for treatments and usage in everyday life has gone up significantly. Going back to the basics, people have realized the threat chemically treated products pose to their life and are rightly so adopting healthier ways of life by including Ayurveda and its principals as the mainstay of their life.

Medicinal Plants and their Uses

English Name	Botanical Name	Uses
Malabar Nut	Adhatoda vasica Nees Pennel	Cough, Asthma, Bronchitis
Pineapple	Ananas comosus Pennel	Sore Throat, Diabetes, Heart Disease, Obesity
Indian Gum	Acacia arabica Willd Pennel	Oral Care, Bleeding Gums, Wounds
Thyme leafed gratiola	Bacopa monniera Pennel Pennel	Enchances Memory, Anxiety

Coriander	Coriandrum sativum Linn Pennel	Indigestion, Flatulence, Controls Spasmodic Pain
Kalmegh	Andrographis paniculata Pennel	Indigestion, Acne, Diarrhea
Garlic	Allium sativum Pennel	Ringworm, Dysentery, Wounds
Nut Grass	Cyperus rotundus Linn Pennel	Fever, Diabetes, Solar Dermatitis
Spreading Hog-weed	Boerhaavia diffusa Linn Pennel	Anemia, Liver Diseases, Wounds
Shal Leafed Bush	Desmodium gangetium DC Pennel	Analgesic, Anti-Inflammatory
Holy Basil	Ocimum sactum Linn Pennel	Indigestion, Heart Diseases, Respiratory Diseases
Elephant Creeper	Argyreia speciosa Sweet Pennel	Diabetes, Skin Diseases, Wounds
Eagle Wood	Aquilaria agallocha Roxb Pennel	Bed-Wetting, Incompetency of Urinary Bladder
Sage leaf alangium	Alangium salvifolium Pennel	Snakebite, Scorpion Bite, Dog Bite
Greater Cardamom	Amomum subulatum Pennel	Bronchitis, Asthma, Appetizer, Digestant
Prickly chaff flower	Achyranthes aspera Pennel	Indigestion, Cough, Asthma, Anemia, Jaundice
Lesser Cardamom	Elettaria cardamomum Maton Pennel	Nausea, Vomiting, Dry Cough
Country Mallow	Abutilon indicum Pennel	Facial Paralysis, Joint Disorders, Increases Strength
Staff Tree	Celastrus paniculatus Willd Pennel	Muscle Cramps, Backache, Osteoarthritis, Paralysis
Margosa Tree	Azadirachta Indica A. Juss Pennel	Leprosy, Eye Disorders, Bloody Nose, Intestinal Worms
Onion	Allium cepa Linn Pennel	Prostate Cancer, Esophageal, Stomach Cancer
Asparagus	Asparagus racemosus Willd Pennel	Infertility, Loss Of Libido, Threatened Miscarriage
Devil's Cotton	Abroma augusta Pennel	Gynaecological Problems, Irregularity In Periods
Camel Thorn	Alhagi camelorum Pennel	Rheumatism, Vomiting, Stomachache, Constipation
Pellitory	Anacyclus pyrethrum Pennel	Toothache, Dryness Of The Mouth, Throat, Catarrh
Winter Cherry	Withania somnifera Dunal Pennel	Stress Tolerance, Immunity, Joint Pains, Skin Sores
Bengal Quince	Aegle marmelos Corr. Pennel	Dysentery And Diabetes, Sunstrokes, Anti-Cancer
Leadwort	Plumbago zeylanica Linn Pennel	Arthritis, Skin Diseases, Menstrual Disorders, Obesity

Benefits and Importance of Medicinal Plants

Ayurvedic herbs are time tested for their health and other benefits. The nutritive value that they pack are highly recommended for their healing powers. Known to induce no side effects, they have a unique aroma and flavor and when consumed regularly, they act as a perfect mechanism to bring about a balanced harmony between mind and body. They rejuvenate the whole system instead of focusing on one specific organ or body part.

Benefits of medicinal plants:

- They have a holistic approach and aid in proper absorption and digestion.
- They are not disease specific but act as a preventive medicine that positively affects the overall health and well-being by boosting the immune system.
- They are at par with allopathic medicines and are at times known to be effective in treating diseases like cancer and autoimmune diseases.
- They are self-contained and nutritive in nature, therefore, are non-toxic and harmless.

- It deals with the overall well-being and aims to bring harmony between mind, body and soul.
- Several metabolic and chronic conditions can be treated without any side effects using Ayurvedic medicines and treatments.

Ayurvedic herbs/spices and their medicinal values:

- Ayurvedic herbs and spices such as black pepper, cinnamon, aloe, sandalwood, ginseng, red clover, burdock, bayberry and safflower are used to heal wounds, sores and boils.
- To reduce fever and the production of heat caused by the condition, certain antipyretic herbs such as chirayta, black pepper and sandal wood are recommended.
- Sandalwood and cinnamon are great astringents apart from being aromatic. Sandalwood is especially used in arresting the discharge of blood, mucus etc.
- Ajwain, amalaki, aswatha etc., serve as antacids and are recommended for healthy gastric acid flow and proper digestion.
- Herbs like cardamom and coriander are renowned for their appetizing qualities. Other aromatic herbs such as peppermint, cloves and turmeric add a pleasant aroma to the food, thereby increasing the taste of the meal.
- Herbs like aloe, sandalwood, turmeric, sheetraj hindi and khare khaskhas are commonly used as antiseptic and have very high medicinal values.
- Camomile, basil, cardamom, ginger, peppermint and coriander are known to promote blood circulation in the body and keep the heart healthy.

Ayurvedic Acupressure

The Subtle body describes a subtle physiology having a number of focal points connected by a series of channels. This kind of medical treatment is also known as Marma Therapy and involves the 10 elements, physical and metaphysical. So, Ayurvedic Acupressure is the energy pathways for healing body, mind and consciousness with knowledge of Ayurveda. And, a 3,000 years old Vedic text, the Suchi Veda, incorporates for the first time the Ayurvedic Acupuncture as another Ayurvedic system. But, it has been practiced as an accessory therapy since it was used in conjunction with other forms to effect healing. And the instruments for applying pressure on the reflex zones of the body are various as the acuball, the energy roller, foot roller or krupa chakra, power mat, spine roller and the Teishein.

Marma Points of Ayurveda

The Marma points are an important element of Ayurveda's healing power. So, the studies of this-points come from India centuries ago. And these energy points affect the body, mind and spirit and ease the deepest levels of healing. Besides, by receiving the name of energy points, these pressure points help in stimulating not only circulation but also improve the mental and emotional outlook. Throughout the body are all the Marma points. The Prana is the current of energy that infuses every cell within the body. The Ayurvedic Acupressure stimulates marmani or energy points directly taps into this reservoir of energy and promotes health. The marma therapy integrates vital knowledge of the energy points with specific techniques of Ayurvedic massage. And this vital knowledge of the points reveals how to do detoxification, acupressure, aromatherapy, yoga practices, meditation and more.

Doshas in the Ayurvedic Acupressure

Pitta and Kapha, the doshas. These doshas support the meridians or marma points. But, the therapy restores the imbalance of the ten elements in the human body with the aid of an entirely newly created set of meridians and their points. So, the ten elements are represented on the ten fingers of the two hands and similarly on the ten toes of the two feet. Hence, Ayurvedic acupressure talks about 10 elements:

- 5 physical elements: Space, Air, Fire, Water and Earth.
- 5 metaphysical elements: Time, Direction, Mind, Soul and Tam.

So, there are thirty basic ayurvedic meridians on each finger and toe including thumb and big toe. That makes it 300 basic meridians on the two hands and 300 basic meridians on the two feet, a total of 600 basic meridians. And, each meridian has ten points corresponding to the ten elements, thus giving us 6000 points. Also, the combination of various basic marma Points develops many secondary meridians that give us more meridians and points running into thousands. In the Ayurvedic Acupressure, we can see that the treatment is done with the help of 14 main meridians only. Hence, the therapy is quite simple and its intricacies can be picked up in a few months as opposed to many years that it takes to get knowledge of allopathic or other alternate medicines.

Effectivity of Ayurvedic Acupressure

The therapy is effective and without side effects, has the potential to revolutionize medical treatment around the world. Our therapies of Ayurvedic Acupressure harmonize the body's vital energy by working on the Governing and Conception Vessels, the mother and father of all the meridian pathways. And, it can reach depths within you when an Acupressure point is hold with just the right amount of pressure. This can help you transcend the limitations and traps of negative thoughts and feelings. All this, instead of closing up in judgment, worry, doubt, or expectation, you can begin to relax and open up. Using this therapy balances your hormones. Also, the chakra centers of your brain to bring more harmony and beauty into your life.

Daily Life with Ayurvedic Acupressure

Every human being has the potential to heal and be healed, as Ayurvedic Medicine explains. It can start with something as simple as practice Pranayama, which can clear your head and make you feel renewed and energized. Or maybe it's through a friendly glance or a smile, or the kindness of going out of your way to help someone, as the Karma Yoga. Besides, beyond these everyday gifts, there are many simple healing methods to help ourselves and others get greater wellness. And this is why Ayurvedic Acupressure is so important you can open your points to feel the healing energy. The acupressure points determinate one of the most powerful ways to do pure energy work and transform physical and emotional problems.

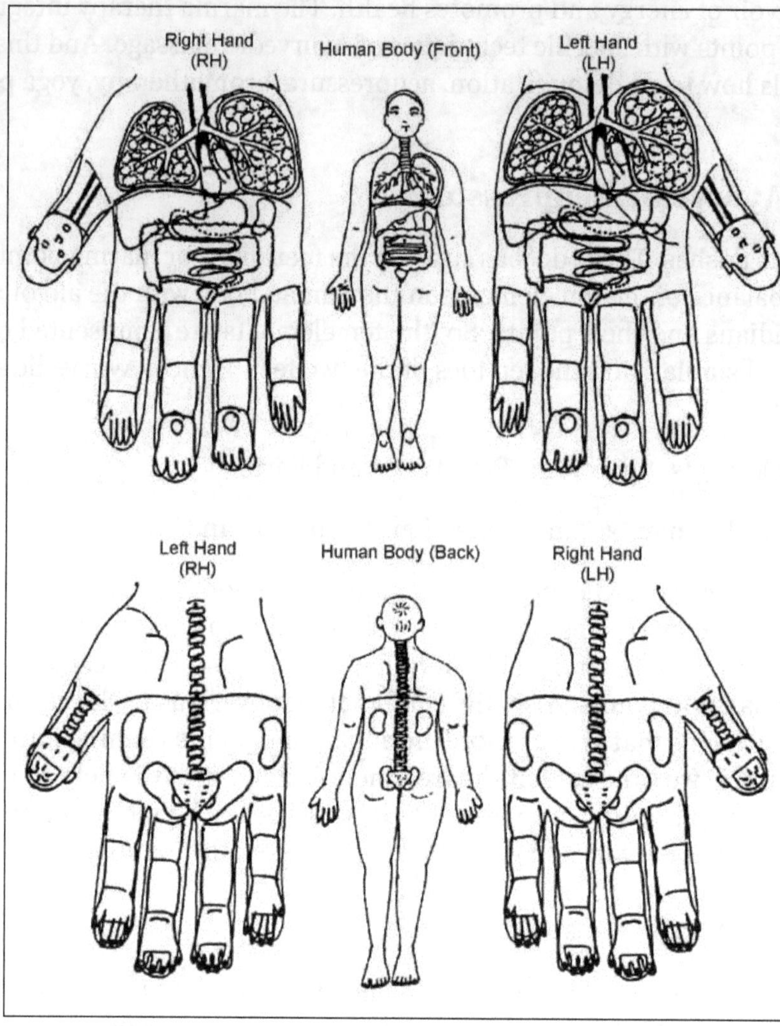

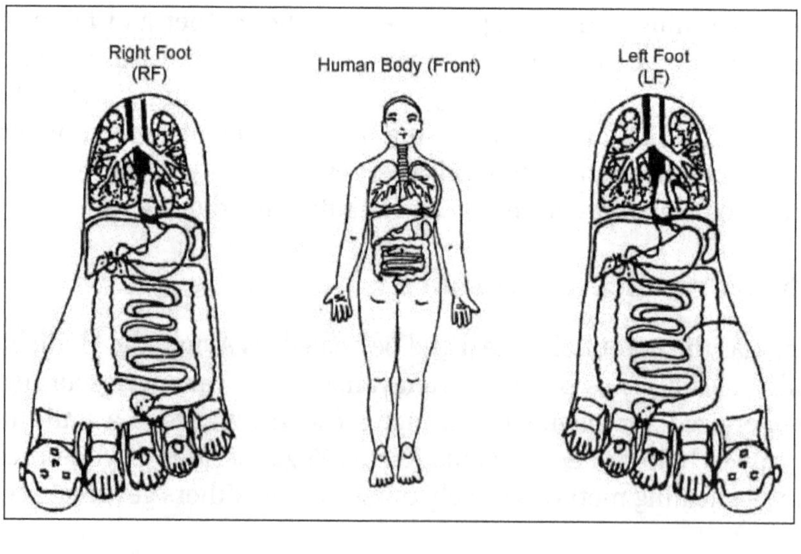

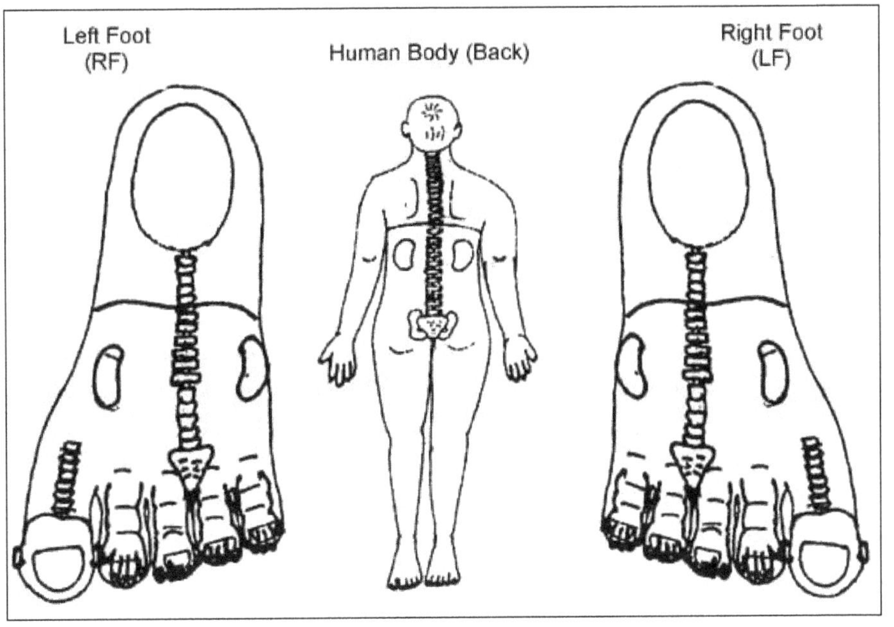

Dinacharya

Dinacharya refers to ayurvedic daily routine recommendations that educate how to live a healthier, happier and longer life and avoid all diseases. Ayurvedic Daily routine helps in maintaining balance and harmony in your body and nature by regulating your biological clock and advocating a healthy lifestyle. It also helps in proper digestion, absorption and assimilation of food. The discipline that you adopt in daily routine also improves self-esteem, brings happiness and promotes longevity. Let's start with the daily routine steps:

Wake Up in Brahma Muhurta

Ayurveda recommends waking up early in the morning. According to ayurveda, you should wake up 96 minutes (around 1.5 hours) before sunrise. It is called Brahma Muhurta in ayurveda and yoga science. This is the perfect time for waking up for a healthy person. However, the time of sunrise may vary according to season and country. So, you should fix your time for waking up for supporting the rhythm of your biological clock. For example, if you are living in India, then 4:30 am is a perfect time to wake up for healthy people. Timings can be changed according to your body's requirement during disease.

- If you suffer from any Kapha Disease, then you must get up by 4 am in the morning.
- If you suffer from any Pitta Disease, then you should wake up before 5 am.
- If you suffer from any Vata Disease, then you should wake up by 5:30 am in the morning.
- Children, pregnant women and aged people may require more rest, so they can get up just before sunrise.

However, if you don't suffer from any disease and want to keep yourself healthy and happy, you should wake up by 4:30 am in the morning. If you cannot get up so early, you should try to wake up as early as possible, but you must wake up at least before sunrise. Don't sleep for a longer duration after sunrise, otherwise, the stool in the bowel starts spoiling your health. It will start causing gas, bloating, acid reflux and several other diseases later in the day. If you don't experience these symptoms yet, they may appear later in your life.

Expressing Gratitude

You should express your gratitude toward God by reciting its name for 1-2 minutes immediately after waking up. You can meditate for 1 – 2 minutes and feel the surroundings and nature. You can also do prayer. If you want to do prayer, it should be in your own words. The most important thing when you do any of these rituals you should feel happiness, peacefulness and kindness in your mind and keep a sweet smile on your face. This thing is more essential for living a stress-free life and improving your memory, intelligence, mental capabilities and analytic skills.

Evacuation

After waking up, you will feel the urge for urination and bowel evacuation. Follow your urge and rush to the toilet for evacuating your bowel and urinary bladder. In most people, this is an autonomic reflex for a bowel movement and urination in the morning. This urge should commence on its own. Do not force to evacuate the bowel. Sometimes, you may need to walk a few steps before getting this urge.

If you suffer from constipation or you don't get the natural urge in the morning, you must treat it with healthy foods and triphala rasayana. In such cases, you should follow the rules of vagbhata's triphala rasayana. According to him, you should take 3 grams triphala churna along with 2.5 grams of ghee and 5 grams of honey in the evening after taking the evening meal. Following this rasayana, you will start getting a bowel evacuation urge in the morning. You can continue this rasayana throughout life. Because triphala contains powder of three fruits: amla, behera and harad, which also provide nourishing and antioxidant benefits like other fruits. It also helps in the prevention of several diseases.

After evacuating bowel and urinary bladder, wash your hands and face with cold water. It can be your tap water or water kept in an earthen pot. Ayurveda also recommends washing face with medicated water or milk. You should also wash your hands before and after eating food, after cleaning nasal discharge and dried rheum from eyes and after touching hair or another person and after returning home.

Wash Hands

Wash your hands after immediately after waking up and after evacuation helps to reduce the likelihood of diseases.

5 Minutes Meditation

After passing the urge for urination and bowel movement, you must meditate for 5 minutes. Our mind has three states:

- Elevated State: Happiness.

- Neutral State: Pure State of Mind.
- Suppressed State: Sadness.

Meditation restores your neutral state. The neutral state is a pure state of your mind. It is beyond happiness and sadness. The best time to restore the neutral state of mind is before sleep at night and after waking up in the morning. Meditation before sleep helps to release whole day stress and restores the neutral state of the mind. It prevents all stress disorders, depression and anxiety in your life. It helps you to sleep better. Psychology says the first-morning thought affects your whole day. So, meditation after waking up helps you to get positive energy and make your day more constructive, joyful and energy fulfilling.

Drinking Water

1. Acamana (Sipping Water): Vagbhata in Ashtanga Sangrah recommends acamana. Acamana is an ancient ritual of sipping water on a specific occasion. He recommends sipping a small amount of water:

- After getting up from sleep.
- After sneezing.
- After taking a bath.
- At the beginning and end of meals.
- At the commencement of worship.
- After traveling.
- After the usual daily activities.

Amount of water you should take for acamana: The water that you can hold in one hand making a concavity with your fingers and palm, you should take it for Acamana.

2. Ushapan (Drinking Water in Morning): Drinking water in the morning in large quantity is not written in Dinacharya by Charak, Vagbhata and Sushruta. Drinking water in the morning is a kind of ayurvedic water therapy, which helps to prevent and manage several diseases. So, it is called Rasayana (rejuvenation therapy). Here is a brief introduction:

Timing of drinking water in the morning	Dawn – a few minutes (about 20-30 minutes) before sunrise.
Water quantity	8 Anjali *
Contraindications	During panchakarma, Chest injuries, excessive hiccup, loss of appetite due to kapha and vata disorders, indigestion, abdominal heaviness or stiffness.

*Anjali means concavity formed by adjoining both hands. 8 Anjali means the quantity of water that you hold 8 times in the concavity formed by adjoining both hands. For example, if you can hold 50 ml water in 1 Anjali, then your drinkable water recommendation is 400 ml. The amount of water varies person-to-person.

Cleaning the Teeth

Use plant twigs or herbal tooth powder. Do not use any toothpaste. Most people are using toothpaste, but ayurveda don't recommend it. Ayurveda recommends the use of plant twigs or herbal powder for cleaning teeth. Ayurveda recommends the use of astringent, bitter and pungent tree stems (twigs). You can use any of the following plant twigs:

Tree twigs	Most suitable for body type
Bargad – Banyan – Ficus benghalensis	Kapha and Pitta
Asana – Terminalia alata	Kapha and Pitta
Arka – Calotropis procera	Kapha
Khadira (catechu) – Acacia catechu	Kapha, Pitta and Vata
Karanja – Pongamia pinnata	Kapha and Vata
Karavira – Nerium indicum	Kapha
Sarja-Vateria indica	Pitta and Vata
Irimeda (Sweet acacia) – Acacia farnesiana	Pitta and Kapha
Apamarga – Achyranthes aspera	Kapha and Vata
Malati – Aganosma heynei	–
Arjuna – Terminalia arjuna	Pitta and Kapha
Babul (Kikar) – Acacia arabica	Pitta and Kapha
Neem – Azadirachta indica	Pitta and Kapha

The twig should be straight, soft and healthy and without knots and leaves. The thickness of twig should be around that of your little finger. Tree twigs should be collected from the unpolluted area. They must not be foul smelling, sticky to teeth or dry.

Khadira stems can be used by anyone. A person with Pitta Body Type can use twigs of neem or arjuna tree. People with Vata-Pitta body type should use a stem of banyan (Bargad) tree. Vata body type people can use Khadira stem or Apamarga twigs. People with Kapha body type should use Karaj stem. You can select the most suitable plant twigs for you according to the above table. Children should use the stem of the licorice (Mulethi) plant. People with Vata and Pitta body type can also use licorice stem. Neem or catechu (Khadira) stems provides additional benefits for people suffering from skin diseases.

Contraindications of Teeth Cleaning with Twigs

Who should not use Tree Twigs?

People suffering from the following diseases should not use plant twigs for cleansing the teeth:

- Indigestion.
- Vomiting.
- Severe breathing trouble.
- Persistent cough.

- Fever.
- Facial paralysis.
- Excessive thirst.
- Mouth ulcers.
- Heart diseases.
- Eye diseases.
- Diseases related to head.
- Ear disorders.

In such cases, tooth powder should be used for cleaning the teeth.

Tooth Powder

We can understand it is not possible for everyone to collect fresh plant twigs on a daily basis. So, ayurveda also provides a solution for it. You can use herbal tooth powder. Please do not use marketed products. It is better to prepare your tooth powder at home. Here is a recipe:

Triphala powder	25 grams
Khadira (Catechu) bark powder	25 grams
Arjuna bark powder	15 grams
Dalchini (Cinnamon)	15 grams
Green cardamom powder	15 grams
Clove powder	5 grams
Trikatu powder	5 grams
Sendha Namak (Rock Salt)	5 grams

In the case of children, you can also add 25 grams of Yashtimadhu (Mulethi) Powder in this formulation.

How to use Tooth Powder?

- Take a small amount of tooth powder in your hand.
- Add some water or honey in it to make a paste.
- Now, do gentle massage of teeth and gums with this paste for 3 to 5 minutes.
- Then gargle with warm water and clean your mouth.
- If you suffer from pyorrhea or any gum or dental problems, then mix this powder in mustard oil instead of water or honey.

How many Times should you Clean your Teeth?

According to Ayurveda, you should clean your teeth 3 times a day.

- In the morning after evacuating bowel and urinary bladder.
- After morning meal.
- After evening meal.

Gum Massage

After cleaning teeth, you should also do massage of gums with the fine herbal powder made of Kuth (Saussurea Lappa), Triphala, Trikatu and Trijataka.

Kuth or Kushta (Indian Costus Root) – Saussurea Lappa	10 grams
Triphala: Amla, Behera, Harad	30 grams
Trijataka: Cinnamon, Cardamom, Indian Bay Leaf	30 grams
Trikatu: Black Pepper, Long Pepper, Ginger	7 grams

How to use Herbal Gum Powder?

- Mix all ingredients in a given ratio.
- Then take 3 grams of this powder and add sufficient honey to it.
- Mix this powder with honey to make a thin paste.
- Apply this paste on gums and do gentle massage with the index finger for 3 to 5 minutes.

Cleaning Tongue

According to ayurveda, you should clean your tongue using tongue scraper made of copper, silver or gold. You can also use tongue cleaner made of wood or plant twig. However, tongue scraper made of gold is considered best, silver is better and copper is good. You can use any. Tongue cleaner made of copper and silver are easily available. You can buy any according to your affordability.

In most case, it is recommended to use a copper tongue scrapper. It helps in removing bad breath, kills microbes and improves the function of taste buds. It is most suitable for Kapha body type people. However, if you suffer from frequent mouth ulcer, sour taste in the mouth, hyperacidity, peptic ulcer, GERD or any acid peptic disorder, then silver tongue scraper is best for you. It is most suitable for people with Vata body type and Pitta body type. Tongue scraper made of gold is more suitable for children and adults who have low immunity and frequently suffer from common cold, cough and fever. Regardless of the body type, anyone can use a gold tongue scraper. It also increases glow on face, improves memory, boosts intelligence and removes all toxins from the mouth.

Benefits of Tongue Cleaning

- Tongue cleaning removes dirt from the tongue.
- It removes bad taste and smell of the tongue, mouth and teeth.
- It produces better taste in the mouth.
- It is also helpful in the prevention and treatment of diseases related to tongue, mouth and teeth.
- After using a tongue cleaner, you will experience the feeling of softness and cleanliness in the mouth.

Splashing Cold Water into Eyes

Vagbhata recommends splashing cold water into eyes in the morning every day during the summer and autumn seasons. It helps to improve vision and reduces tension and tiredness of the eyes. But he did not talk about what should be done in other seasons. So, splashing water into the eyes is only recommendable for two seasons – summer and autumn. In other seasons, you must avoid it.

How to Splash Water into Eyes?

- Take water into your mouth.
- Keep the mouth filled with water.
- Now, take drinkable cold water (kept in the earthen pot overnight) in hands and splash water into the eyes.
- Repeat this process 5 times.

Precautions while Splashing Cold Water into Eyes

- Polluted or contaminated water can cause an eye infection. Therefore, water should be drinkable water and free from germs and dirt.
- In ayurveda, cold water does not mean water kept in the refrigerator. It means water kept in the earthen pot overnight and this pot is kept in a place where natural air circulates. So, you must not use chilled or cold water kept in the refrigerator.
- Splash water into eyes only in recommended seasons – summer and autumn. Don't do it in other seasons. Some suggest splashing warm water into eyes during winter, but the use of warm water for eyes is not recommendable. It can cause harms to eyes instead of any benefits. If you require splashing water into eyes due to any reason in other seasons, use drinkable water with normal temperature.

Nasya (Nasal Therapy)

Charak Samhita recommends putting a few drops of Anu Thailam in each nostril every day in the morning. This process is called Nasya or nasal therapy in ayurveda. Charak advocates it during three seasons: Raining season, autumn and spring. He further advises that Nasya should be done during clear weather when there is no cloud in the sky.

How to do Nasya?

- Lie down with straight back and tilt your head slightly back, so your nose opens towards the sky.
- Instill 3 drops of Anu Thailam in each nostril. Put drops lateral side of each nostril so that drops move into the nose through the lateral wall of each nostril.
- Inhale or sniff deeply for 1-2 times. Then take rest for about 5 minutes in the same position.

Benefits of Nasya

- It helps in the prevention of diseases of eyes, ears and nose.
- If you take nasya on a regular basis, it will help to prevent white or grey hair and hair fall. It also promotes hair growth.
- It is highly useful in the prevention and treatment of headache, torticollis, facial paralysis, lockjaw, rhinitis, hemicrania and tremors.
- It improves the strength of the neck.
- It provides nourishment to blood vessels, joints, ligaments and tendons of head and neck.
- Your face will become more cheerful and plumpy.
- The voice becomes sweet and more stabilized.
- Sense organs become clearer.
- People who regularly take Nasya never suffer from head and neck diseases even in old age.

Precautions and Contraindications of Nasya

A person should not administer Nasya in the following conditions:

- Immediately after drinking water.
- After drinking alcohol.
- After eating food.
- After head wash.
- After blood donation or blood-letting therapy.
- For the first 4 days of the common cold (acute phase).

- Patients with asthma and cough.
- When the weather is not clear.
- People who stop the natural urge of urination and bowel movement should not take Nasya.

Gandusha (Ayurvedic Mouth Wash)

After nasya, Vagbhata recommends Gandusha. Gandusha is an ayurvedic mouth wash. It has 3 types:

- Oil Gandusha (Oil Pulling).
- Decoction Gandusha.
- Warm Water Gandusha.

Type of Gandusha	Indications & Benefits
Oil Gandusha or Oil Pulling (Oils: Coconut Oil, Sesame Oil or Arimedadi Thailam).	The roughness of lips, Cracking of lips, Dryness of mouth, Diseases of Teeth and disorders of the voice.
Decoction Gandusha (Herbs for decoction: Khadira and Irimeda).	Loss of appetite, bad taste and excessive salivation.
Warm Water Gandusha.	Make the mouth clear.

Oil pulling is originated from ayurveda and become famous in the West due to its huge beneficial effects in oral hygiene. Gandusha also alleviates throat irritation caused by Nasya.

How to do Gandusha and Oil Pulling?

- Take warm Arimedadi Thailam or coconut oil into your mouth.
- Keep the mouth filled with it for a while.

Abhyanga (Body Massage)

According to ayurveda, morning massage helps to delay aging, reduces tiredness, prevents Vata disorders, improves eyesight, nourishes the body, increases lifespan and improves sleep quality. Abhyanga mitigates vata dosha, promotes strength, improves sleep quality and increases the firmness of the hairs and boost growth in children. It also improves skin tone and tactile sensation. Therefore, you must massage your body on a daily basis. It is also useful in the prevention and treatment of body pains, tiredness, debility and old age disability.

Which Oil Should we use for Massage?

- Sesame Oil.
- Castor Oil.
- Mustard Oil.

- Coconut Oil.
- Ayurvedic Medicated Oils.

1. Sesame Oil: According to Sushruta Samhita, sesame oil is beneficial for the skin. He uses the word "TWAK PRASAADANAM", which means it is soothing and gratifying for the skin. So, it has demulcent (emollient) action on the skin. You can take sesame oil internally and apply externally.

2. Castor Oil: Then Sushruta has written about castor oil. He uses word TWACHYAM, which means beneficial for the skin. It also means restorative for the skin. So, it restores the natural health of the skin.

3. Mustard Oil: Then Sushruta has talked about several oils including Mustard Oil. For mustard oil, he says KRIMIGHANAM, which means anthelmintic (kills parasites), KANDU KUSTHA HARAM, which means antipruritic (reduces itching) and treating skin diseases. According to the description, mustard oil is highly useful for people suffering from itching and skin infections with Kapha dosha dominance. You should also note it has warming nature. Therefore, mustard oil is not suitable for people with Pitta Body Type and Pitta Dosha dominance in their skin. It is recommended to use of mustard oil, fragrance oils and ayurvedic medicated oils for Abhyanga or any of medicated ayurvedic oils.

4. Medicated Oils: Some of the most useful oils include:

- Maha Narayan Oil.
- Dhanwantharam Oil.
- Maharajaprasarini Thailam.
- Balaswagandhadi Thailam.
- Chandanadi Thailam.

However, you can use any oil according to your personal needs. However, mustard oil is best for daily Abhyanga. Before using mustard oil, boil it once then added a pinch of turmeric powder in it when it is hot. Leave it for 24 hours. After 24 hours, filter the oil and use this oil for daily massage. This process is not required for medicated oils.

How to take Abhyanga?

- First, apply oil to the head and ear. Do a gentle head and ear massage for 5 minutes.
- Then apply oil on feet and get proper feet massage of about 5 minutes.
- Then apply oil to other parts of the body and get a gentle massage for every organ. This process may take 20 to 30 minutes.

Contraindications of Abhyanga or Massage

People suffering from the following health conditions should not get oil massage or abhyanga:

- Kapha disorders.

- Fever.
- Indigestion.
- Ama Dosha.
- After taking purgatives or emetics.
- Obesity.

Pre-Workout Massage

Ayurveda recommends both pre-workout (before exercise) and post-workout (after exercise) body massage. First, discuss the pre-workout massage. Pre-workout massage helps in warming up the muscles and makes them more flexible. It prevents muscle tension and strengthens the body. Gentle massage with medicated ayurvedic oils also helps to prevent muscle soreness that can occur after a workout in a few people, especially sportspeople. It further speeds up cell recovery and reduces inflammation. However, massage should be gentle. Deep tissue massage is not recommendable before a workout.

Exercise

Your body is not made for a sedentary lifestyle. Due to the current scenario, most people are suffering from lifestyle disorders. These diseases are a result of a sedentary lifestyle and unhealthy eating. You eat more than you require and do no physical activity that produces sweating. Therefore, daily exercise becomes more important for everyone. You must do the exercise according to your physical capacity. Normally, 45 minutes of daily exercise helps in the prevention of lifestyle diseases. If you never did any exercise or physical work before, you should gradually increase the duration of exercise to 45 minutes over several weeks.

In ayurveda, exercise is termed as Vyayama. Activities that produce tiredness in the body are known as Vyayama. So, you should stop doing exercise when you feel tired. In winters (cold season), people who eat more fatty foods must exercise half of their capacity. Half of the capacity means when they start feeling the dryness of the mouth and get sweating on the forehead, nose, axillae and joints of the limbs. It is the time when you should stop exercising in winters. Whatever the recommendations, you must listen to your body and stay within your limits.

Benefits of Exercise

- Exercise increases work capacity.
- It produces a sensation of lightness in the body.
- It aids in improving and having a good appetite.
- It reduces excess body fats.
- Your body becomes firm and you gain more strength in your muscles.
- It helps to prevent constipation, diabetes, high blood pressure, hormonal imbalance, obesity, osteoporosis, respiratory diseases and several other diseases.

Who should not Exercise?

- People suffering from Vata and Pitta disorders should avoid exercise.
- Young children.
- Old persons.
- Patients suffering from indigestion.

Side Effects of doing Exercise beyond Limits

If you do exercise beyond your limits, you may suffer from the following health conditions:

- Excessive thirst.
- Emaciation.
- Breathing difficulties.
- Exhaustion.
- Fatigue (even without doing anything).
- Cough.
- Fever.
- Sometimes, excessive exercise also leads to vomiting.

Post-Workout Massage

After exercise, you must get a body massage. Ayurveda strongly recommends getting full body oil massage after exercise. In ayurveda, oil massage before exercise and after exercise both are equally important. Post-workout massage helps to speed up muscle recovery. It also improves flexibility and strength. It reduces muscle soreness, which may occur when you exercise. It relieves soft tissue tension.

Udvartana Massage

Massage with a fine powder of astringent herbs is called Udvartana. This type of massage is helpful for liquefying fats underneath the skin. It also mitigates the Kapha Dosha. It is highly recommendable for over-weight and obese people.

Bath

After the massage, take rest for a few minutes (around 15-30 minutes). Then you can take a bath. In ayurveda, the bath is termed Snana. It improves appetite, vigor, lifespan and strength. It alleviates itching and removes dirt and sweat.

- Hot or warm water should not be poured on the head. Too cold water should also be avoided.

According to ayurveda, hot or warm water head bath diminishes vision and strength of hairs.

- The warm water bath is suitable for the lower body – below the neck. Water should not be too hot.

How to take a Bath?

Ayurveda does not recommend the use of soap for taking bath. Instead, it recommends using Amla in place of soap.

- Take 5 grams of amla powder. Mix it in lemon juice. Add some water to make it thin.
- Apply and gently rub it on the head and your body. In a similar way, as you were taking a bath with soap or shampoo.
- Then take a shower and wash away the amla lemon from your head and body with water.
- Pat dry your body with a soft towel.

Alternatively, you can also use gram flour instead of amla. You can also use Amla water for taking bath.

How to make Amla Water for Bath?

Amla water is recommended for a bath.

- For making amla water, take 1280 ml water. Add 10 grams coarse powder of amla fruit pulp.
- Boil water with Amla and then filter it.
- Add this water in your bathtub with 30 liters of water. Take a bath with this water. While taking a bath, you should rub all parts of the body with your palms.

Who should not take a Bath?

People suffering from the following diseases should not take bath:

- The acute phase of facial paralysis.
- Acute diseases of the eyes, mouth and ears.
- Diarrhea.
- Abdominal distension.
- Runny nose.
- Indigestion.
- Soon after taking a meal.

20 Minutes Meditation

After following above routines, the next step is meditation or chanting mantra for 108 times. Vagbhata recommends repeating the name of god for 108 times and ask to do Pranama to god and elder members of the family. You can recite any name of a god or any mantra that provides you feeling of peacefulness, kindness, gracefulness and joyfulness. Instead of chanting mantra, you can also meditate for 20 minutes. 20 minutes meditation provides excellent results in the prevention of neurological disorders and psychosomatic diseases.

Meditation or chanting mantra may or may not relate to god, but it surely relates to mental health. It is also important to feel and understand the surrounding Mother Nature. Several research studies have shown positive effects of meditation and mantra chanting in the prevention and treatment of stress disorders, depression and anxiety. In breathing meditation, you just need to watch the process of inhaling (breathe in) and exhaling (breathe out) for a couple of minutes. If you cannot do this, you can practice deep breathing. Take a deep breathe in and hold it in the abdomen for a few seconds and release the breath out. You should also express your gratitude toward mother nature by saying thank you for a wonderful life, thank you for a wonderful day or anything that you want to say to express your gratitude.

During meditation, chanting mantra or deep breathing or while expressing your gratitude toward mother nature, keep a smile on your face and feel joyfulness, gracefulness, kindness and peacefulness in your mind. It is more important than anything else.

Pranama

You should also Pranama to your elders in your family. They could be your parents and grandparents. Pranama is a respectful salutation, which is done by adjoining both hands bowing the head and saying Pranama, Namaskar or Sat Shri Akaal. Whichever tradition you follow, you can do it accordingly. Pranama helps in better communication in the family and improves the relation between family members. It also makes a person feel connected with each other and their importance and respectfulness in the family. It is most important in terms of social health.

Diet Plan

Ayurvedic diet principles are basic dietary guidelines for living a healthier, happier and longer life. Ayurveda is a stable science. Whatever it recommends keeping you healthy, it is still valid. Here we will discuss healthy eating habits based on ayurvedic principles of eating. These healthy eating habits will help you to prevent and get rid of almost all diseases in your life.

Food Ratio

Solid Foods	1/2 part of the stomach
Liquid Foods	1/4 part of the stomach
Keep Stomach Empty	1/4 part of the stomach

- Solid foods: Whole grains, lentils, fruits, vegetables, seeds and nuts are solid foods.

- Liquid foods: Fruit juice, vegetable juice, lemon water, coconut water, coconut milk, water, etc. are liquid foods.
- Keep stomach empty: You should always eat less than your appetite. It means you must keep 1/4th part of your stomach empty.

You should not take liquid foods with fruits and raw vegetables because they are already water-rich foods fulfilling the criteria for both solid and liquid foods. During the main meals, you should adjust liquid intake accordingly. Sometimes, it is difficult to judge the quantity of food. You should always check the signs of healthy eating. Signs of healthy eating:

- Focus on your feelings after having a meal. You will feel fresh and active after eating healthy food. You will feel restless, nauseous and uncomfortable with the abdomen after eating junk and unhealthy food.
- You still feel lightness in the abdomen even after eating.
- You are comfortable with your stomach.
- Your stomach never reminds you that something went wrong, or you have overeaten.
- You do not experience any fullness or heaviness in the abdomen after eating.

Ayurveda Mealtimes

Ayurveda recommends two types of meal plans:

Meal Plan	Best Timings
One Main Meal	12:00 pm to 2:00 pm
Two Main Meals	First Meal: 8:00 am to 10:00 am & Second Meal: 3:00 pm to 5:00 pm

Ayurvedic texts also suggest eating whenever you feel hungry. So, you can also eat fresh fruits and raw vegetables any time whenever you feel hungry in addition to scheduled timings.

- The above timings apply to the main meals only.
- This rule applies to grains, lentils (beans) and cooked foods (including cooked vegetables). You can eat fruits and vegetable salad any time whenever you feel appetite. You can also drink water whenever you feel thirsty.
- In a one-time meal plan, you can eat cooked food one time a day.
- In two times meal plan, you can eat cooked food 2 times a day.

Ashtanga Sangrah has not given any timing for a meal, but it has only mentioned morning meal and evening meal. The above timings are recommended by Sushruta Samhita.

Table: One main meal diet plan.

8:00 am to 9:00 am	Fruits
12:00 pm to 2:00 pm (main meal)	Raw Vegetable Salad, Grains, Lentils, Seeds and Nuts

Table: Two main meals diet plan.

8:00 am to 9:00 am	Fruits
9:00 am to 10:00 am (main meal)	Grains with Steamed Vegetables
3:00 pm to 5:00 pm (main meal)	Raw Vegetable Salad, Grains, Lentils, Seeds and Nuts

You need to select a suitable meal plan for you. So, your body adjusts its biological clock according to your circumstances.

What Should we do if we do not Feel an Appetite for the Second Meal?

Ayurveda recommends whenever you do not feel an appetite for the second meal, it is okay to eat an evening meal at the scheduled time even if you have not digested the morning meal. But you must not eat the morning meal if you have not digested the previous day's evening meal. Because during nighttime digestion capacity reduces 3 hours after sunrise, digestive capacity increases. So, if you fast for a few hours in the morning, then it will help to digest the food properly. Eat when you feel appetite in the morning and your bowel gets clear. You can take your evening meal as per your scheduled time. But remember the following things:

- Do not eat before the scheduled time.
- Do not overeat.
- Eat less keeping at least ¼ part of the stomach empty.
- Keep a minimum of 16 hours fasting period after the evening meal. So, you must not eat anything after taking the evening meal. It will help to digest the food taken in the day properly.

If you follow the above points, then there is no harm to eat the second meal at the scheduled time.

What Should we do if we Feel Appetite after Eating the Main Meal?

Some people feel appetite again after eating a primary meal. In most cases, it occurs within the first 2 hours after eating a primary meal. Pitta dosha increases after eating food. It is a natural pitta cycle in your body. It is a false appetite. In reality, Pitta is digesting the food previously eaten. If you feel appetite even after eating a good amount of food, then it could be a false appetite. False appetite pacifies itself after a few minutes. If it is not a false appetite, then you can eat the healthiest foods keeping a minimum of two hours' gap from a primary meal. The healthiest foods include:

- Fruits.
- Uncooked vegetables (raw vegetables or salad).
- Fresh vegetable juice. (Do not take fruit juice, instead eat fruits).

These foods are easy to digest, full of nutrients and suitable for all people.

What do Research Studies say about 2 Times Meals a Day?

Research studies have shown that eating frequent meals causes insulin resistance and people who eat frequent meals will develop diabetes and other lifestyle diseases later in their life. People who eat 2 times a day have no insulin resistance in their body. Another study also confirms this. According to the study the secretion of gastric acid decreases during sleep. Sleep is directly linked with low production of acid secretion in the stomach. Waking in the morning is linked with an increase in gastric acid output.

Most people suffering from the acid peptic disease have aggravated symptoms in the morning and evening. It indicates an increase in acid secretion in the stomach in the morning and evening. They also feel significant relief from symptoms at night. So, acid secretion diminishes at night. Therefore, you should eat 2 primary meals a day. Two primary meals a day is an ancient concept of ayurveda. In India, taking meals is compared with Agnihotra Yagya, which is done two times a day. Agnihotra Yagya is done two times a day. You should also take food 2 times a day.

In villages in Punjab, India, some families still follow this tradition. They eat only 2 times a day. They are healthier than people who are eating 3 to 6 times a day. However, 2 times the meal tradition is disappearing because of the adoption of western culture – breakfast, lunch and dinner.

Appetite Rule

You should respect your appetite and hunger and eat food accordingly.

- Do not suppress appetite.
- Eat whenever you feel hungry.
- Do not overeat.

Do not Suppress Appetite

Do not suppress your appetite. If you suppress appetite, the following disease may occur:

- Body ache.
- Loss of interest in food.
- Fatigue.
- Laziness.
- Vision Weakness.
- Loss of tissues.
- Loss of strength.
- Loss of Appetite.

A few health conditions are given above. But if you suppress appetite and do not eat when you are hungry, it is dangerous for your overall health. If you still feel hungry even after eating one or two main meals a day then you should eat fresh and healthy foods – fruits, uncooked vegetables, salad and nuts and seeds. You can eat coconut and drink coconut water or vegetable juice.

Eat whenever you Feel Hungry

After proper digestion and utilization of food in your body, you also require eating food. Your body itself tells you when you need to eat. When you need to eat, your stomach will ask for it. So, eat whenever you feel a real appetite. Eat whenever your stomach asks you to eat. Do not listen to your tongue. Do not eat just for taste. Of course, eat delicious food, but when you feel a real appetite.

- The golden role of healthy eating and stay healthy is to eat only when you are hungry. Drink water only when you are thirsty.
- When you are thirsty, do not eat food. You should drink water at this time.
- When you are hungry, do not drink water. You should eat food at that time.

Benefits of Eating Food when you Feel Appetite

If you eat when you have an appetite, it provides the following things to your mind and body:

- Joyfulness.
- Strength.
- Excellent Memory.
- Longevity.
- Endurance and Tolerance.
- Good Complexion and Glowing Skin.
- Immunity.
- Vitality.
- Gracefulness.

Difference between Real Appetite and Food Craving

Real Appetite	Food Craving
Your stomach demands food. It is empty and you have not eaten anything for hours.	Your tongue demands food even when your stomach is full and satisfied.
You never overeat.	You overeat.
You eat for energy as per your physical and mental requirements.	You do not need to eat for energy. You just eat for taste.
You stop when you feel full.	You continue to eat regardless of the stomach is full or not.
Your abdomen has a feeling of lightness even after eating.	You feel heaviness in the abdomen after eating.

It is the main and first most important principle of the ayurvedic diet, eat when you feel appetite and avoid eating when you do not have hunger. All other principles come after this. If you are healthy, you will feel appetite after digestion and utilization of the previous meal. So, do not eat if you don't feel appetite. Eat when your stomach asks for food.

Signs of Proper Digestion of Previous Meal

- Proper evacuation of bowel and urinary bladder.
- Clear burp. Or no burp or belching with abnormal taste or taste of food previously eaten.
- Lightness in the body.
- Feeling thirst and appetite or hunger.
- Feeling of lightness in the heart, chest and abdomen.
- Feeling an increase in digestive fire and your stomach ask for food.
- The clarity in senses and mind.

Do not Overeat

Keep your abdomen ¼ part empty. Avoid overeating. You should not feel heaviness in the abdomen after eating any food. However, eat in a sufficient amount that satisfies your hunger. Ayurveda also recommends keeping ¼ part of the stomach empty. It provides a ratio according to solid and liquid foods and an empty part of the stomach.

Eat Food in their Natural Form

Eat foods in their natural form as you get from nature. Do not cook foods, which you can eat without cooking. It includes fruits, vegetables, nuts and some seeds. Eat them in their natural form. Foods that are cooked excessively have no life in them. It means that cooked foods have fewer nutrients than uncooked foods.

- Eat food based on quality, not quantity.
- Meals should be juicy and there should not be an excess of oil to improve the absorption rate of nutrients.
- One should avoid too dry food items.
- Cooking should be lighter as much as possible.

Balanced Ayurvedic Diet according to Taste

Ayurvedic diet does not mean eating only rice, boiled vegetables and salad, it follows specific principles and can be applied to any type of cuisine. Ayurveda recognizes mainly six tastes and these tastes include sweet, salty, pungent, sour, astringent and bitter.

Sweet taste	Fruits
Salty taste	Seaweed, Sea Vegetables, Salty foods

Pungent taste	Chili and ginger
Sour taste	Lemons and vinegar
Astringent taste	Pomegranate and lentils
Bitter taste	Turmeric (Curcuma Longa).

Food is digested in a particular order and these six tastes should be included in your daily diet to feel satisfied. So, you should add some spices like turmeric, cumin, cinnamon, cardamom and fresh spices like fresh ginger, fresh coriander or cilantro in each recipe. The foremost step towards following Ayurvedic Diet is to get to know your constitutional type or dosha with the help of the ayurvedic dosha test. Vata, pitta and kapha dosha are the energies responsible for various physiological functions in the body of an individual. Take your time to set a particular schedule for meals every day.

Eat Sattvic Foods

It is time to be familiar with the principle of 'GUNAS' and to know the difference between sattvic, rajasic and tamasic foods.

- Generally, SATTVIC foods are juicy, tasty, organic and easy to digest.
- RAJASIC foods are freshly canned foods, cooked foods, eggs, caffeine, etc.
- TAMASIC foods are leftovers, frozen foods, fermented foods and all food items obtained from animals including meat and milk products etc.

You should include more sattvic foods in your daily diet to live a healthy life. Many people include cow's milk and ghee in sattvic foods, but I disagree with them. Sattvic foods always come from plant sources with the absence of five evils:

- Kama (lust).
- Kroth (anger).
- Lobh (greed).
- Moh (attachment).
- Ahankar (ego).

Around 95% of plants have no such evil and all animals including cows have the first four evils in them. If you consume any food products from animals, they will contribute to the manifestations of these evils in you. Therefore, these foods should be considered tamasic foods. However, plants also have Kama characteristics for reproduction, but it is different from animals because they do not have lust and desire. Their reproduction is very natural and nature assists them to reproduce.

Eat Fresh

- Eat food within 48 minutes of cooking: Ayurveda recommends eating foods within 48 minutes of cooking them. You can maximum store food for 3 hours. Shree Krishna in Bhagavad Gita says food should not be kept more than 3 hours. After three hours, food is considered stale food. You must eat within 3 hours. Do not keep them in the refrigerator for the next time or the next day. Cook the food amount, which you and your family can easily consume immediately.

- Eat Food Cooked at Home: Eat food cooked at home. Do not eat readymade food sold in shops and restaurants. Cook food for yourself and your family at home. You should not eat food that is sold in restaurants, shops and packaged foods.

Eat Food with a Calm Mind

Do not eat in a hurry. In ayurveda, taking a meal is like worship.

- Your mind should be calm.
- You should sit in a cross-legged posture on the floor. You can sit on the floor mat.
- Before start eating, express gratitude toward nature for food. Feel joyfulness, calmness and kindness in your mind.
- Before you eat food, first provide food to poor people if they are on the door to asking for food. Then serve foods to guests, elders and children. Then you should eat food. You should eat food with your family members.
- Always eat in a calm and comfortable environment.
- Stay away from distractions like TV and mobile phone while having food.
- It is important to be present while eating. This means one should take time to appreciate the taste, look, texture, flavor and smell of food using all five senses.

All these rituals help in the prevention of Alzheimer's disease, depression, anxiety and other psychological diseases. It is most important to eat with your family members. Research studies concluded people who eat a meal with their parents and children are less likely to suffer from mental diseases later in their life.

Rules of Drinking Water

Drinking water in the morning can prevent and help to manage abdominal disorders including constipation, malabsorption and piles. It also helps with urinary disorders and blood disorders. It is also beneficial in diseases of upper parts of the body including head, nose, ear and throat. It is highly useful in the prevention and treatment of skin diseases.

Ushapan Vessel

There are mainly three types of vessels are used for keeping water overnight for Ushapan.

- Golden Vessel.

- Earthen Pot.
- Copper Pot.

Thin people and people with Vata body type and Pitta body type should drink water kept in a golden vessel. If you cannot afford a golden vessel, then you can drink water kept in the earthen pot overnight. Overweight or obese people or people with Kapha body type should drink water kept in a copper vessel overnight. Alternatively, you can drink warm water. Warm water and water kept in a copper vessel also help to reduce weight in addition to other benefits.

How much Water should we Drink in Ushapan?

The amount of water varies person-to-person. It depends on how much water you can hold in 8 Anjali. Anjali is a Sanskrit word, which means concavity formed by adjoining both hands. 8 Anjali means the amount of water that you can measure 8 times in the concavity formed by adjoining both hands. For example, if you can hold 100 ml water in 1 Anjali, then your drinkable water recommendation is 800 ml. So, you have to measure the water quantity suitable for your body yourself. The water that you can hold in 8 Anjali, you should drink in the morning.

Right Time for Ushapan

When should we Drink Water in the Morning?

Ushapaan consists of two words–Usha and Paan. Usha means dawn and Paan means taking or drinking. It occurs just a few minutes before sunrise when light becomes visible all around, but the sun does not appear in the sky yet. This is a perfect time. Ayurveda recommends waking up in Brahma Muhurta, which is around 96 minutes before sunrise. Usha means dawn, which is nearly just before sunrise. So, there is around 60 minutes gap between the time of Brahma Muhurta and Dawn. There is no specification mentioned in ayurveda literature that you should drink water before or after cleaning teeth and tongue. Morning saliva has some healing properties if it is applied externally on the skin lesion.

The flow of saliva reduces significantly during sleep, which allows microbial growth in the mouth. This process also results in bad breath in the morning. However, lysozyme, an enzyme, present in saliva prevents microbial overgrowth. But bacterial growth due to the diminished flow of saliva during sleep still causes bad breath in the morning.

When you follow Dinacharya, you can see, most of the morning activities get completed until dawn if you wake up in Brahma Muhurta. So, if we follow the definition of Ushapan, then you should drink water after all morning cleaning activities. you should drink water after cleaning your teeth and tongue. Still, it's your personal decision when you want to drink water in the morning. You can also drink water before bowel evacuation or after cleaning your teeth and tongue.

Benefits of Ushapan

Drinking water in the morning prevents and cures almost all diseases. Especially, it is helpful in piles, Grahani disease (irritable bowel syndrome), fever, obesity, diseases of organs located in the upper part of the body (above the neck). It helps in diseases of the ear. It improves longevity. It is also useful in urinary disorders and blood disorders.

- Cleanses Stomach and Intestine: Ushapan cleanses the stomach and intestine. Water enema cleans the colon and large intestine. Enema has no reach to the stomach and small intestine. For detoxifying stomach and small intestine, Ushapan is the best technique. It removes the undigested or poorly digested food particles from the walls of the small intestine and improves nutrients absorption and digestion of food that you eat in the following meal. Because the undigested food particles are the main cause of constipation, indigestion and acid peptic disorders. So, Ushapan benefits in the prevention and treatment of these diseases.
- Irritable Bowel Syndrome: In ayurveda, Ushapan is recommended for Grahani Rog, which is correlated with irritable bowel syndrome. In Grahani Rog, Ama Dosha is the main cause. Ama dosha is formed due to undigested or poorly digested food particles. it removes undigested food particles from the walls of the small intestine, so it ultimately eliminates the cause of irritable bowel syndrome. Thus, it helps in the management and treatment of irritable bowel syndrome.
- Reduces Weight: During Ushapan, if you drink water kept in a copper pot, it aids in reducing weight. Copper charged water has additional properties that reduce Kapha Dosha in the body, which induces fat loss.
- Cleanses Kidneys and Urinary Bladder: Ushapan benefits in cleansing the kidneys and urinary bladder. If you suffer from kidney stone or debris in the urinary bladder, its cleansing effects are very beneficial for removing the stone from the kidney and debris from the urinary bladder. It also prevents frequent urinary infections (UTIs).

Ushapan Contraindications

Ushapan is not suitable for all people. It has a few contraindications.

When Should we not Drink Water in the Morning?

- A person who undergoes for Oleation Therapy should not drink water in the morning.
- You should not drink water after eating oily and fatty foods.
- If you have any chest injuries, you should avoid drinking water in large amount in the morning.
- During Panchakarma: While undergoing any of panchakarma procedure, drinking water in the morning is contraindicated.
- Excessive Hiccup: If you are suffering from excessive hiccup, you should not drink water in the morning.
- Loss of appetite due to any Kapha and Vata disorders.

- If you suffer from abdominal heaviness or stiffness in the abdomen or distension of the abdomen, then you should also not drink water in the morning.

Rasa Shastra

The famous Rasa Shastra formed about 7 Cen as a branch of the Ayurveda. While the theme of Rasa Shastra can be traced back to the Vedic period where noble metals are meant to derive from the holy fire (yangyan) for the well-being of human society, the methods or art or science are not clearly defined or well known today. In the Samhita time, the materials related to Rasa Shastra are contained in a dispersed manner by means of a detailed explanation of their therapeutic application, but without a definition of their mode of care. The Middle Ages claim to be the golden age of Rasa Shastra; the explanation of the raw materials manufacturing processes, along with the therapeutic and alchemical usage of the finished product, can be found in various literatures of this era. Every research has its own vocabulary of speech and its own basic values.

Principles of the Fundament

Values/concepts/phenomenons that are necessary within a given discipline or method are known to be the basic principles of that discipline or method. These are important for a detailed and proper comprehension and creation of subjects or programs. Topics, manufacturing processes, raw materials evaluation, product validation, harmful effects and their remedies, etc., are defined in ancient Rasa literature, which are very useful for a better understanding of the subject matter. The following points may be considered to be the basic concepts of Rasa Shastra.

Technical Terminologies (Paribhasa)

- Mana (Measurement).
- Yantra, musha (Tools and devices).
- Puta,kosthi (Heating arrangements).
- Dravyapariksha (Identification of materials).
- Rasashala (Setup of Ayurvedic pharmacy).
- Processing technologies & their sequence (Shodhana, marana).
- Aushadhipariksha (Techniques of assessment of finished product).
- Dose determination.
- Therapeutic uses.
- Knowledge of adverse effect of Rasaushadhies and their remedies.

As other philosophy, Rasa Shastra has its own vocabulary of speech and comprehension. The literatures for the same are also enriched with so many technical terms which are practically difficult to understand by common people and scientists of other discipline. Hence, it is very much necessary to explore these technical terms, conveying principles of working, appraisal of products, references and meaning of, hidden/partially explored concepts, for its better understanding and cross disciplinary study, for development of the system in particular and wellbeing of the society in general.

Measurement (Mana)

Rasa Shastra is the topic of medicinal diagnosis, dosage calculation and clinical usage of Rasaushadhies (Herbo-mineral preparation) and thus proportions are important instruments to use. As the measuring form of ancient India (e.g. rati, tola, pala, sana, etc.) was specific in relation to the modern period, the correct translation of such measures must be understood to those concerned. The raw materials used in the manufacture of medicinal goods are manufactured into a number of folding techniques involving many similar materials of specific origin (mineral/herbal/animal) and hence, in each and every phase, the appropriate quantity of measurement plays a significant role in the excellence of the finished product. Rasaushadhies contains drugs made from Hg, As, Pb, Sn, Cu etc. Thus, the utmost precaution must be taken with respect to the assessment during the determination of the medication, since the actual dosage type is to be given to the human body. E.g. 1 Rati of 125 mg. 1 tola of 12.5gm, 1 pala of 50gm, etc.

Tools and Devices (Yantra, Musa)

Tools and equipment are important for the development of some form of medication. These not only serve as the keeper of raw materials during manufacturing, but are often constructed in such a way that, depending on the raw materials to be handled, these induce an improvement in the potency of the prepared drugs and at the same time decrease the toxic impact of the so-called doshas of the raw materials. These are also used to control the material during dealing with them. According to the nature of raw material to be processed, working principle for particular processing, requirement of the quality of the finished product to be achieved, arrangement of heating devices to be employed, the yantra (different kinds of instruments) and musas (different kinds of crucibles) are constituted and designed. Hence, these are the fundamentals of all personals associated with Ayurvedic drug manufacturing. E.g. Dolayantra for swedana, damaruyantra for hingulothaparada, kachhapayantra for gandhakajarana, musa for sattvapatana, etc.

Heating Arrangements (Puta, Kosthi)

These are heating systems used for the processing of pharmaceutical items, primarily of metallic/mineral type. Among them, puta is the main note for the preparation of bhasma and kupipakvarasayana.It is the quantity of heat needed to achieve the desired quality product in the cycle of marana (inceneration) with the warning that more or less quantum results in the spoilage of medicinal goods. Puta induces apunarbhava, varitara, laghutva and deepana consistency in the prepared bhasma. This also allows the drug to circulate rapidly through the micro-circulation of the body. Puta also induces a decrease in dose and introduction of medicinal efficiency and eventually causes mrita (bhasma) of the raw material extracted in this scheme.

It is very necessary, since without its awareness, the bhasma and hence the Rasaushadhies cannot be prepared. Once, it is important as the utmost precaution must be taken to include a particular volume of heat over a specified duration of time for the development of a diligent substance that should be therapeutically successful with little to no negative effects on the human body. For processing of different raw materials an understanding regarding the putas is indispensable. Every kind of puta offers three phases of the temperature cycle, i.e. the cycle of the increasing temperature, the pattern of the maximum temperature range and the pattern of self-cooling. Both three of these formulations yield the desired result. High temperature range (absolute temperature level measured over overall period of time) and self-cooling play a more critical part in the processing and compounding of products.Different putas described in variousliteratures are mahaputa, gajaputa, varahaputa, kukkutaputa, balukaputa, bhandaputa, gorbaraputa etc. for marana of different materials as per need.

Kosthi is a particular scale and form of heating device used for the extraction and purification of sattva. Kosthi is constructed in such a manner that a sufficient volume of oxygen is supplied to the furnace during the cycle to ensure a high temperature for the content being treated. It is used primarily for the extraction of sattva. Any mineral sattva extraction is required therapeutically because sattva bhasma is more effective than bhasma of the same raw material. Sattva is an important prerequisite throughout any alchemical cycle (abhraka sattva &makshika sattva for dvandana). For sattva patana, therefore, knowledge of kosthi is necessary and is integrated into the fundamentals of Rashastra.

Identification of Materials (Dravyapariksha)

Raw materials are the foundation of an appropriate and honorable formulation in some type in care technique. The recognition of raw materials is an essential step for GMP (Good Industrial Practices). So, it is only by deliberately choosing the raw material; the Rashastra moto can be accomplished. If the raw material is not up to the mark and according to the GrahyaLakshana (acceptable features) mentioned in different Rasa literature, then all subsequent attempts to prepare the medication to cure a specific disease will not be effective. There are several products that appear somewhat identical in their organoleptic properties but behave differently after processing. The supplier and all relevant staff must be informed of the main features for the differentiated recognition of such products, for the planning of appropriate medicines. Until the processing of raw materials, the following may be confirmed:

- Understanding the Grahya Lakshana of the raw materials in the literature.
- By questioning local and field experts where the document is silent on the correct features.
- Polan by matching the marker compounds and the various analytical fingerprints produced by an authoritative entity for a specific item. For other products where the raw material recognition requirements are provided for the product, but the manufacturing procedures to be practiced, such as the form of puta, no. of puta, no. of bhavana, etc, They are not described; in this circumstance there is a chemical structure such as MP, solidity, Sp. Gravity, stiffness, interaction with specific maraka drugs (associated substance used during the incense phase) in various conditions should be understood to start the process.

Establishment of Ayurvedic Pharmacy (Rasashala)

In ancient India, Rasa sala was designed to create Rasaushadhies, both for alchemical and therapeutic purposes and was regulated by Acharya. They were architect the Rasashala and placed the needful equipment's, raw materials, finished product and cited proper manufacturing area with respect to different techniques like firing, washing, drying, grinding etc. in such a way so as to maintain the balance with the magnetic and cosmic resonance of the nature e.g. the jobs related with fire like putapaka, heating etc. are supposed to be done in Agneya corner, job related to air like drying etc. are done in Vayavya corner. The positioning of students, scholars and support staff was often used to position them in the right location in order to promote better coordination and successful performance. The Deity Rasa bhairava was also an essential edifice of the ancient Rasashala and was put in the East corner so that all could believe that God is watching after individual success and giving mental calm and attention to the work that should be performed.

Processing Methods and their Sequence

The core aspect of Rasashstra is the refining of raw materials into medicinal dosage type. As a consequence, the various methods and strategies introduced have their own interpretations in order to increase the consistency of the drugs to be prepared. Alsostepwise processing proves more effective & logical to the nobleness of the finished products, instead of by passing certain intermediary processes which is sometimes seen in practice by certain manufacturers. There is not much processing mentioned in Rasa's literature on the essence of the raw material to be handled, but some processing is very important and sometimes happens in most Rasa shastra raw drugs. They are sanskara, shodhana, jarana, marana, amritikarana and sattvapatana.

Sanskara

Sanskara is a method that causes the necessary properties of the raw material to be used for various purposes. According to Acharya Charakasanskara, it is achieved with the aid of water/fire or by adding/subtracting any necessity, or by executing other procedures, such as churning, crushing or automated time development. In Rasa shastra sanskara, Parada is conducted with the intention of obtaining medicinal and alchemical results. 08 sanskaras are made for the first purpose and 18 sanskaras are made for the latter. Growing sanskara is performed only after the previous one has been successfully completed. Today, 18 sanskaras are hardly in action. Sanskara may allow trace elements to be incorporated to certain specific materials used in the procedure which can enhance Parada's therapeutic progress.

Shodhana

It is a primary method for all raw products, irrespective of their type, such as plant, mineral or animal. Shodhana can be characterized as Ayurvedic treatment of raw drugs that reduce doshas (impurities)/toxic effects and induce therapeutic properties by means of a variety of techniques, such as wet trituration (bhavana), pounding/grinding (mardana), fomenting (swedana), heating (roasting/frying), heating/quenching (nirvapa), etc., not just material purification. Shodhana signifies:

- Reduction of doshas (impurities)/toxic effect.

- Induction of therapeutic property.
- Reduction of size of raw drugs.
- Facilitation of marana (incineration) process.
- Probably addition of certain necessary trace elements.

Marana

This is the key method used to adopt the effective dosage type of Ayurvedic Therapeutics for the preparation of bhasmas. Marana can be defined as a process in which the shodhita material is subjected to bhavana with certain herbal juices/decoctions with or without addition of certain other mineral/animal originated materials followed by burning in different types of puta system of heating with the rich involvement of oxygen. Puta is the usual device used for marana. Types of puta are chosen according to the quality of the substance to be handled. The text has immense instructions for the collection of a kind of puta for a specific item. But, practically a particular bhasma is hardly prepared as per exact type and no.of puta described for the same in the texts. Nevertheless, the signs are reasonably available and performed with some adjustment by examining the substance from time to time and studying the expert opinion. Throughout the case that no sign is detected, the procedure is started by a professional opinion on the chemical and physical properties of the material. Marana signifies:

- Conversion of components into compounds and current substances in raw materials into some other substances for planned medicinal usage known as bhasma.
- Reduction of particle size.
- Approximate introduction of some trace elements to the final product and are known to be helpful to the human body for medicinal usage.

Amritikarana

Amritikarana is a specific pharmaceutical treatment conducted in some products, such as Tamra, Abhraka, etc., after marana, to eliminate residual toxicity when current, with the intention of ensuring the best quality of bhasma with no or reduced toxicity. Ancient Acharyas were well aware of the toxic existence of Tamra and hence explicitly identified amritikarana for this content, which is also shown in a scientific analysis that Tamara bhasma contains highly toxic mercury oxide compounds, while amritikarana does not contain any mercury oxide compounds. Therefore, amritikara is an integral operation.

Jarana

Once gandhaka and other items are digested by various methods in the procession, the method is known as jarana. Yet in the case of putilohas (Pb, Sn & Zn), jarana is the medium of bhasmikaranaIn-putilohasjarana is achieved after shodhana, by rubbing with various organic alkali materials (Apamargakshara, Ashwatthakshara etc.) in the presence of heat to turn it into powder shape in order to promote the cycle of marana. This is very relevant for both the medicinal and alchemical processes.

Sattvapatana

The method in which the substance is mixed with mitrapanchaka/dravakagana drugs stored in musa and shot in an extreme fire in kosthi with the intention of removing the metal essence is regarded as sattvapatana. Sattvapatana is important for both alchemy and therapy since it is believed that sattva bhasma is more therapeutically active than bhasma of a particular substance. Abhraka sattva and makshika sattva are necessary criteria for dvandana (amalgamation) in Paradajarana during alchemical production.

Aushadhipariksha

Upon production, it is really important to determine the consistency of the final product before it is planned for human use. There are so many quality assurance metrics for bhasmas of various materials recorded in ancient Rasa texts. These are varitara, rekhapurna, apunarbhava, nirutha, niswadu etc.

References

- Ashtang-ayurveda-eight-branches-of-ayurveda: ayurtimes.com, Retrieved 23, January 2020
- Herbal-medicinal-plants, science-of-ayurveda: dabur.com, Retrieved 10, March 2020
- Ayurvedic-acupressure: maayogashram.com, Retrieved 13, June 2020
- Ayurvedic-accupresure-figures: acusansthan-ald.in, Retrieved 20, August 2020
- Ayurvedic-diet-principles: ayurtimes.com, Retrieved 17, February 2020

Chapter 4

Alternative Medical Therapies

Some of the important alternative therapies are acupuncture, acupressure, apitherapy, hydrotherapy, halotherapy and animal assisted therapy. Acupuncture is practiced to attempt pain relief and involves inserting thin needles into the body. The topics elaborated in this chapter will help in gaining a better perspective about these various alternative therapies.

Acupuncture

Acupuncture is the practice of penetrating the skin with thin, solid, metallic needles which are then activated through gentle and specific movements of the practitioner's hands or with electrical stimulation.

Acupuncture is part of the ancient practice of Traditional Chinese medicine. Traditional Chinese medicine practitioners believe the human body has more than 2,000 acupuncture points connected by pathways or meridians. These pathways create an energy flow (Qi, pronounced "chee") through the body that is responsible for overall health. Disruption of the energy flow can cause disease. By applying acupuncture to certain points, it is thought to improve the flow of Qi, thereby improving health.

Studies have shown that acupuncture is effective for a variety of conditions. Acupuncture is not for everyone. If you choose to see an acupuncturist, discuss it with your doctor first and find a practitioner who is licensed as having proper training and credentials.

What does Acupuncture Feel Like?

Acupuncture is done using hair-thin needles. Most people report feeling minimal pain as the needle is inserted. The needle is inserted to a point that produces a sensation of pressure or ache. Needles may be heated during the treatment or mild electric current may be applied to them. Some people report acupuncture makes them feel energized. Others say they feel relaxed.

Improper placement of the needle can cause pain during treatment. Needles must be sterilized to prevent infection. That is why it is important to seek treatment from a qualified acupuncture practitioner. The FDA regulates acupuncture needles just as it does other medical devices under good manufacturing practices and single-use standards of sterility. Instead of needles, other forms of stimulation are sometimes used over the acupuncture points, including:

- Heat (moxibustion),
- Pressure (acupressure),
- Friction,

- Suction (cupping),
- Impulses of electromagnetic energy.

How does Acupuncture affect the Body?

Acupuncture points are believed to stimulate the central nervous system. This, in turn, releases chemicals into the muscles, spinal cord, and brain. These biochemical changes may stimulate the body's natural healing abilities and promote physical and emotional well-being.

Acupuncture is an effective treatment alone or in combination with conventional therapies to treat the following:

- Nausea caused by surgical anesthesia and cancer chemotherapy.
- Dental pain after surgery.
- Addiction.
- Headaches.
- Menstrual cramps.
- Tennis elbow.
- Fibromyalgia.
- Myofascial pain.
- Osteoarthritis.
- Low back pain.
- Carpal tunnel syndrome.
- Asthma.

It may also help with stroke rehabilitation.

What Conditions may benefit from Acupuncture?

Many people seek acupuncture treatment for relief of chronic pain, such as arthritis or low back pain. Acupuncture, however, has expanded uses in other parts of the world. Before considering acupuncture, talk to your doctor. Conditions that may benefit from acupuncture include the following:

Digestive	Emotional
Gastritis Irritable bowel syndrome Hepatitis Hemorrhoids	Anxiety Depression Insomnia Nervousness Neurosis

Eye-Ear-Throat	Gynecological
Rhinitis Sinusitis Sore throat	Menstrual pain Infertility
Musculoskeletal	Neurological
Arthritis Back pain Muscle cramping Muscle pain and weakness Neck pain Sciatica	Headaches Migraines Neurogenic bladder dysfunction Parkinson's disease Postoperative pain Stroke
Respiratory	Miscellaneous
Allergic rhinitis Sinusitis Bronchitis	Irritable bladder Prostatitis Male infertility Some forms of impotence Addiction

Considerations when Choosing Acupuncture

Because scientific studies have not fully explained how acupuncture works within the framework of Western medicine, acupuncture remains a source of controversy. It is important to take precautions when deciding about acupuncture as follows:

- Discuss acupuncture with your doctor first. Acupuncture is not for everyone. Discuss all the treatments and medicines (dietary supplements, prescription and over-the-counter) you are taking. If you have a pacemaker, are at risk for infection, have chronic skin problems, are pregnant, or have breasts or other implants, be sure to tell your doctor. Acupuncture may be risky to your health if you fail to mention these matters.
- Do not rely on a diagnosis of disease by an acupuncture practitioner. If you have received a diagnosis from a doctor, you may wish to ask him or her whether acupuncture might help.
- Choose a licensed acupuncture practitioner. Your own doctor may be a good resource for referrals to a licensed or certified practitioner. Friends and family members may also be good sources of referrals. You do not have to be a doctor to practice acupuncture or to become a certified acupuncturist.

The number of acupuncture points was originally established to correlate with the number of days in the year – 365, but because acupuncturists in all parts of Asia came to identify points on the body differently, there was never an exact standard number. However, the World Health Organization (WHO) Scientific Group met in 1989 to adopt a proposed standard acupuncture nomenclature for international use, and it was then that 361 points were agreed upon.

The WHO also identified an additional 48 points that are included in the international standard. The criteria for including the extra points were: common usage, considered clinically effective, had a clear anatomical location and were at least 0.5 centimeters from a classical point. While there are multiple acupuncture locations on the body, most acupuncturists still look to the traditionally identified points. The acupuncture points are mapped to 14 main meridian channels. In Chinese medicine, a meridian channel is also known as a Jing Iou through which Qi (vital life energy) Xue (blood), Jinye (body fluids), Jing (essence) and Shen (spirit) flow. One meridian channel relates to each of the 12 inner organs. The two additional channels relate to "extraordinary vessels" – the interior of the spine (governing vessel) and another along the midline of the abdomen (conception vessel).

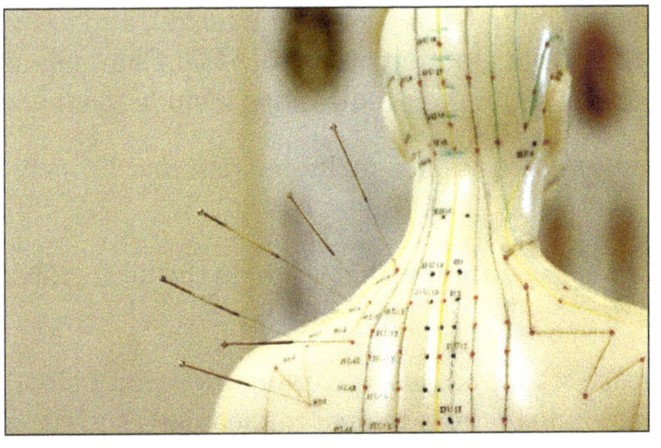

Meridians are like a network and can be compared to the circulatory system in Western medicine; however, meridians are not visible, but rather energetic. Each of the 14 meridian channels has a specific number, and acupuncture points meanings. Those include:

Lung (1); Large intestine (20); Stomach (45); Spleen (21); Heart (9); Small intestine (19); Bladder (67); Kidney (27); Pericardium (9); Triple energizer, an organ recognized in Chinese medicine, but not Western medicine (23); Gallbladder (44); Liver (14); Governing Vessel (28, also known as the sea of yang); and Conception Vessel (24, also known as the sea of yin). Each acupuncture point can treat a multiple list of disorders.

Commonly used points and acupuncture treatments include:

- Stomach Channel (ST36): Located on the front of the leg and below the knee, this point treats digestive disorders, immune deficiency, fatigue and a variety of other illnesses. It is also emotionally and physically grounding.
- Spleen Channel (SP6): Located on the inner side of the leg above the ankle, this point treats hormonal disorders like irregular menstruation, digestion and immune disorders.
- Liver Channel (LV3): Located on the top of the foot and between the second and first toes, this point treats headaches, is used to balance emotional energy, regulate menstruation and reduce high blood pressure.
- Governing Vessel (GV20): Located on top of the head, this point treats vertigo, ear and nasal disorders and various mental disorders.
- Conception Vessel (CV12): Located midway between the breast bone and the navel, this point treats digestive disorders and harmonizes the intestines.

- Conception Vessel (CV6): Located approximately 1.5 inches below the navel, this point treats exhaustion, weak Spleen Qi and the energy of the low abdomen and organs.
- Large Intestine Channel (LI4): Located on the back side of the hand between the thumb and first finger, this point activates the immune system and helps pain, especially in the face.
- Kidney Channel (KI3): Located behind the inner ankle, this point treats asthma, insomnia, sore throat and lower back pain. On the back of the body, there are several acupuncture points along both sides of the spine that connect to the yin organs (solid organs). These acupuncture points are considered to be very powerful in strengthening the heart, liver, lung, kidney and pericardium (sack around the heart), and are very important in Chinese medicine. Many of the points located on the Bladder Channel can treat a variety of conditions. The common points and their indications include the following:
    - BL13: Treats all lung-related issues, including asthma, bronchitis, nasal congestion and sore throat.
    - BL14: This point can help conditions that relate to the pericardium, including palpitations, anxiety and stress, depression and panic attacks.
    - BL15: Treats all heart-related issues, including blood and circulatory problems. It is the main point for all emotional issues related to the heart, such as palpitations, anxiety, fear, stress and poor memory. It can also help with insomnia and night sweats.
    - BL18: Main point for all physical liver conditions, such as hepatitis, jaundice and cirrhosis. It is an important point for relieving emotional issues like depression, anger, irritability and stress.
    - BL21: This point can help alleviate problems associated with the spleen. Some physical spleen issues include distention, abdominal pain, bloating and poor appetite.
    - BL23: This point treats the entire kidney system. It can improve sexual deficiency problems in men, such as impotence, as well as female sexual and reproductive disorders like irregular menstrual cycles and infertility. It is also a main point for lower back pain and sprains, and is useful for ear-related issues like tinnitus and deafness.

Acupressure

In its literal sense - acupressure is acupuncture with no needles. It refers to the practice of applying manual pressure to specific energy points of the body. Acupressure finds its roots in the principle of Chinese medicines that say – human body consists of invisible lines of energy flow called meridians or "qi." It is said that there are at least 14 meridians that connect our organs to other parts of the body. Also, it is believed that acupuncture and acupressure are performed on these meridians.

These meridians begin at your fingertips and connect to the brain and then are connected to organs rather a network of organs – creating a channel of communication. Blocking the flow of energy at any point on a meridian can cause different types of symptoms and health conditions. Acupressure helps to restore the energy balance by applying pressure on specific points along these meridians.

The Difference between Acupressure and Acupuncture

Often people tend to get confused between acupressure and acupuncture. Both use the technique of applying pressure on several points on our body, but the way it is done differs. In the case of acupressure, the pressure is applied manually by a practitioner on several body points. It is usually applied through fingertips, elbows, knuckles, etc. Whereas in acupuncture, the pressure is applied using specially designed needles, which are placed strategically on several pressure points on the body.

How can People take Advantage of Acupressure?

Acupressure can offer an array of benefits to older adults as it helps in releasing endorphins, a hormone produced by our body that assists in relieving several ailments. Its use can prove to be advantageous in many ways such as for:

- Cancer: Apart from relieving nausea caused by chemotherapy, acupressure can also help reduce stress, relieve pain, and improve energy levels.
- Soothing the pain from an injury: By easing muscle tension and improving blood circulation, acupressure can help reduce pain significantly.
- Arthritis: Acupressure helps promote anti-inflammatory effects, which in turn reduce the pain caused by arthritis.
- Improving sleep: It is said that acupressure helps the body to relax and rest, thereby improving sleep quality.
- Reducing digestive issues: Acupressure regulates the flow of energy throughout the body, making sure all systems are working smoothly. It also helps improve the functioning of the digestive system.

Acupressure Precautions

Acupressure, in itself, is pretty safe. If you're planning to opt for acupressure treatment in case of cancer, arthritis, heart disease, or a chronic condition, then you must consult your doctor. Another important thing is to check whether the acupressure practitioner is licensed and certified.

Avoid acupressure if you are:

- Required to undergo treatment for a cancerous tumour or in case cancer has made its way to the bones.
- Suffering from rheumatoid arthritis, a spinal injury, or a bone disease that could worsen if manipulated physically.
- Someone with varicose veins.

Some Facts about Acupressure

- Acupressure is often used as a diagnostic tool. If you press the right point on your hand

and it feels tender or painful, then there's a chance that the organ represented by that point needs repair. Because of this, it is possible to diagnose a condition in the early stages of its onset.

- Acupressure can be cost-free since it can be practiced at home. Moreover, practicing it doesn't need a lot of space either. Therefore, it can prove to be advantageous for people of all ages, and it doesn't consume much time.
- By unblocking several nerve impulses, acupressure reduces stress and tension. Practicing it on a daily basis will help the body recover and relax.
- It is believed that women wear ornaments on specific pressure points on the body. For example, rings and nose pins are worn on locations associated with fertility and the proper functioning of the uterus.

Things to Consider before Buying an Acupressure Product

- Consult your doctor or the acupressure specialist before purchasing any acupressure product. For example, check whether you need a mat or a massager of a particular type.
- Purchase the product from a reliable and trustworthy source - you can even compare the options available and make the right choice.
- Understand your health requirements and check whether the products align with those.
- Try opting for products that can be cleaned quickly and require low maintenance.
- Ensure that the products are slip-free and made of durable material, especially if you're purchasing a mat.
- Make sure that the product you buy doesn't lead to any pain - if it does, you need to consult your doctor right away.

Some of the acupressure products are:

- Health Mat: Health Mat provides relief against aching feet and back. These ergonomically engineered mats absorb shock and promote perfect posture. They also help in reducing fatigue, relieving strain, and preventing the resultant health disorders.

  Features:

  - Water resistance.
  - High resistance to temperature.
  - Pet and child-friendly.
- Acupressure Massager Set for the Whole Body: This massager set identifies the most critical pressure points of the body to provide relief against pain. Using this set will have a therapeutic effect and increase the circulation of blood throughout the body.

Features:

- Stimulates blood circulation.
- Helps relieve muscle pain.
- Helps improve concentration.

- Thermal Belt: This belt is studded with the miraculous stones called Tourmaline. It helps you feel relieved from pain, achieve your weight-loss goals, and provides various other wellness benefits too.

  Features:

  - Makes you feel relaxed.
  - Regulates nervous system.
  - Cell stimulation.

- Island Therapy Acu Roll Massager: This massager set is beneficial for the entire body as it identifies the most important pressure points. It provides relief against stiffness and pain.

  Features:

  - Relaxes muscles and joints.
  - Helps relieve muscle pain.
  - Handcrafted with wood.
  - Helps improve concentration.
  - Helps with cramps, migraines, sinus, insomnia, and stress.

- Acupressure Dot Slippers: These slippers target organs of the body by applying pressure to the energy points related to those organs. They help in curing insomnia, neck pain, back pain, arthritis, lower energy levels, etc. These come in a universal size and fit men and women both.

  Features:

  - Reduces the effects of depression and anxiety.
  - Helps with headaches and migraines.
  - Increases energy levels.
  - Develops a positive mental outlook.
  - Improves digestion, solves eye problems effectively & improves concentration.

Acupressure, if used for the right ailment at the right time, can prove to be very beneficial. You just need to consult a doctor before opting for it. If you don't have any ailments, that shouldn't be a worry – you can view this as a therapy for stress relief and better mental health.

Pressure Points

You can use pressure points for good or evil. Practitioners of some martial arts exploit the body's most vulnerable pressure points by striking them during battle. Hitting certain points with force can knock a person out or make someone stop and gasp for air.

For healing purposes, practitioners apply pressure to points near an afflicted area. For instance, pressure on many points on the head is helpful for ailments of the mind, like anxiety. Other times, the most useful points, called distal points, are on the opposite end of the meridian or opposite part of the body from the area of pain or discomfort. Stimulating these points opens the entire channel of energy.

Don't expect the average medical doctor or insurance company to endorse acupressure anytime soon. The metrics of Western medicine — clinical trials — are dull tools for measuring energetic nuance. But that doesn't mean it's not effective, especially for people with tough-to-treat conditions such as fibromyalgia, chronic fatigue, and addiction recovery.

Acupressure is safe for almost everyone, and basic techniques are easy to learn. Whether you are looking for a basic tune-up or hoping for something more give it a try.

Top Ten Acupressure Points

You could spend years memorizing the location of the body's hundreds of acupoints, but some are considered power players. Many lie at the crossroads of more than one meridian and, therefore, are believed to have widespread benefits across multiple organ systems. Each point has an assigned letter and number combination that corresponds to its location on the body (a standard referencing system used by professional acupressurists and acupuncturists), as well as a more poetic name, derived from its Chinese character and offering insight into the point's location or benefit.

Acupressure Points for Arm Pain and Digestion

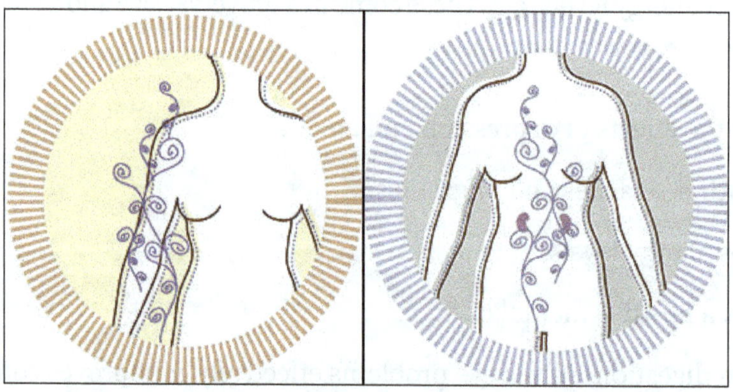

Pool at the Crook (Li 11): As its name suggests, this point is in the crook of the elbow. Hold your left arm in front of you at a 90-degree angle, as if it was in a sling. Turn the left palm up. Place your right thumb at the outside end of the elbow crease. Press firmly. Switch arms.

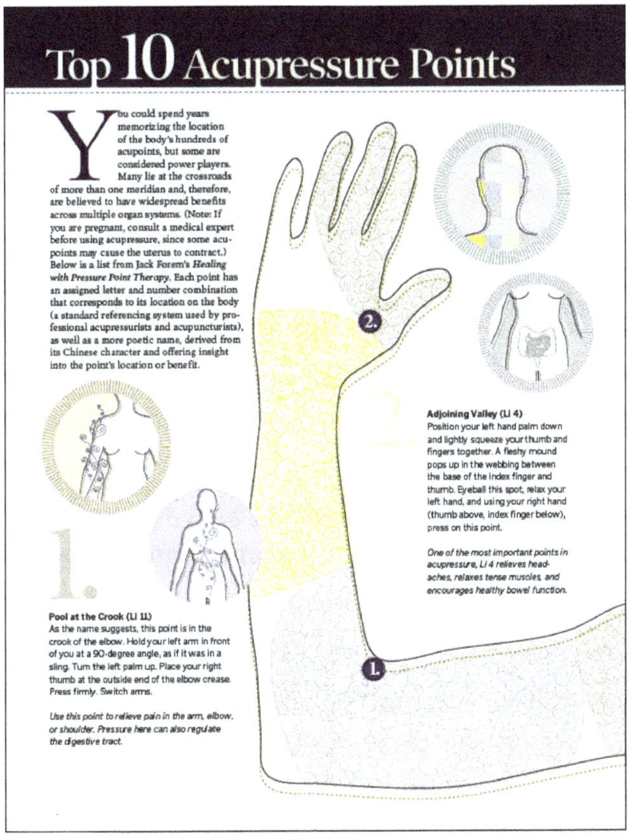

Top 10 Acupressure Points

You could spend years memorizing the location of the body's hundreds of acupoints, but some are considered power players. Many lie at the crossroads of more than one meridian and, therefore, are believed to have widespread benefits across multiple organ systems. (Note: If you are pregnant, consult a medical expert before using acupressure, since some acupoints may cause the uterus to contract.) Below is a list from Jack Forem's *Healing with Pressure Point Therapy*. Each point has an assigned letter and number combination that corresponds to its location on the body (a standard referencing system used by professional acupressurists and acupuncturists), as well as a more poetic name, derived from its Chinese character and offering insight into the point's location or benefit.

1.

Pool at the Crook (Li 11)
As the name suggests, this point is in the crook of the elbow. Hold your left arm in front of you at a 90-degree angle, as if it was in a sling. Turn the left palm up. Place your right thumb at the outside end of the elbow crease. Press firmly. Switch arms.

Use this point to relieve pain in the arm, elbow, or shoulder. Pressure here can also regulate the digestive tract.

2.

Adjoining Valley (Li 4)
Position your left hand palm down and lightly squeeze your thumb and fingers together. A fleshy mound pops up in the webbing between the base of the index finger and thumb. Eyeball this spot, relax your left hand, and using your right hand (thumb above, index finger below), press on this point.

One of the most important points in acupressure, Li 4 relieves headaches, relaxes tense muscles, and encourages healthy bowel function.

Acupressure Points for Headache, Muscles and Bowel Movements

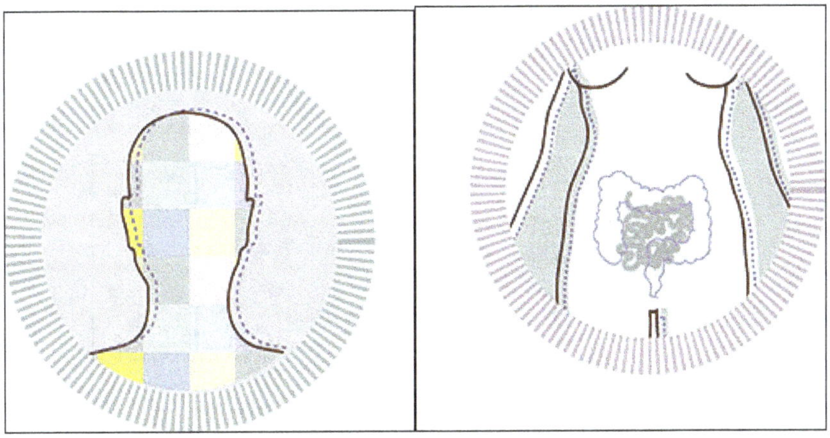

Figure: One of the most important points in acupressure, Li 4 relieves headaches, relaxes tense muscles, and encourages healthy bowel function.

Adjoining Valley (Li 4): Position your left hand palm down and lightly squeeze your thumb and fingers together. A fleshy mound pops up in the webbing between the base of the index finger and thumb. Eyeball this spot, relax your left hand and using your right hand (thumb above, index finger below), and press on this point.

Acupressure Points for Skin Problems

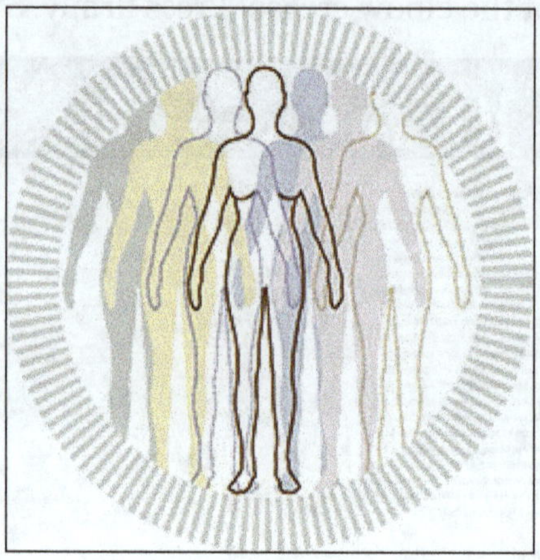

Figure: These points cleanse the blood and nourish the skin.

Sea of Blood (Sp 10): To find these two points, sit in a chair with your feet flat on the floor. Feel for a bulge in your thigh muscles about two thumb widths above the top edge of your knee. The bulge is on the top inside portion of the leg. Press on the points firmly with your thumbs or the knuckle of your middle finger.

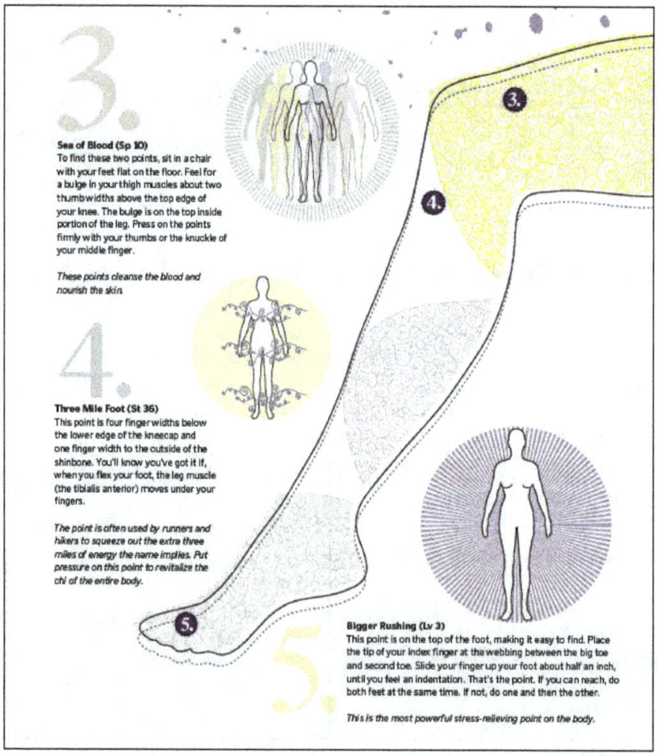

Acupressure Points for Energy

Three Mile Foot (St 36): This point is four finger widths below the lower edge of the kneecap and one finger width to the outside of the shinbone. You'll know you've got it if, when you flex your foot, the leg muscle (the tibialis anterior) moves under your fingers.

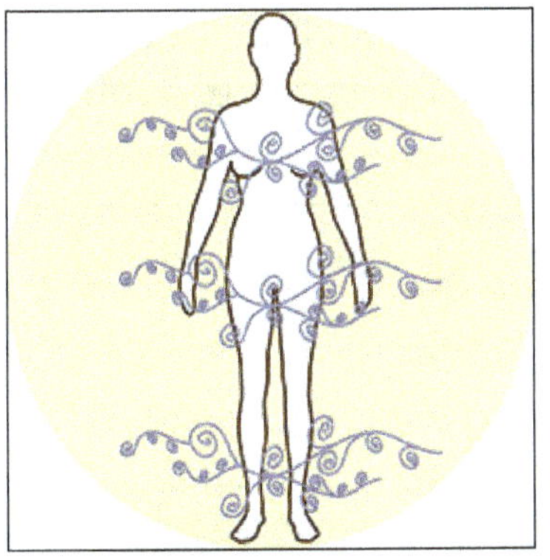

Figure: The point is often used by runners and hikers to squeeze out the extra three miles of energy the name implies. Put pressure on this point to revitalize the chi of the entire body.

Acupressure Points to Relieve Stress

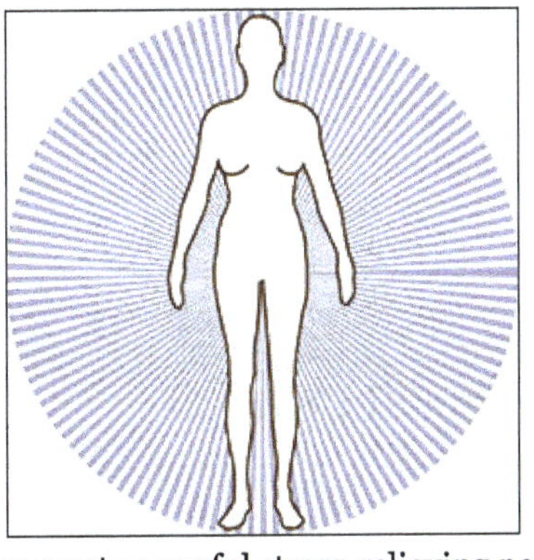

Figure: This is the most powerful stress-relieving point on the body.

Bigger Rushing (Lv 3): This point is on the top of the foot, making it easy to find. Place the tip of your index finger at the webbing between the big toe and second toe. Slide your finger up your foot about half an inch, until you feel an indentation. That's the point. If you can reach, do both feet at the same time. If not, do one and then the other.

Acupressure Points for Sinus Congestion

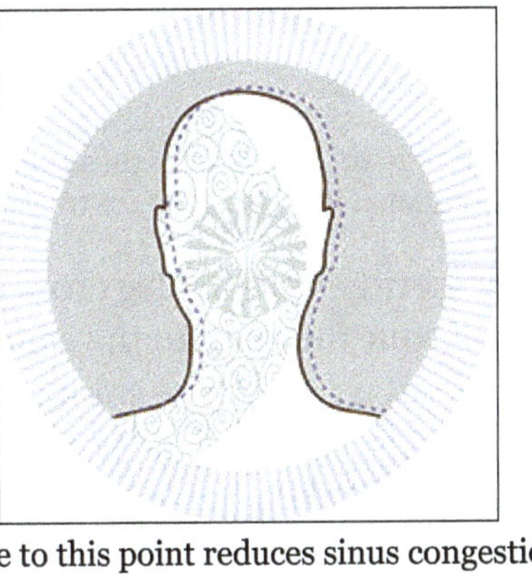

Figure: Applying pressure to this point reduces sinus congestion and mucus buildup.

Abundant Splendor (St 40): A bit hard to find, this point is worth the hunt. It lies on the outside of the leg, halfway between the anklebone and the center of the kneecap. Take a seat. Wrap your fingers around the back of the shin at the middle of the leg. Using your thumb, press into the shinbone (tibia), and then slide your thumb two inches or so off the bone toward the outside of the leg. Press firmly.

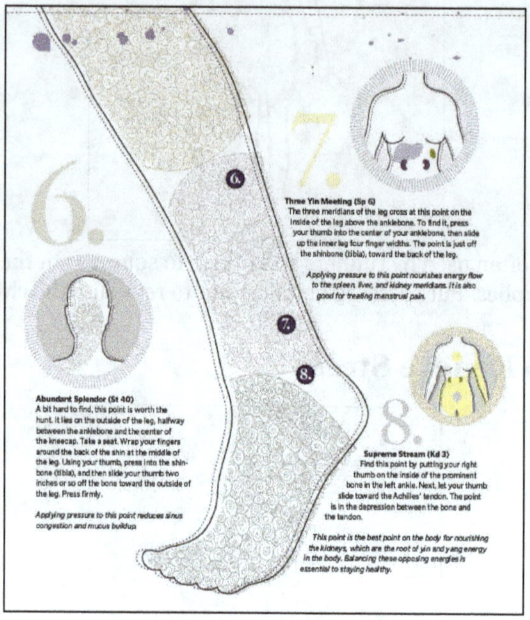

Acupressure Points for Menstrual Cramps

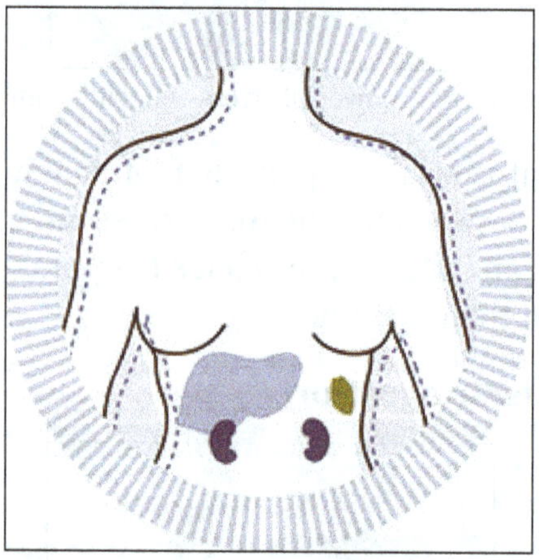

Figure: Applying pressure to this point nourishes energy flow to the spleen, liver, and kidney meridians. It is also good for treating menstrual pain.

Three Yin Meeting (Sp 6): The three meridians of the leg cross at this point on the inside of the leg above the anklebone. To find it, press your thumb into the center of your anklebone, then slide up the inner leg four finger widths. The point is just off the shinbone (tibia), toward the back of the leg.

Acupressure Points for Kidney Health

Supreme Stream (Kd 3): Find this point by putting your right thumb on the inside of the prominent bone in the left ankle. Next, let your thumb slide toward the Achilles' tendon. The point is in the depression between the bone and the tendon.

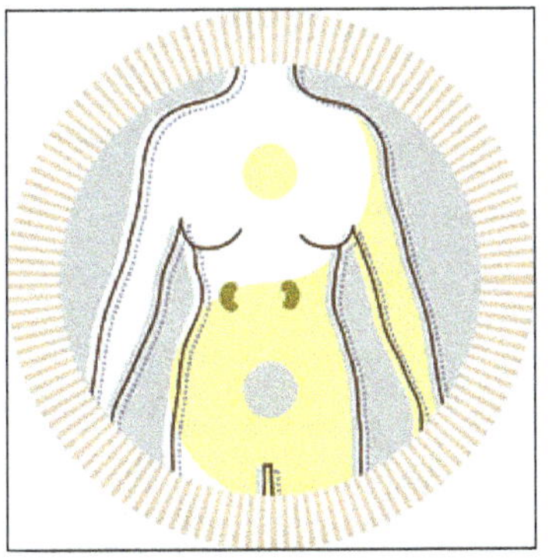

Figure: This point is the best point on the body for nourishing the kidneys, which are the root of yin and yang energy in the body. Balancing these opposing energies is essential to staying healthy.

Acupressure Points for Migraines, Colds and Neck Stiffness

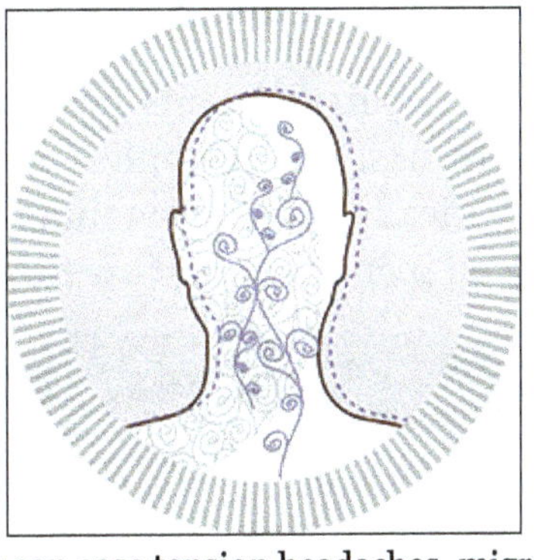

Figure: Pressure to these points can ease tension headaches, migraines, colds, and neck stiffness.

Wind Pool (Gb 20): Corresponding with the gall bladder meridian, these two points are found along the ridge of the occipital bone. Place your thumbs on the base of your skull near the hairline. Slide your thumbs along the bony ridge of the base of your skull until each thumb is midway between the spine and the ear. The points lie there, between the two neck muscles that come together where the neck meets the skull.

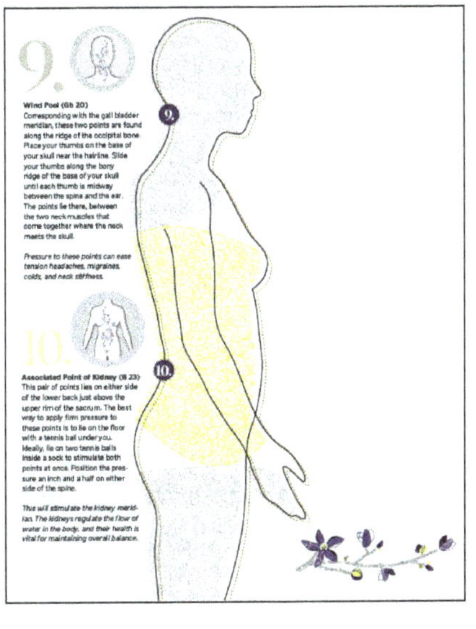

Acupressure Points to Stimulate the Kidney Meridian

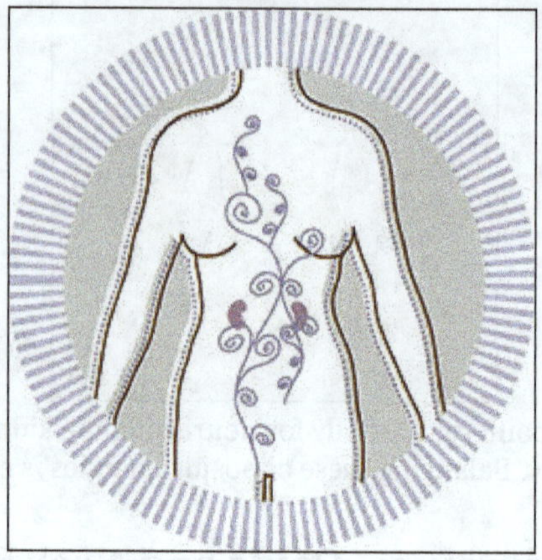

Figure: This will stimulate the kidney meridian. The kidneys regulate the flow of water in the body, and their health is vital for maintaining overall balance.

Associated Point of Kidney (B 23): This pair of points lies on either side of the lower back just above the upper rim of the sacrum. The best way to apply firm pressure to these points is to lie on the floor with a tennis ball under you. Ideally, lie on two tennis balls inside a sock to stimulate both points at once. Position the pressure an inch and a half on either side of the spine.

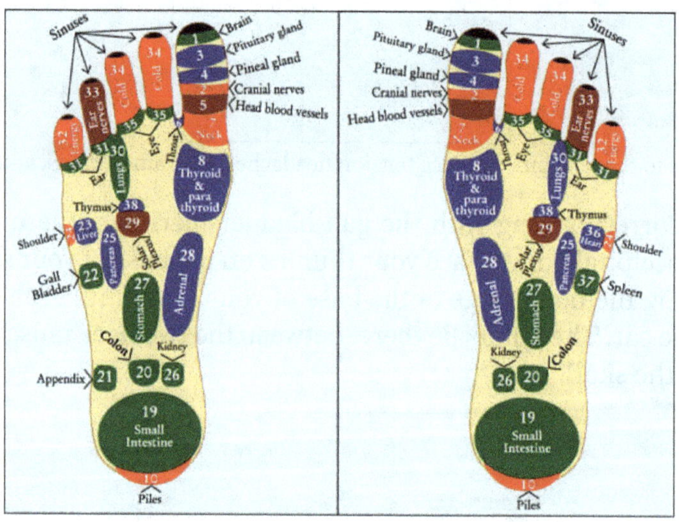

Apitherapy

Honey

Mature honeybees collect nectar from plant blossoms. Nectar is 80 to 95 per cent water and 5 to 20 per cent sucrose (table sugar). As the bee transports the nectar back to the hive, a protein enzyme in her honey stomach, called invertase, breaks the sucrose down into the two simple sugars, fructose and glucose.

Young bees remove water from the sugar solution using two methods. They pass the nectar from bee to bee and 'drink' the water out of the nectar by absorbing it through their stomach wall. They also create heat and air flow in the hive by vibrating their wings and flight muscles, thus evaporating water out of the nectar which has been stored in open cells.

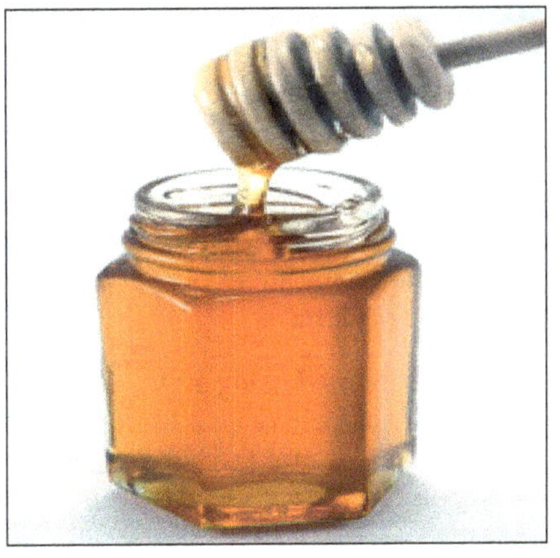

When most of the sucrose has been converted to fructose and glucose AND enough water has been dehydrated out of the mixture to bring it approximately 17.8% water content, we have a delicious sticky mixture, called honey. After honey is made, bees cap it with beeswax to maintain the low moisture content.

Honey Processing

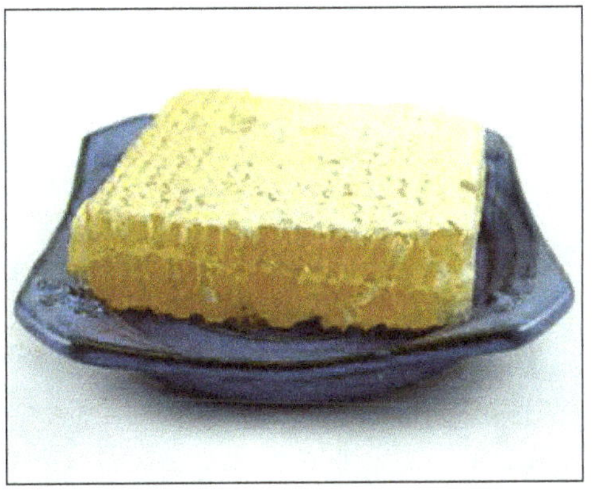

Many years ago, beekeepers crushed honeycomb to get liquid honey! That method of honey processing produces less honey for the beekeeper as it forces bees to spend time and resources building replacement comb rather than making more honey. Honeybees consume 7 kilograms of honey to produce 1 kilogram of beeswax. The advent of the centrifugal extractor, allowed beekeepers to 'scratch' or 'slice' off a thin layer of wax from the surface of the comb and spin the honey out using centrifugal force. The integrity of the comb is maintained and the bees have far less work to do to repair any cracks or shallow spots in the comb.

Whole honeycomb is available for people who want to enjoy honey completely untouched by human hands. They cut off a bite size portion of wax and chew the honey out of it. Wax will dissolve if chewed for about 15 minutes, but most people discard chewed wax like they would gum.

The vast majority of people prefer liquid honey, so extractors are used to remove honey from the comb. Freshly extracted honey contains bits of wax and the odd bee knee or elbow. Honey may be cleaned by allowing it to settle in a holding tank for a day or two, or by pumping it through a filter.

What is the Best Type of Honey?

Honeycomb	Untouched by human hands. Contains all the goodness that nature has put into the honey. Bit awkward to chew.
Raw Honey	Extracted and cleaned using a settling tank at room temperature. Contains virtually all the goodness that nature put into the honey. Will granulate quickly and may separate in the jar with liquid fructose on top and granular glucose on the bottom.
Liquid Honey - Filtered with minimal heat	Extracted and cleaned using a 50 micron filter. Honey is heated to the same temperature inside a hive on a hot day. Contains a great deal of the goodness that nature put into the honey. Will granulate in two to six months, depending on the type of flowers the bees visited to gather the honey.
Creamed Honey	Creamed honey is made from pure liquid honey through a controlled crystallization process to produce very fine uniform crystals, thus resulting in a creamy smooth consistency. Creamed honey has nothing added and has the same nutritional value as its liquid counterpart.
Liquid Pasteurized Honey	Extracted and cleaned using flash heating to a high temperature, super filtered through a 1 to 5 micron filter, and quickly cooled. Looses much of the goodness that nature provided, but will last over 9 months on the store shelf without granulating.

Varieties of Honey

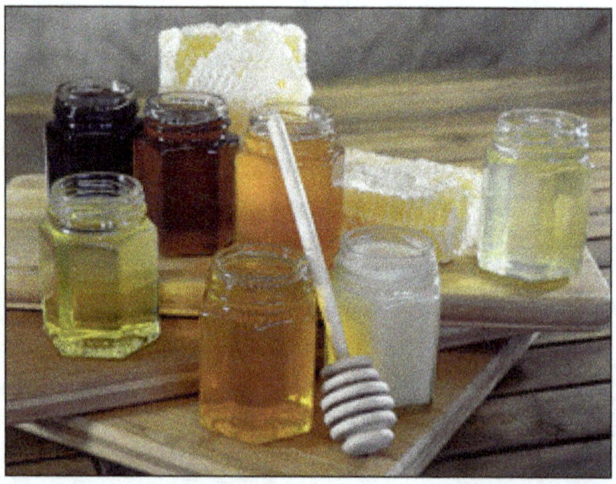

The flavour, colour, texture, and aroma of honey depends on which plants the bees gathered nectar from. Blueberry blossom honey is made with the nectar from blueberry blossoms, is dark amber in colour, and has a brown sugar after taste. Raspberry blossom honey is extra light in colour with a slight fruity taste, and buckwheat honey is almost black in colour with a heady, pungent odour and flavour. Generally, a dark honey will have a higher nutritional content than a light honey.

There are hundreds of flowering plants in the world that produce nectar, thus providing the potential to have hundreds of types of honey. Wild flower honey represents a blend of flowering plants and varies in colour and flavour depending on region and season.

The Nutritional Value of Honey

Average Composition of Honey

Honey is primarily fructose (38%), glucose (31%), water (17%), maltose (7%), and small amounts of trisaccharides, other higher carbohydrates, sucrose, minerals, vitamins, and enzymes.

- Vitamins - trace amounts: Thiamin, Riboflavin, Niacin, Pantothenic acid, Vitamin B-6, Vitamin B-12, Folate, Vitamin C, Vitamin A, Vitamin D, Vitamin E, Vitamin K.
- Minerals - trace amounts: Calcium, Copper, Iron, Magnesium. Manganese, Phosphorous, Potassium, Sodium, Zinc.
- Antioxidants - enzymatic and non-enzymatic: Catalase, ascorbic acid, flavonoids.

Standard Nutritional Information

Nutritional Facts (per 20 g serving)		
Label	Amount	Daily Value
Calories	60	
Fat/Lipides	0 g	0 %
Carbohydrates/Glucides Sugars	17 g 16 g	6 %
Protein	0 g	0 %

Honey Crystallization

Crystallization is the formation of monohydrate glucose crystals from a super-saturated sugar solution (i.e. honey). The rate of crystallization increases with:

- Lower water content.
- Higher glucose content.
- Presence of solid particles (i.e. pollen grains & honey crystals).
- Temperature close to 14° C (Temperatures above 28° C and below 5° C result in very slow crystallization).
- Stirring.

The slower crystallization produces larger and more irregular crystals. Crystallization of honey is completely normal and does not damage the honey. In most cases the crystallization process can be reversed by gently warming the honey to "melt" the crystals.

How to Decrystalize Honey

Honey that has started to crystallize, characterized by glucose crystals forming on the bottom of the container, can be easily melted. Simply put the honey container (with the lid on) into a warm water bath on the stove at approximately 45 C for a couple hours, or as necessary. Stirring the honey, or turning the container upside down occasionally to break up the crystals, will speed the process.

Storing Honey

Honey is a very robust food product, and if stored properly, will last years if not decades. In fact, honey has been found perfectly preserved in tombs of the Pharaohs in Egypt.

The quality of honey may be damaged by the following factors:

Excessive moisture	Ideally the moisture content of honey should be less than 17.8%. If the moisture content is too high, say greater than 20%, the honey may ferment due to yeasts in the honey. Since honey is hygroscopic, if it is not in a sealed container, it will attract moisture from the air.
Excessive heat	Honey loses many of its' health benefits with the combination of heat and time. The following is a rule of thumb storage time vs. temperature to retain most of its' health benefits: • 4 °C for 30 days. • 3 °C for 6 months. • 2 °C for 4 years. • 1 °C for 35 years.
Prolonged exposure to sunlight	Honey loses many of its health benefits with prolonged exposure to sunlight.
Noxious elements in its environment	Honey is hygroscopic and takes on odours from its environment. It is also acidic, so it can dissolve metal if stored in metal containers.

Honey Storage Guidelines

- Store honey in a sealed non-metallic container.
- For normal use, store the container in a cupboard (away from direct sunlight) at room temperature (21 °C).
- For prolonged storage of honey (> 4 years), store at refrigerator temperature (4 °C).

Honey and Infants

The bacterium, Clostridium botulinum is very common in nature and any raw food, including honey, may contain Clostridium botulinum spores.

A fully developed digestive system will protect a person against ingested C. botulinum. However, the digestive system of an infant under the age of 12 months is not fully developed, and thus cannot deal with many kinds of antigens, including C. botulinum. The toxins produced by C. botulinum are extremely dangerous and present a very serious condition for infants.

Honey is a raw food and is not recommended for infants less than 12 months of age. It is extremely rare to find C. botulinum in honey, but there have been a hand full of documented cases over the last 40 years. In these cases it is thought that the bacteria came in contact with the honey somewhere during honey processing.

Due to honey's bacteriostatic properties, bacteria, including C. botulinum, will not grow nor produce toxins in honey. C. botulinum spores are very resilient and can withstand harsh conditions, including the honey pasteurization process. If an infant were to ingest honey that was contaminated with C. botulinum spores, the honey would become diluted in the infant's intestinal tract, and the spores would have suitable conditions to be activated, thus providing the conditions for botulism. The honey pasteurization process does not destroy C. botulinum spores in honey.

Health and Healing with Honey

For thousands of years, the unique antimicrobial and antioxidant properties of honey have been valuable for healing cuts, scapes, burns, and even open wounds.

Apitherapy is the use of honeybee produced substances for health and healing.

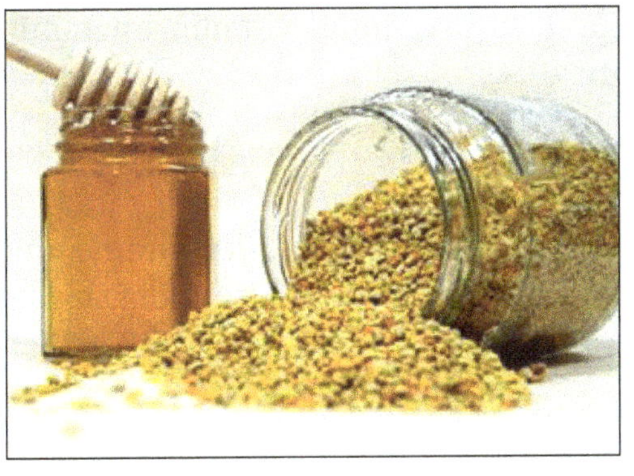

Honeybees produce honey, pollen, propolis, royal jelly, and beeswax, all of which are used by people for nutrition, immune system support, and treatment of a variety of ailments, skin care, and healing of open wounds. Even bee venom is used to treat many chronic conditions.

Honeybee Produced Substances used for Apitherapy

Bee Pollen

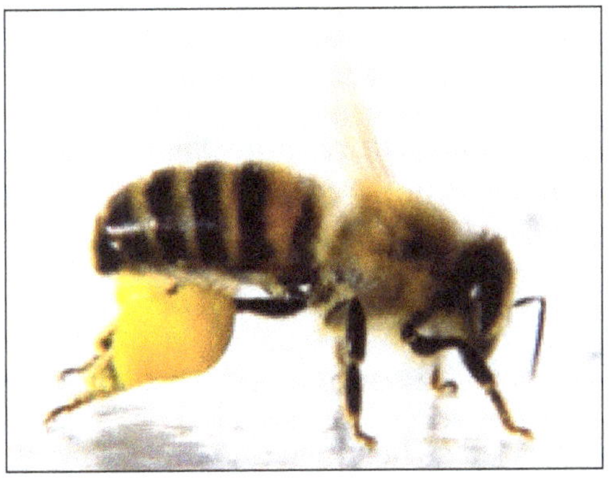

Bee Pollen is the male reproductive material of plants used by bees to feed their larvae. Pollen is the honeybee's exclusive source of protein, containing all the essential amino acids that people require. People use bee pollen as a multi-vitamin, energy booster, and/or to build up their resistance to air-borne (hay fever type) allergens.

Propolis

Propolis is a combination of beeswax, honey, and tree resins mixed with bee-produced enzymes, used to protect the bee hive from bacteria, fungus, and viruses. Propolis has natural anti-bacterial, anti-viral, anti-fungal, anti-oxidant, and anti-inflammatory properties. People use propolis as a remedy for colds & influenza, and to boost the immune system. The antibacterial and anti-fungal properties of propolis make it an ideal topical ingredient for treating various skin conditions.

Royal Jelly

Royal Jelly is an enzyme enriched food, produced by young worker bees and fed to a queen bee for her entire life. People use royal jelly as a multi-vitamin, an immune system booster to promote longevity, and for mental clarity.

Honey

Honey is plant nectar, converted to simple sugars, dehydrated, and used for energy and winter food. People use honey as a natural sweetener, as a sore throat remedy, cough suppressant, and for healing wounds.

Bee Venom

Bee Venom is produced by worker female bees to defend themselves and their colony. People use bee venom to treat over 40 illnesses, including warts, arthritis and multiple sclerosis.

Beeswax

Beeswax is produced by worker female bees for building the honeycomb structure that is used for brood rearing and storing of honey & pollen. People use beeswax for a number of items including candles, cosmetics, and furniture polishes.

Health and Nutrition

Bee Nutraceutical products are pure and natural honeybee products used as dietary supplements to promote good health. The products produced by the honeybee are Royal Jelly, Pollen, Propolis, and Honey. These products may be taken separately in their native form or mixed into blends to provide the right balance in an easy to take mixture.

Natural Body Care

Honey, beeswax, and propolis are used as healing and pampering agents in a number of body care products including soap, lip balm, cremes, salves and lotions.

Honey in Wound Care

Honey has been used in treating open wounds for centuries. Until the development of antibiotics in the mid-1900s, honey was the primary treatment for wounds on the battlefield. For the next 50 years, the use of honey in wound care, especially in western countries, lost favour. However, in the past 20 years there has been renewed interest in using honey, driven in large part by the concern of the rapid development of antibiotic resistant strains of bacteria.

There has been a large number of peer reviewed scientific studies that have shown the efficacy of using honey, particularly manuka honey, in the treatment of severe chronic wounds such as diabetic foot ulcers. Honey can be used to treat open wounds, burns, and skin ulcers. Results from studies have shown that honey used on open wounds has the following results:

- Inflammation, swelling and pain are quickly reduced.
- Unpleasant odours cease.
- Wound dressings can be changed painlessly with no damage to re-growing tissue.
- Minimal scarring occurs.

Honey has been shown to prevent the growth of wound bacteria and to protect the wound from getting infected. Honey also provides a moist, nutrient rich environment that actually assists the natural healing process of the body.

Anti-Microbial Properties of Honey

Unlike antibiotics that have a single mode of action against bacteria, honey has multiple modes of action that attack bacteria in different ways:

Anti-Microbial Properties of Honey	
Mode	Description
Osmotic Effect	Honey is over 80% sugar and leaves few water molecules available for micro-organisms.
Acidity	The pH level for honey is between 3.2 and 4.5, which is inhospitable for most wound bacteria that can tolerate a minimum pH level of approximately 4.0 to 4.5.
Hydrogen Peroxide	Honey contains glucose oxidase, an enzyme which facilitates a reaction that produces a slow release of hydrogen peroxide. The low levels of hydrogen peroxide produced are sufficient to kill bacteria without damaging tissue.
Phytochemical Factors	Some honey contains other plant chemicals with anti-microbial properties. These are not available in all types of honey. The best known, and most widely researched honey with phytochemical anti-microbial properties, is manuka honey.

Honey has been shown to be effective against species of bacteria most commonly involved in wound infection. This includes several studies showing honey being effective against "super bugs" such as Methicillin-resistant-Staphylococcus aureus (MSRA) and Vancomycin-resistant-Enterococci (VRE).

Not all Honeys are Equal

All honey has anti-microbial properties. However, the anti-microbial activity can range up to 100 times, i.e. one honey may be up to 100 times more effective than another honey. Different honeys also have differing anti-microbial activities against various strains of wound bacteria.

Manuka Honey

Manuka honey is produced from nectar from the manuka bush (Leptospermum scoparium), a member of the tea tree family, native to New Zealand. Manuka honey is known for its highly active antibacterial properties, far beyond those of normal honeys.

The special antibacterial properties of manuka honey, also referred to as the Unique Manuka Factor (UMF), are due to phytochemicals in the manuka nectar. The UMF activity of manuka honey is highly stable compared to the hydrogen peroxide antibacterial mode, which deteriorates with high temperatures and over the span of 6-12 months.

Manuka honey is clearly the honey of choice in modern honey wound care dressings. It is recommended that only medical grade honey is used in the care of open wounds, as the honey has been sterilized to ensure that it contains no active pathogens.

Manuka honey is also widely used to assist in the treatment of gastrointestinal problems, such as peptic ulcers. The belief is that the UMF antibacterial activity of the manuka honey works against harmful bacteria in the digestive tract. Anecdotal evidence appears to support this theory but peer reviewed scientific evidence is still lacking.

Bee Venom Therapy

Bee Venom Therapy (BVT) is the use of bee venom to treat human and animal disorders using a live bee or bee venom injection. BVT is used to treat people, horses, dogs, and cats. Over 40 different illnesses are treated with BVT including arthritis and multiple sclerosis.

BVT practitioners need to be careful because bee venom is histamine (poison) and it may cause a person to have an allergic reaction, which may vary from slight reddening of the skin to a life threatening situation with difficulty breathing.

Before a person starts with a BVT treatment schedule, he/she should conduct thorough research, consult a physician, and have an EpiPen nearby.

BVT is not for everyone. It is sometimes difficult to obtain bees and a treatment is painful.

The old fashioned method of applying a bee sting caused the bee to die. New methods consist of stinging through a stainless steel micro mesh, which allows the venom to enter the skin but prevents the stinger barb from attaching. Thus, the bee is not harmed and her venom regenerates within one or two days.

Immune System Dysfunction or Problems	Genital Apparatus Diseases (Gynecology)	Skin Diseases (Dermatology)
Multiple Sclerosis (Ms)		Acne
Arthritis	Cervix Erosions	Bedsores
Hay Fever	Hypofoliculinic Dysfunctional Syndromes	Breast Skin Sores
Neurologic Problems	Irregular Periods	Bruises ("Blue" Skin After Contusion)
Als (Lou Gehrig's Disease)	Leucorrhoea	Burns And Scalds

- Multiple Sclerosis (Ms)
    - Shingles
    - Scar Pain
- Musculoskeletal Problems
    - Arthritis
    - Gout
    - Tendonitis, Bursitis
    - Spinal Pain
- Infectious Problems
    - Bacterial, Viral, And Fungal Illnesses
    - Lyme Disease
- Traumas
    - Wounds, Acute And Chronic
    - Burns
    - Sprains
    - Fractures
- Tumors
    - Benign
    - Malignant (Cancer)
- Allergies (Allergology)
    - Bv Allergy
    - Bee Pollen Allergy
    - Hay Fever
    - Ragweed Polinosis
- Cardiovascular Diseases (Cardiology)
    - Acute Rheumatic Carditis
    - Angina Pectoris
    - Arrhythmias
    - Artheritis Obliterans
    - Artheriosclerosis
    - Atherosclerosis
    - Menstrual Cramps
    - Menstrual Cramps
    - Mood Swings
    - Premenstrual Syndrome (Pms)
    - Sexual Dynamic Weakness
    - Trichomonas Vaginalis
    - Vaginal Sores (Post-Surgical)
    - Vaginitis
    - Vegetations
    - Wounds (Hardly Healing) After Gynecological Surgical Operations
- Immune System Diseases (Immunology)
    - Aids
    - B-Cell Enhancement
    - Multiple Sclerosis (Ms)
    - Systemic Lupus Erithematosus
    - T-Cell Suppression
- Kidney Diseases (Nephrology)
    - Chronically Kidney Insufficiency
    - Kidney Diseases (Non-Specific)
- Mental Diseases (Psychiatry)
    - Alcohol Addiction
    - Oligophrenia
    - Schizophrenia
- Musculoskeletal System Diseases (Rheumatology, Myology, Osteology)
    - Acute And Chronic Bursitis
    - Ankylotic Spondyilarthritis
    - Ankylotic Spondylitis Deformans
- Canker Diseases
- Chronic Furuncles
- Decubitus Ulcer
- Degranulated Wounds
- Eczema
- Epidermophyses
- Erysipelas
- Folliculites
- Furunculosis
- Hair Loss
- High Sensitiveness
- Hydradenites
- Hyperkeratosis
- Infected Skin Lesions
- Intertrigo (Infants)
- Low Sensitiveness
- Lupus Erythematosus
- Melanoma
- Moles
- Mycosis Fungoides
- Neurodermitis
- Parasitory Sicosis
- Psoriasis
- Pyodermites
- Radiodermatitis
- Scars
- Scleroderma
- Seborrheic Dermatitis
- Shank (Calf) Chronic Ulcers
- Skin Tuberculosis (Adjutant)
- Spots Alopecia
- Total Alopecia
- Topical Ulcers

Atherosclerotic Arteritis Of The Inferior Limbs	Arthritis	Tricophysis
Capillary Fragility	Arthrosis	Trophic Ulcers
Cardiac Diseases (Non-Specific)	Fibrositis	Varicose Ulcer
Cerebral Atherosclerosis		Warts
Cerebral Trombosis		Wounds
Coronary Heart		Zona-Zoster
		Sexual Diseases (Sexology)
		Benign Prostatic Hypertrophy
		Chronic Prostatitis
		Insufficiency Of Sexual Hormones.

Hydrotherapy

Hydrotherapy, earlier called the hydropathy, is defined as the use of water to treat a medical condition or to maintain the general health. The therapy belongs to conventional medicine as well as alternative medicine. It is said to be used in naturopathy, physiotherapy, and occupational therapy. The treatment involves the therapeutic use of water to provide healing effects.

Many prefer hydrotherapy or Aqua therapy as it is a natural way of treatment and the results are approving. Water has many properties that aid in providing relief. It improves blood flow and has a soothing, calming, and relaxing effect on the patient. Certain postures when done in water are easier to do and provide immense relief to painful joints. The increase in buoyancy allows for more degrees of activity and hence exercises done in water are more effective than when done on land. Different temperature conditions inside the water also play a role in this therapy. The increase in temperature and hydrostatic pressure increases blood circulation and the body's flexibility and decreases swelling.

Hydrotherapy differs from swimming because this constitutes specific postures and exercises and is commonly administered in a hot water pool. The water temperature of such a pool is usually maintained between 33-36 °C. which is warmer than a typical swimming pool.

Types of Hydrotherapy Treatment

Types of hydrotherapy include:

- The Kneipp system: In this system both hot and cold water is used. This involves methods like snow walking, dew walking, and water-treading. The Kneipp system helps in building the immune system of the body also increases the physiological response in the individuals.
- Sitz bath: There is a use of both hot and cold water simultaneously and people are given adjacent bath one with cold and one with warm water. This bath helps in relaxing the body by sitting alternative in both the baths.

- The Baleno therapy: This helps in healing the conditions like arthritis, skin allergies and fibromyalgia. This bath is given using both hot and cold water but particularly hot water springs and natural spas are used. The bath includes minerals like sulfur, silica, radium thus benefiting the treatment.
- The hydro massage technique: In this hot water is used for the therapy so as to inculcate thermal and mechanical massage. This therapy is very useful and boosts the blood circulation on the body, helps in relieving the pain and tension of the joints and knots.
- Steam, sauna and compresses: In these techniques hot or warm water is used for the healing treatment. Steam treatment is done by boiling the water beyond the boiling point which then vaporizes to form steam and detoxifies the body. Sauna treatment is done with dry heat and it detoxifies the body and also relieves the pain. Compress treatment is done with the towels in which the towels are dipped in very hot or very cold water and then placed on the painful body part to bring relief.

How does Aqua Therapy Work?

Hydrotherapy primarily includes anything from floating in the water and directly benefiting from the increased temperature and relaxation properties to highly intense exercise sessions. The form of hydrotherapy used will depend entirely on the conditions of the individual undergoing treatment. Many land-based exercises can be therapeutically used in the water. Walking in a pool is easy on the joints due to the buoyancy. Some state-of-the-art facilities may even have underwater treadmills! Other exercises such as squats and lunges can also be done inside the pool.

One method of hydrotherapy is also known as the Bad Ragaz Ring Method. It is a form of muscle re-education where the patient is kept afloat and specific patterns of resistance, endurance, elongation, relaxation, a range of motion, and tonal reduction techniques are applied. All the exercises are progressed by increasing the speed of the movement or the turbulence of the water. Other methods of increasing difficulty include increasing surface area. This can be achieved for example by holding something wide in hand when moving it through the water.

The buoyancy of the water acts as either a tool to assist movement or to increase the difficulty of an exercise. For example, when using the shoulder, the water can be used to help in lifting the arm upwards from by the side. Also, the water will provide some resistance against pushing the arm back down. This resistance can be increased further by attaching a float to the arm.

Who would see a Hydrotherapist?

Hydrotherapy is used in many illnesses and medical conditions. It is effective in most cases of arthritis and rheumatic illness. It is also advised to asthma patients and a range of problems such as cold, depression, stomach problems, nerve problems, headaches, and sleep disorders. It is also used by many to maintain overall health.

The treatment is most effective for Stage-1 patients. In the case of higher severity of illness, it is used along with other treatments. Statistics says that hydrotherapy has a very high success rate when it is used for a prolonged time. It shows satisfying results in most cases. However, the severity assessment is the primary criteria for the effectiveness of the treatment.

Who is not Eligible for the Treatment?

Hydrotherapy is advisable to everyone, however, under certain circumstances, hydrotherapy is not recommended. The therapy is not recommended for persons with:

- Acute injuries with redness still visible on the injury.
- High temperature.
- Heart disease - Increased blood flow may put stress on the heart.
- Hypertension - Increased blood flow may place stress on the heart.
- Vascular conditions - Extensive circulation is not advised in such a situation.
- Kidney problems.
- Cancer.
- Haemorrhage.

What are the Side Effects of Aqua Therapy Treatment?

Hydrotherapy is safe if it is administered correctly. Several people may react differently to the extent and magnitude of treatment. Some people may have headaches, aches and pains, sleep problems, nausea, chilliness, and faintness. It is important to discuss the physical condition and medical history with the doctor or physical therapist before trying hydrotherapy.

Always tell the doctor if an alternative therapy is already on. It is not safe to forgo conventional medical treatment and rely only on an alternative treatment. Invasive hydrotherapy techniques like enemas, douching, and colonic irrigation is not well accepted by medicinal science because these internal cleansing methods can cause damage to an individual by interfering with the natural balance of the digestive tract.

Hydrotherapy often puts on a risk of allergic reaction known as "contact dermatitis" for some patients using essential herbs and oils in their bath water. Overheating is one of the most common side effects of hydrotherapy, which can be very harmful. This may occur when an individual spends too much time in a hot tub or pool.

What are the Post-treatment Guidelines?

There is no specific post-treatment instruction after undergoing hydrotherapy. Though it should be kept in mind that to maintain the patient at ease for a few hours after the treatment. Laborious works should not be undertaken. It should also be borne in mind that the patient is kept warm after the treatment or else there arise chances of catching a cold.

How much Time does it take for the Recovery?

There is no fixed recovery time for this treatment. The individual can walk out if he or she feels comfortable in doing so. Though, it depends on the practitioner who accesses the conditions of a severity of the ailments and decides the recovery time.

Benefits of Hydrotherapy

These are the benefits of hydrotherapy:

- Boosts the immune system: Hydrotherapy helps in the increases in the flow of blood in the body and there is also increased circulation of white blood cells around the body which helps the lymph to move around the body efficiently thus making the immune system strong. It also helps in fighting sickness and cold.
- Rehabilitation of injured muscles: Warm or hot water helps to raise the temperature of the body which increases the flow of blood around the circulatory system thus helps in elevating any kind of pain present in the damaged muscles or joints.
- Relieves pain and muscle tension: Hydrotherapy is very helpful in relieving muscle pain and tension. Because with the help of hydrotherapy there is a release of endorphins which are the natural pain reliever of the body. They also reduce the soreness in the muscles.
- Relieves stress: Hydrotherapy is very helpful in relieving the stress of the body by reducing the stress-causing blood pressure. Anxiety is also released by hydrotherapy and the release of endorphins which is a natural stress buster helps the body to relax.
- Encourages detoxification: Hydrotherapy detoxifies the body as the sauna and steam induce the sweat from the body thus flushing out all the impurities.

The results of hydrotherapy are not permanent as it gives temporary relief from the ailment by increasing the flow of blood. Though prolonged used of hydrotherapy have shown instances of permanent cure in arthritis and asthma.

Precautions for Hydrotherapy

These are the precautions which should be taken before hydrotherapy:

- The temperature of the water must be minded as it can cause severe burns.
- The temperature of the water must be checked and should be regulated up to the tolerance level.
- The tolerance level of the water must be changed according to the treatment, body temperature and the injury or illness.
- If the water is very hot or very cold it should not be directly applied to the skin but must be applied with a towel or barrier to prevent the skin.

Hydrotherapy Contraindications

These are the contraindications of hydrotherapy:

- Active infections.

- Altered sensations.
- Poor balance.
- Intolerance of heat or cold.
- Open wounds.
- Hydrophobia.

What are the Alternatives to Aqua Therapy?

Some common alternatives of hydrotherapy are:

- Steam bath.
- Sauna Bath.
- Spa therapy.
- Sitz bath.
- Wet sock treatment.
- Hot fomentation.

Halotherapy

Salt has been used for millennia in different parts of the world by different cultures because of its health benefits and therapeutic effect, but this was initially proved in 1843 by the Polish therapist Feliks Boczkowski. He noticed that people working in the salt mines in Poland enjoyed excellent health despite the harsh working conditions and the lack of sufficient food. In addition to this, they almost never suffered from colds or any respiratory diseases, which were frequently observed among the rest of the population. This prompted the physician to conduct research by which he established that all this was due to the saturated with salt air that the miners breathed daily. Thus, salt mines in Poland and Eastern Europe gradually became popular sanatoriums, attracting visitors from all over the world. A new method of treatment was established – Halotherapy (salt therapy). Lately, in many places, predominantly in Eastern Europe, artificial salt rooms and caves have been established, because of uncomfortable feelings when visiting salt mines, their difficult accessibility and too high expenses for their visitation.

In the last decades halotherapy has gained the trust of more and more people around the world and has been spreading quickly to Western Europe, Canada, Israel, North America, and many other countries. Lots of studies that prove its effectiveness and application with different diseases are published.

Halotherapy and Salt Therapy

Salt therapy can be dry or wet. Halotherapy is a dry salt therapy that is provided in environments, supplied with special equipment called a halogenerator. The halogenerator disperses a precise dry salt aerosol into the salt chamber. There are two types of salt rooms – active and passive. Active salt room is supplied with a special piece of equipment known as a halogenerator where pure sodium chloride is placed and dispersed into micro-sized particles into the air of the salt room. This kind of salt therapy is called halotherapy. Wet salt therapy includes gargling, drinking salt water, bathing in salt water or nasal irrigations.

On the other hand in many SPAs there are rooms filled with large amounts of varying types of salt such as Dead Sea, Himalayan, rock salt, Mediterranean, Caribbean, etc. There is no halogenerator in these chambers and they are created to look like salt caves but they do not provide the same salt air particles present in natural salt caves. They are known as passive salt rooms. The temperature, humidity and airflow are controlled but the concentration of sodium chloride is smaller than in dry salt rooms and the stay in these rooms is not considered to be halotherapy. Passive salt rooms provide an environment suitable for relaxation, meditation and improve the psycho-emotional condition of a person. As a result of many scientific searches it is proven that salt therapy is based on the inhalation of salt particles into the upper and lower parts of the respiratory system and penetration through the skin of micro-sized particles. This is possible to happen only by using halogenerators. That clarifies the difference between active and passive salt therapy, and halotherapy and salt therapy.

Technology of Halotherapy

At the base of this technology is the Halocomplex. The Halocomplex consists of a chamber with a halogenerator, and walls and floor covered with salt. In most of the cases the walls and floors are made of sea salt, and do not provide the real treatment. The special salt covering on the walls and floor acts as a buffer for air. Dry sodium chloride is produced in this room by a special nebulizer – halogenerator, which brings a flow of clean, dry air, saturated with highly dispersed negatively charged particles of sodium chloride into the salt room. The halogenerator is supplied with microprocessor that monitors the temperature, relative humidity and mass concentration of aerosol in the chamber.

Application Method

When conducting the procedure, the patients are left in the salt room or cave for 45 minutes and breathe the saturated with salt air, which is transported to the smallest of the bronchi as well as to the sinuses and the nasal cavity. The halotherapy rooms have air with low humidity and a temperature in the comfort zone – 22-24°. The low humidity in the room is of vital importance. There are no requirements for special clothing or other equipment. Benefits are better if patients are barelegged. The number of sessions depends on the patient's condition and the disease treated. Twelve to twenty sessions for 45 minutes each and for a short period of time are recommended for patients with chronical pulmonary diseases like asthma, bronchitis, sinusitis, COPD, allergic disease.

The mechanisms of action of halotherapy are manifold:

- Mucolytic.

- Antibacterial.
- Anti-inflammatory.
- Immunomodulating.
- Hyposensitizing.

Halotherapy is a natural and safe treatment without serious side effects. This method is very beneficial for the overall wellness of a person by improving function and removing toxic substances from respiratory system, improving the function and appearance of the skin, boosting the immune system and reducing stress.

There is evidence from several scientific researches that inhaled dry salt particles have bactericidal, moistening and anti-inflammatory properties, which may reduce inflammation in the entire respiratory tract and widen the airway passages. Salt inhalation leads to a quicker improvement of the parameters of respiratory failure, which can be observed in the worsening of obstructive pulmonary diseases. Dry salt particles accelerate the transportation of mucus, the elimination of residual toxic substances and foreign allergens. The application of salt therapy thus results in a clean respiratory system with higher oxygen intake, increases energy and improves the immune system.

Scientific researchers have confirmed that halotherapy has an influence over superficial and deeper skin layers providing healing and cosmetic effects. This increases activity of the skin cell ion channels, activates electrophysiological activity and improves skin's protective properties. Halotherapy leads to pH normalization and stimulates reparative and regenerative processes in the epidermis and derma, increasing skin rigidity. Dry salt improves skin microcirculation and cellular membrane activity, enhances skin regeneration and elasticity, and reduces wrinkles and edema.

The Positive Effects of Halotherapy

The efficiency of salt therapy is mainly due to three reasons:

- Salt has an antibacterial, antimycotic sand anti-inflammatory effect (it has been established that the environment in salt rooms is three times more sterile than the cleanest operating room).
- Salt has a natural ability to emit negative ions, neutralizing a positive charge.
- Salt is superabsorbent when it is dry.

Indications for Use

Halotherapy is indicated in most respiratory diseases, including:

- Respiratory tract infections.
- Asthma.
- Allergic and chronic bronchitis.
- Frequent colds.

- Pharyngitis.
- Sinusitis.
- Rhinitis.
- Tonsillitis.
- Pneumonia, after an acute stage.
- Cystic fibrosis.

It has been proven that this is a highly effective way of positively influencing numerous respiratory diseases with a prompt resolution of symptoms, improvement of pulmonary ventilation and tolerance of physical strain, as well as increase in the immunity and protective capacity of the organism.

Because of the influence of halotherapy over superficial and deeper skin layers which increases the activity of the skin cell ion channels, activates electrophysiological activity and improves skin's protective properties this treatment can provide healing and cosmetic effects. Halotherapy leads to pH normalization. It stimulates restorative and regenerative processes in the epidermis and derma, resulting in an increase in skin rigidity. Dry salt improves skin microcirculation and cellular membrane activity, enhances skin regeneration and elasticity, and reduces wrinkles and edema. Halotherapy can be applied in some skin diseases such as:

- Psoriasis.
- Eczema.
- Dermatitis.
- Acne.
- Rosacea.
- Onychomycosis.
- Skin aging.

Halotherapy is conducted in a pleasant and cozy environment, which has a beneficial effect on the psycho-emotional state of the patients. This treatment can be used with some psychosomatic conditions including:

- Stress and fatigue.
- Headache.
- Increasing immune reactivity.

Salt therapy is recommended as an additional treatment for some pediatric diseases. It is safe, noninvasive, with no side effects and potential health risks. Clinical researches have proven that children react quicker and more intensively. There is evidence about the high effectiveness of halotherapy for prophylaxis in frequently ill children and the possibility of its use for the treatment of acute respiratory diseases with children affected with chronic ears, nose and throat (ENT) disorders, respiratory and skin problems. This treatment is easily workable with children. There are special salt rooms supplied with toys and occupational appliances which make children feel calm and comfortable.

Side Effects

During the treatment itself, certain side effects might be observed, such as increased coughing and more abundant secretion, which is actually considered a positive effect because it leads to respiratory tract clearing and it is a signal for a change and adaptation of the organism to the specific irritant.

Skin irritations are rare side effects and are normally resolved by the third or fifth session. Conjunctivitis as result of irritation of the mucoid membrane is rarely observed. It is not a reason to interrupt the sessions. In such cases, it is recommended to keep the eyes closed when spending time in the salt room.

Contraindications include hyperthyroidism, active tuberculosis, high-grade hypertension, cardiovascular and respiratory failure, acute-stage blood disorders, contagious diseases, fever, open wounds and malignant diseases. Caution should be exercised when prescribing this therapy to patients with claustrophobia.

Animal Assisted Therapy

Animal-Assisted Psychotherapy (AAP) or Animal-Assisted Therapy (AAT) is a modality of therapy and counseling wherein a qualified and trained mental health professional incorporates one or more animals, into the therapeutic process, with specific, planned goals in mind; the animal(s) are an essential part of the treatment, and the therapist is practicing within the scope of his/her specialty or field.

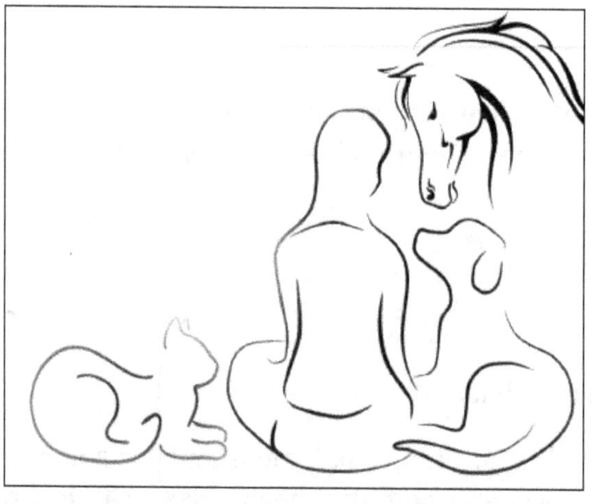

AAT is defined as "a structured, a goal-directed intervention in which an animal is incorporated as an integral part of the treatment process. AAT is delivered and/or directed by a professional health or human service provider who demonstrates skill and expertise regarding the clinical applications of human-animal interactions."

There are other terms used in conjunction with, and often confused with Animal-Assisted Therapy. Pet Partners defines them as below:

- Animal-Assisted Activities (AAA) provides opportunities for motivational, educational, therapeutic and/or recreational benefits to enhance quality of life. AAA are delivered in a variety of environments by a specially trained professional, paraprofessional, and/or volunteer in association with animals that meet specific criteria. Detailed note taking and developing specific goals are not required in AAA, and they often constitute simple visits where the animal meets, greets, and spends some time with the person.
- Animal-assisted education (AAE) is a goal oriented, planned and structured intervention directed by a general education or special education professional. The focus of the activities is on academic goals, pro-social skills and cognitive functioning with student progress being both measured and documented.
- Animal-Assisted Interventions (AAI) is goal oriented and structured interventions that intentionally incorporate animals in health, education and human service for therapeutic gains and improved health and wellness. AAT, AAA, and AAE all fall under the umbrella of AAI.

What does AAT Involve?

Animal-Assisted Therapy looks and works almost like any other therapy session, with the exception of the animal component. That is to say, AAT is first and foremost psychotherapy, of any style (client-centered, play-based, psychodynamic, cognitive-behavioural, or even eclectic), depending on the inclination or training of the therapist, applied in concurrence with the benefits and advantages the presence and involvement of an animal brings to the process.

AAT involves the therapist and the therapy animal, often referred to as a co-therapist or therapy partner, working as a team to help the client meet their need-based, specific goals. This is done through different means and methods, depending on what instruments or modality the therapist utilizes. For example two different therapists could be trying to achieve the same goal; one through animal-assisted play therapy, the other through animal-assisted client-centered therapy, or even through cognitive-behavioral techniques.

The therapy animal is chosen based on predetermined criteria that help decide the suitability of the animal for therapy. Some criteria, among others, include a basic obedience training (like sit, down, stay etc.), having a welcoming and sociable temperament, enjoying human interaction, and being at least a year old. The therapy animal usually belongs to the therapist themselves, which helps lay the foundation for the duo's working partnership.

The therapist-therapy animal bond is the key in the therapeutic process, for multiple reasons. Having a thorough knowledge of one's therapy animal, her personality traits, stressors, and individual quirks helps the therapist keep the environment safe & comfortable for both the client, and the animal, during session. It enables the therapist to pre-empt any negative interactions between the client and the animal, and facilitate a positive connection and experience between the two.

Aside from physical and emotional safety of all involved, a deep understanding of one's therapy animal aids the therapist in gleaning additional therapeutic 'raw material' to work with; this refers to any responses or behaviors of the animal that may indicate any emotion, or concern that the client is experiencing.

Therapy animals can be a dynamic and animated medium for the client, through which they are able to get in touch with their own inner world, express the contents of the same, to themselves, and to the therapist, without feeling judged or compelled to do so. The animal can serve as a sensory medium (sound, touch, sight, movement), as well.

For the psychodynamic animal-assisted therapist, the animal can perform the function of an entity to project upon. Clients, especially children, often tend to project their thoughts, emotions, and cognitions onto the animal, offering the therapist a perspective of what their internal state of mind may look like. This helps provide an opportunity to begin a dialogue about the same, and to examine, explore, and process any past traumas, lingering emotions or fears and anxieties the client has.

From an attachment theory standpoint, the animal can also play the role of a transitional object, for clients; an object (or in this case a relationship) that provides the client comfort, and helps ease the stress of normal development and separation from the primary caregiver.

Animals can also fulfil humans' needs for love, affection, and belongingness (analogous to Maslow's hierarchy of needs in some manner), and in that way, enhance and uplift one's psychological well-being.

How does AAT help?

AAT has numerous benefits, ranging from physical and physiological, to psychological and social. Animals often have a positive, motivating effect, and this has been harnessed before to help patients in physical exercise & rehabilitation, movement therapy and physiotherapy. It has also shown some amount of success in the case of persons with muscular dystrophy, cerebral palsy and other conditions involving lessened motor skills and control. It helps to improve their balance and mobility.

Studies have even shown that the simple act of petting/touching/handling a dog can lower one's blood pressure and decrease a person's risk for cardiovascular disease. It also reduces stress and anxiety and can help manage behaviors that stem from the same.

Meaningful relationships with animals can moderate or diminish feelings of isolation, and improve one's self-esteem, self-efficacy and confidence. Moreover, clients' attention-span, and concentration skills also increase.

Perhaps one of the most profoundly felt effects of AAT, however, is that interacting and working with an animal can help foster empathy within a client, and improves their socializing abilities and reinforces appropriate social behavior, especially since animals can provide a sort of "instant feedback" with their responses, in a non-judgmental, non-punitive manner.

For example, a dog that has been subject to rough handling by a child (hitting him hard, pulling his tail or scratching his face) will slink away from the child, and avoid further aversive interactions.

On the other hand, a dog that is treated with kindness and love, and whose boundaries are respected, will want to keep interacting with the child, and probably return the same affection he received. This helps the child understand what is acceptable and appropriate through an immediate cause-and-effect method.

Who benefits from AAT?

Animal-Assisted Therapy can be employed to help individuals of all ages, with a range of different issues. AAT is not necessarily limited only to individuals, but also to groups, couples, and families.

AAT is often applied in settings where children are involved. This is because animals have a way of lowering children's defenses (usually against adults), and gaining their trust with their unquestioning acceptance of the child, and unconditional affection for them. This helps children feel safe enough to delve into their problems and work through them, while feeling supported and loved. Animals tend to also naturally be spontaneous, energetic, and sometimes creative, making them great agents to facilitate play, which is the child's innate means of processing any event/trauma/ unresolved emotion they are experiencing.

AAT has been extensively used with individuals on the Autism Spectrum. Animals have helped persons on the spectrum to improve their social skills (e.g. eye contact, verbal communication), their empathetic abilities, to learn and reinforce appropriate, acceptable behaviors through structured and organized agenda, and even helped soothe clients with sensory issues, especially those with high tactile sensitivity. AAT is also beneficial to individuals dealing with depression, anxiety, cancer, substance addictions, and post-traumatic stress disorder (PTSD), behavioral concerns, or even emotional disorders.

There is a small fraction of the general population that may not be suitable for AAT, and these include people who are severely phobic of animals, gravely allergic to their fur or hair, and/or have a history of abuse or violence towards animals.

AAT at Direct

At Direct, the therapist creates a treatment plan based on the needs of the client, in collaboration with the other expert therapists working with the client. This ensures that common goals are worked on together, which guarantee consistency and reinforcement of positive outcomes for the client.

Based on the goals of the client, their level of functioning, and ability to interact safely with the animals, the therapist determines which animal(s) will be best suited to help the client achieve his objectives for therapy. Goals are re-assessed regularly, and added or edited, as needed.

References

- Acupuncture, wellness-and-prevention, health: hopkinsmedicine.org, Retrieved 17, May 2020
- Acupuncture-points: woninstitute.edu, Retrieved 03, February 2020
- Acupressure-for-seniors-everything-you-need-to-know: seniority.in, Retrieved 24, April 2020
- Find-your-pressure-points: experiencelife.com, Retrieved 12, August 2020

- All-you-want-to-know-about-acupressure-points-on-the-feet-bd-15: powermaxfitness.net, Retrieved 21, May 2020
- Apitherapy-Holistic-Healing-Through-the-Honeybee-and-Bee-Products-in-Countries-with-Poor-Healthcare-System-278698896: researchgate.net, Retrieved 11, January 2020
- HALOTHERAPY-BENEFITS-AND-RISKS-331996764: researchgate.net, Retrieved 26, June 2020

Chapter 5

Naturopathy and Homeopathy

A form of alternative medicine that makes use of an array of pseudoscientific practices that are natural and promote self-healing is termed as naturopathy. There are various types of treatments in naturopathy such as fasting therapy, mud therapy, masso therapy and magnet therapy. This chapter discusses in detail these significant types of treatments in naturopathy.

Naturopathy

Naturopathy is a distinct system of primary health care-an art, science, philosophy, and practice of diagnosis, treatment, and prevention of illness. Naturopathy is distinguished by the principles upon which its practice is based. These principles are continually re-examined in the light of scientific advances. The techniques of naturopathy are a blend of modern and traditional, scientific, and empirical methods.

Naturopathy is a holistic system of healing that incorporates a range of treatments and natural therapies, with the underlying belief that your body is able to fight infection and disease itself, given the right support. While conventional medicine is preoccupied with treating the symptoms of a disease or illness, naturopathy takes a more holistic approach to health care with a patients overall health a priority. Naturopathy believes that if one restores or maintains the equilibrium of the body, our immune system is better placed to defend itself against infection and disease. There is therefore no use of or reliance on medication, which would only serve to suppress the symptoms of an illness. Naturopathy is more likely to recommend a programme of exercise, a change in diet or a natural treatment. Natural treatments and therapies are used to ensure that the body and mind are able to remain resilient, and recover promptly. When we do succumb to an illness and contract a fever this is viewed as the body dealing with the source of the problem. The fever is therefore not viewed as a negative event, rather as part of the body's natural defence mechanism. The naturopathy is able to make use of different natural treatments together to allow the patient to have optimal health. Some of these are detoxification, hydrotherapy, physical medicine and lifestyle, and psychological counselling. Detoxification is the process of eliminating toxins and other harmful chemicals from the body through fasting, drinking high volume of water and using enemas. Hydrotherapy or water therapy where the patient is recommended to take certain baths, water exercise, alternate hot and cold applications and drink natural spring water. Physical medicine is healing with the involvement of touch therapy and cold compresses as well as electric currents and sound waves in manipulating spine, bones and muscles. Lifestyle and psychological counselling includes guided imagery, hypnosis and many counselling methods in the treatment program. Naturopathy has addressed many conditions so that there is no limitation to what illnesses it can treat. This is because of the many therapies under this alternative medicine; acute to chronic conditions can be helped by the naturopath. Naturopathic medicine aims to heal the whole body and not just one area of it. It is best to allow nature to do the treatment and to enhance the capability of the body to heal itself. Doing this will not only get relief from a certain disease but also boost the immune system of the body.

Principles of Naturopathic Medicine

Some of the basic principles of naturopathic medicine are discussed below:

- The Healing Power of Nature: Human organism has a unique capacity to heal itself and that such healing is only aided, not accomplished, by a physician. The incredible bimolecular complexity of the numerous cyclic, cybernetic processes of the organism is believed to account for this capacity.
- First Do No Harm: Hippocratic concept would be that sometimes harmful therapies are needed but they should be reserved for the last resort and, if at all possible, avoided. This principle does not mean harmful therapies should never be used.
- Health workers as Teacher: One of naturopathy's primary roles is to educate the patient. This means that, to the extent possible and appropriate, information sharing with the patient should take place so that they are able to make informed decisions about their health care. Since the creation of a healthy lifestyle often rests on the choices and decisions the patient makes, this principle also implies that the patient has a responsibility to assist in the restoration of their own health. Another way to think about this that the "healing power of nature" can be constrained if significant obstacles are not addressed or if the patient is ignorant of their own self-healing processes. One of the naturopathic physician's key tasks as a teacher is to empower the patient to appreciate and accept this responsibility.
- Prevention and Wellness: Whenever possible, naturopathic physicians work to prevent illness rather than waiting until invasive treatment is required. Naturopathic physicians also strive to maintain wellness in all aspects rather than simply helping to prevent and treat illness. This principle implies that naturopathic medicine acknowledges the social and cultural antecedents of disease, since economic, cultural, and political factors can play as much of a role in determining one's health as the better established mental, emotional and physical causes of illness.
- Treat the Cause: Naturopathy typically strive to determine the underlying causes of illness and to address these to the extent that it is feasible. Naturopathy physicians also work to relieve suffering and palliate disease. Sometimes this may be all that as possible if the causes of illness cannot be identified in an individual patient, though the cause can often be treated while suffering is simultaneously alleviated. The naturopathic healthcare model holds, however, that it is imperative to avoid suppressing symptoms in most cases without addressing the cause of the dysfunction. It is believed that if this clinical guideline is not observed, the potential for even greater pathology may ultimately be created.
- Treat the Whole Person: Naturopathy focus on taking into account the totality of the human individual. Even a relatively minor physical ailment affecting one organ system may actually be a clue to larger pathology. The mind, body, and environment form an ecological

whole that requires them to be considered together in the process of assessing health and disease.

Naturopathic Approaches

Naturopathic treatment can take the form of a variety of therapies and approaches, including:

- Dietary advice: A balanced diet is an essential component for a healthy body.
- Herbal remedies: Traditional remedies utilized for hundreds of years for healing.
- Hydrotherapy: The healing power of water.
- Iridology: Analysis of the iris for diagnosis of health issues.
- Massage: The manipulation of the tissues of the body for healing and relaxation.
- Nutritional supplements: Especially useful when immunity is compromised by illness.
- Osteopathy: Manipulation therapy concerned with the musculo-skeletal system.

Treatments in Naturopathy

Fasting Therapy

Fasting is primarily the act of willingly abstaining from some or all food, drink, or both, for a period of time. The word id derived from the old English, 'Feastan' means to fast, observe, be strict. In Sanskrit 'Vrath' means 'determination' and 'Upavasa' means ' near to God'. A fast may be total or partial concerning that from which one fasts, and may be prolonged or intermittent as to the period of fasting. Fasting is an important treatment modality for health preservation. In fasting, mental preparedness is an essential pre-condition. Prolonged fasting should be done only under the supervision of a competent Naturopath.

The duration of the fast depends upon the age of the patient, the nature of the disease and amount and type of drugs previously used. It is sometimes advisable to undertake a series of short fasts of two or three days and gradually increase the duration of each succeeding fast by a day or so. No harm will accrue to fasting patient provided they take rest and are under proper professional care.

Methods of fasting are water, juices or raw vegetable juices. The best, safest and most effective method is lime juice fasting. During fasting, the body burns up and excretes huge amounts of accumulated wastes. We can help this cleansing process by drinking alkaline juices. Sugars in juices will strengthen the heart, juice fasting is therefore the best form of fasting. All juices should be prepared from fresh fruit immediately before drinking. Canned or frozen juices should not be used. A precautionary measure, which must be observed in all cases of fasting, is the complete emptying of the bowels at the beginning of the fast by enema so that the patient is not bothered by gas or decomposing matter formed from the excrements remaining in the body. Enemas should be used at least every alternate day during the fasting period. The total liquid intake should be approximately six to eight glasses. A lot of energy is spent during the fast in the process of eliminating accumulated poisons and toxic waste materials. It is therefore, of utmost importance that the patient gets as much physical rest and mental relaxation as possible during the fast.

The success of the fast depends largely on how it is broken. The main rules for break in the fast are: do not overeat, eat slowly and chew your food thoroughly and take several days for the gradual change to the normal diet.

Benefits and Physiological Effects of Fasting

Physicians of most cultures, throughout history, have recommended extended fasting as therapy for various conditions from ancient to modern. Though earlier observations were studied without scientific methodology or understanding they still point to utilization of fasting as a therapeutic modality. Earlier observations were based on animal behaviour but today they are based on animal physiology.

Prominent among the physiological effects conferred by fasting (Calorie Restriction and Intermittent Fasting) are the following: increased insulin sensitivity that results in reduced plasma glucose and insulin concentrations and improved glucose tolerance, reduced levels of oxidative stress as indicated by decreased oxidative damage to proteins, lipids and DNA, increased resistance to various types of stress including heat, oxidative and metabolic stresses and enhanced immune function.

Both gross and cellular physiology is profoundly affected by caloric restriction (CR) or intermittent fasting (IF) regimes. With respect to gross physiology there is of course a significant reduction of body fat and mass, which supports a healthy cardiovascular system and reduces incidents of myocardial infarction. In addition to cardio protection a greater tolerance to stress is induced in the liver, the nutrient core of Homo sapiens. The presence of alternative energy stores such as ketone bodies (e.g. β-hydroxybutyrate) enables Homo sapiens to survive additional stresses of life. Excessive and deleterious blood glucose is curtailed by an enhanced sensitivity to insulin (Ins) and glucose and its utilization as an energy source.

Mud Therapy

Mud therapy is very simple and effective treatment modality. The mud used for this should be clean and taken from 3 to 4 ft. depth from the surface of the ground. There should be no contamination of stone pieces or chemical manures etc. in the mud.

Mud is one of five elements of nature having immense impact on the body both in health and sickness.

Advantages of using Mud

- Its black color absorbs all the colors of the Sun and conveys them to the body.
- Mud retains moisture for a long time, when applied over the body part it causes cooling.
- Its shape and consistency can be changed easily by adding water.

- It is cheap and easily available.

Before using, mud should be dried, powdered and sieved to separate stones, grass particles and other impurities.

Mud Pack-local Application

Keeping soaked mud in a thin, wet muslin cloth and making it into a thin flat brick depending on the size of the patient's abdomen, apply it. The duration of the mud pack application is 20 to 30 minutes. When applied in cold weather, place a blanket over the mud pack and cover the body as well.

Benefits:

- When applied to abdomen it relieves all forms of indigestion. It is effective in decreasing intestinal heat and stimulates peristalsis.
- A thick mud pack applied to head in congestive headache relieves the pain immediately. Hence this is recommended whenever there is necessity for a prolonged cold application.
- Application of the pack over the eyes is useful in cases of conjunctivitis, hemorrhages in the eyeball, itching, allergy, errors of refraction like short sight and long sight and especially useful in glaucoma where it helps to reduce eyeball tension.

Mud Pack for Face

Soaked mud is applied on the face and allowed to dry for 30 minutes. This is helpful in improving the complexion of the skin and removing pimples and open skin pores which in turn facilitate elimination. This also is helpful in eliminating dark circles around the eyes. After 30 minutes, face should be washed thoroughly with cold water.

Mud Bath

Mud may be applied to the patient in sitting or lying position. This helps to improve the skin condition by increasing the circulation and energizing the skin tissues. Care should be taken to avoid catching cold during the bath. Afterwards, the patient must be thoroughly washed with cold water jet spray. If the patient feels chill, warm water should be used. The patient is, then, dried quickly and transferred to a warm bed. The duration of mud bath may be 45 to 60 minutes.

Benefits:

- The effects of mud are refreshing, invigorating, and vitalizing.
- For wounds and skin diseases, application of mud is the only true bandage.
- Mud therapy is used for giving coolness to body.
- It dilutes and absorbs the toxic substances of body and ultimately eliminates them from body.

- Mud is used successfully in different diseases like constipation, headache due to tension, high blood pressure, skin diseases etc.

Masso Therapy

Massage is an excellent form of passive exercise. The word is derived from the Greek word 'massier' which means to kneed, from French "friction of kneading", or from Arabic massa meaning "to touch, feel or handle" or from Latin massa meaning "mass, dough". Massage is the practice of soft tissue manipulation with physical (anatomical), functional (physiological), and in some cases psychological purposes and goals. If correctly done on a bare body, it can be highly stimulating and invigorating.

Massage is also a modality of Naturopathy and quite essential for maintaining good health. Massage involves acting on and manipulating the body with pressure – structured, unstructured, stationary, or moving – tension, motion, or vibration, done manually or with mechanical aids. Target tissues may include muscles, tendons, ligaments, skin, joints, or other connective tissue, as well as lymphatic vessels. Massage can be applied with the hands, fingers, elbows, knees, forearm, and feet. There are over eighty different recognized massage modalities. It aims at improving blood circulation and strengthening bodily organs. In winter season, sun bath after massaging the whole body is well known practice of preserving health and strength. It is beneficial to all. It bestows combined benefits of massage and sun rays therapy. In disease conditions, necessary therapeutic effects can be obtained through specific techniques of massage. Massage is a substitute of exercise for those who cannot do the same. The effects of exercise can be derived from massage. Various oils are used as lubricants like mustard oil, sesame oil, coconut oil, olive oil, aroma oils etc. which also have therapeutic effects.

There are seven fundamental modes of manipulation in massage and these are: Touch, effleurage (stroking), friction (rubbing), petrissage (kneading), tapotement (percussion), vibration (shaking or trembling) and Joint movement. Movements vary according to disease condition and parts applied.

Another form of massage helpful in most ailments are the vibratory massage, Powder massage, Water massage, Dry massage. Powders of neem leaves, rose petals and are also used as lubricants for massage.

Physiological effects of Massage

- Reflex Effects (responses mediated by the nervous system):
    - Vasodilation of arteries.
    - Stimulation of peristalsis (aids in digestion).
    - Increase or decrease in muscle tone.
    - Increases activity of the organs in the abdominal cavity.
    - Triggers the relaxation response.

- Soothing or stimulating effect on muscles.
- Stimulates the heart, increases strength and rate of contraction.
- Increases efficiency of the immune system.

- Mechanical Effects (responses resulting from directly applied manual pressure):
    - Increased venous return.
    - Increased lymphatic flow, Lymphatic drainage.
    - Circulatory efficiency.
    - Loosening of mucous (respiratory system).
    - Breakdown of fibrosis/adhesions.
    - Stretch to shorten muscles/ loosens muscle fibres.
    - Increased muscle temperature.
    - Increased metabolic rate locally and gaseous exchange.
    - Stretches scar tissue.
    - Decreased muscle tone/increased muscle tone.
    - Increased range of Motion.
    - Restoration of proper joint mechanics/biomechanics.
    - Elimination of muscle imbalances.
    - Strengthen weakened muscles.

Benefits of Massage

The general massage, dealing with all parts of the body, is highly beneficial in many ways. It tones up the nervous system, influences respiration and quickens the elimination of poisons and waste material from the body through the various eliminative organs such as the lungs, skin, kidneys and bowels. It also boosts blood circulation and metabolic processes. A massage removes facial wrinkles, helps to fill out hollow cheeks and neck and eases stiffness, sore muscles and numbness.

Peer-reviewed medical research has shown that the benefits of massage include pain relief, reduced trait anxiety and depression, and temporarily reduced blood pressure, heart rate, and state anxiety. Theories behind what massage might do include blocking nociception (gate control theory), activating the parasympathetic nervous system which may stimulate the release of endorphins and serotonin, preventing fibrosis or scar tissue, increasing the flow of lymph, and improving sleep but such effects are yet to be supported by well-designed clinical studies.

Magnet Therapy

Using magnets for healing pain is increasingly popular with the public. However, despite this popularity, there is a lack of scientific evidence to prove magnets have any therapeutic benefit. Traditional physicians remain, in general, very skeptical of magnets' benefits. Despite this justified mainstream skepticism, we seek to provide members of the public who are seeking information on magnets with balanced, factual information.

When referring to magnets, we are not talking about the type of magnets found on refrigerator doors - but biomagnets - those magnets manufactured for physical and mental healing. Biomagnets are named after biomagnetism, the science of magnetism.

As children in school we learned that magnetism is an energy force on earth. Each atom has a nucleus around which spins positively charged protons and negatively charged electrons that generate a magnetic field. For thousands of years ancient civilizations studied the positive and negative magnetic forces. For example, in Traditional Chinese Medicine (TCM) it is believed that a balance of these positive and negative forces referred to as Yin and Yang represents good health.

Theory

Although not scientifically proven and controversial, theories suggest biomagnets alone do not heal but rather stimulate the body to heal naturally. Some of these scientifically unproven claims include:

- Restoration of cellular magnetic balance.
- Migration of calcium ions is accelerated to help heal bones and nerve tissues.
- Circulation is enhanced since biomagnets are attracted to the iron in blood and this increase in blood flow helps healing.
- Biomagnets have a positive effect on the pH balance of cells.
- Hormone production is influenced by biomagnet use.

Polarity

Theory aside, an important aspect of biomagnet use is magnet polarity. This relates to the direction in which the magnet is placed. The North Pole corresponds to TCM Yin, or negative polarity. The South Pole corresponds to TCM Yang, or positive polarity. Below, the magnetic influences of the South and North Poles are shown by example.

North Pole Characteristics: Sedating Cooling.

- Negative: Yin.
- Low back pain.
- Arthritis.
- Inflammation.

- Acute headaches.
- Sharp pain.

South Pole Characteristics: Stimulating, Heating.

- Positive: Yang.
- Tingling.
- Numbness.
- Weak muscles.
- Paralysis.
- Scars.

If the body appears to lack both positive and negative energies to heal, the therapist may apply both the North and South Poles (known as Bipolar) simultaneously. Bipolar biomagnet therapy may be used to heal fractures or treat chronic pain.

The type of ailment determines the type and power of the biomagnet to be used, the length of time the patient has had the problem, its severity, if the ailment is superficial or deep, the area of the body to be treated, and the patient's sensitivity.

Some patients are sensitive to biomagnet therapy. The therapy may temporarily make the condition worse as toxins are released. Light-headedness, headache, sleepiness, and itching are some of the side effects.

Biomagnets not for Everyone's Use

As with any treatment, there are cautionary measures to follow. For example, biomagnets should not be used during pregnancy, on patients with a history of epilepsy, while taking blood-thinning medications, on bleeding wounds, or if internal bleeding exists.

Biomagnets should never be used on a patient with a pacemaker or who have metal implants that could be dislodged by magnet use. In infants and children care should be taken as well as use on the eyes, brain, or over the heart at any age.

Biomagnet Power Measured

Biomagnet power is measured in terms of gauss, the line of force per unit area of the pole. The earth's surface is approximately 0.5 gauss. Many manufacturers rate their products using internal gauss and external gauss to indicate strength. Listed below are typical magnetic strength classifications:

- Low gauss (g) = 300 - 700 g
- Medium gauss = 1000 - 2500 g
- High gauss = 3000 - 6000 g
- Super gauss = 7000 - 12000 g

Surface gauss rating also refers to the external strength of the magnet. This measurement is dependent on the size, shape, polarity, and grade of the magnetic material.

Some experts in biomagnet therapy begin treatment at low gauss and gradually increase strength as necessary. We recommend you consult with a specialist who is skilled in administering biomagnet therapy first.

Types of Biomagnets

There are about as many types of biomagnets as there are body parts! Magnetic mattresses and pads are designed to be slept on, magnetic insoles fit inside shoes, block magnets can be placed under mattresses, pillows, or seat cushions, back supports are even available with slots for magnet insertion. Others are made as body wraps with Velcro closures, jewelry, and magnetic foil.

Caring for Biomagnets

Most biomagnets are made of ferrites, which are iron oxides combined with cobalt, nickel, barium and other metals to make a ceramic-like material. The flexible types of magnets are combined with plastic, rubber or other pliable materials. The strongest biomagnets are those made from neodymium (rare earth element).

However, just because biomagnets are strong does not mean they are indestructible! When subjected to intense heat (400+ degrees F) a magnet will lose all its energy. Also, don't drop magnets. And remember, magnets can damage CDs, computer hard drives, credit cards, and other devices with metal components.

Homeopathy

Homeopathy is an effective and scientific system of healing that assists the natural tendency of the body to heal itself. It recognizes that all symptoms of ill health are expressions of disharmony within the whole person and that it is the individual person who needs treatment, not the disease. The homeopathic principles constitute a unified hypothesis whose validity is tested empirically: cured patients confirm the hypothesis. Homeopathic medicines are prepared in a pharmacy or a laboratory, using a technique subject to precise and clearly stated controls. The preparation and administration of homeopathic medicines does not involve mysterious processes.

Homeopathy is an increasingly popular alternative system of medicine whose basic philosophy is viewed skeptically by the orthodox medical profession because it is difficult to understand within accepted scientific theories. Its success with patients, however, has led to its continual growth and development over the past 200 years, culminating in resurgence in recent years partly owing to increasing dissatisfaction with the side effects of modern medicines.

Homeopathy is based on the principles of similars. The standard medical assumption is this: if the body produces a symptom, the appropriate treatment is an antidote, or opposite medicine, whose purpose is to overcome that symptom. For example, a conventional doctor will treat constipation with a laxative, which produces diarrhoea. The premise of the law of similars is this: any substance that can cause symptoms of disease in a healthy person can cure a sick person who manifests a similar symptom profile. A homeopathic practitioner treats constipation by giving a homeopathic medicine that has produced symptoms of constipation in a healthy person.

Treating "like with like" was described by Hippocrates in the 5th century BC; the "father of medicine," and people throughout the world have employed this principle of healing with "similars" for many hundreds of years. It was the German doctor Samuel Hahnemann, however, who discovered this basic approach through an experiment he conducted on himself, in an attempt to understand how medicines worked. Questioning the basis for treating malaria with quinine, Hahnemann ingested Cinchona bark (from which quinine is derived) in order to find out how it might affect a healthy person. After a number of days, he started to experience symptoms of fever (typical of malaria), which cleared up once he stopped taking the medicine.

Hahnemann next experimented with Cinchona bark on family and friends, with similar results. This led him to experiment with many other substances in order to discover what symptoms of illness they could produce in healthy individuals. He called these tests provings and meticulously recorded individual reactions as well as any common themes or patterns of illness produced by each substance—including sensations and feelings. These provings formed the basis of a new system of healing Hahnemann called homeopathy, from the Greek homoios (similar) and pathos (suffering or disease), in order to differentiate it from orthodox medicine, which he called "allopathy," meaning "opposite suffering".

Hahnemann then used the "symptom pictures" he assembled as the basis for his prescriptions. He gave a single medicine at a time, as opposed to the medical practice of his time, which involved mixtures containing many medicines. His departure from "accepted" medical practice attracted much derision, especially from the apothecaries, but the successes he achieved with patients verified his theory, and he continued to develop his system.

Hahnemann experimented with diluting his medicines to minimize side effects but found that simple dilution (with stirring) caused the medicine to lose its efficacy altogether, so he developed a new method of dilution whereby he diluted the substance in carefully measured steps, shaking it vigorously in between each dilution. This shaking he called "succussion" and the resultant liquid a "potentized remedy." He found that this new remedy lacked side effects and had a stronger curative reaction. In fact, he discovered that the more he diluted and successed a substance the stronger it became. This dilution-and-potency issue has become "one of the main areas of controversy in the homeopathic system".

This process of dilution consistently incurred skepticism from the medical establishment which could not explain, and therefore could not accept, how anything so dilute could have an effect. Despite such opposition, homeopathy survived because it worked, and patients who were helped spread the word. Some of those patients were doctors and many of them, having experienced the gentle yet effective healing power of homeopathy themselves, then trained under Hahnemann and took his teachings out into the world, to South and North America, India and Europe.

The Principles

Simillimum

The homeopathic remedy is selected on the basis that it causes similar symptoms in a healthy person, as documented in experiments that are called provings. This remedy is known as the simillimum.

Minimum Dose

Dilution with succussion releases the strength or "potency" of any substance and makes it a more effective medicine while eliminating potential side effects. Homeopathic medicines are made from a wide variety of substances—animal, vegetable, and mineral. Because a homeopathic remedy is diluted beyond the point where there is anything measurable of the original substance—at a molecular level—absolutely anything can be used, including some which are toxic at a material dose, such as acids and snake venoms.

The starting remedy—a tincture or mother tincture—is made by steeping soluble substances in alcohol and then straining them. Insoluble substances are ground for several hours with a pestle and mortar until they are rendered soluble. This process, called trituration, is used for metals and other substances that do not dissolve easily in order to prepare them for dilution and succussion.

There are two scales for diluting substances: the decimal and the centesimal. For the decimal scale, one tenth of the tincture is added to nine tenths alcohol and shaken vigorously; this first dilution is called a 1X. The number of a homeopathic remedy reflects the number of times it has been diluted and succussed: for example, Sulphur 6X has been diluted and succussed six times.

The centesimal scale is diluted using one part in a hundred of the tincture and the letter C is added after the number. Paradoxically, a 6X is called a low potency and 200C a high potency; the greater the dilution, the greater the potency, the stronger the curative potential of the medicine.

The most commonly used potency in the decimal scale is the 6X, although the 9X, 12X, 24X, and 30X are used by some. In the centesimal scale, those potencies most commonly used are the 6C, 12C, 30C, and 200C.

Single Remedy

Remedies are tested, or proven, one at a time and prescribed on an individual basis. Combination remedies (including several remedies that are strongly indicated in a particular disease) are widely available in this country, although results are likely to be disappointing if the single remedy a person needs is not included in a particular mixture.

Whole Person

Every human being should be viewed as a unique individual, whole and complete, functioning as a totality in relation to the surrounding environment; in this context, the only way to cure illness is to increase the health of the afflicted person. Based on this philosophy, alternative treatments look at the disease within the "whole person context." They take into account the person who has become ill, and their treatment is designed to stimulate that person's own self-healing abilities. Alternative health care practitioners believe it is important to explore both how a person has become ill, as well as the known stressors in their lives, especially those that have led up to illness and will take these into account when planning a course of treatment. Many people find this a relief and are grateful to be treated as a whole rather than having to separate themselves into "parts" to be handed over to a host of "experts."

Vital Force

The human organism has a unique relationship with its environment, which biologists refer to as "homeostasis." As such, a healthy living being is self-regulating, with an innate (protective) tendency to maintain its equilibrium and compensate for disruptive changes. Hahnemann believed that an energetic substance, independent of physical and chemical forces, exists and that this "vital force" gives life and is absent at death. It is also known as chi or prana by Eastern medical practitioners. This vital force acts in predictable ways and operates both in sickness and in health, by producing coping mechanisms to counteract stressors. Disease is the body's way of coping with stress. Homeopaths credit this balancing mechanism for the maintenance of health, provided that the stresses on the mind and body are neither too prolonged nor too great.

Susceptibility and Constitutional Treatment

Susceptibility is simply the degree to which a person is vulnerable to an outside influence. Not everyone who goes for a walk in a cold wind will be affected, but some are "susceptible." Their predisposition is due to an underlying constitutional weakness, which is either inherited or due to past and/or current stress (mental, emotional, or physical).

Many people consult a homeopath to receive "constitutional treatment" for chronic complaints that have not been alleviated through other forms of treatment. The value of such treatment is that it boosts the weak constitution and decreases its susceptibility to disease. This type of intervention requires specialized education and training.

How does Homeopathy Work?

Although homeopathy has been compared to vaccination, they are very different practices. Vaccines stimulate the immune system directly to produce specific antibodies to a particular disease. They are tested on animals and then on humans to verify their safety; even then side effects are common. Most vaccines are introduced directly into the bloodstream, bypassing the body's natural defense system and stimulating it in a way that is not fully understood.

Homeopathic medicines are administered orally in safe, diluted, and succussed doses; they are tested on healthy humans (not on animals), and when used correctly have no side effects. They work on an individual's energy patterns, by stimulating the immune system generally.

Homeopathic Dilutions

The founder of homeopathy, Samuel Hahnemann found that undiluted doses caused reactions, sometimes dangerous ones, so specified that preparations be given at the lowest possible dose. To counter the reduced potency at high dilutions he formed the view that vigorous shaking by striking on an elastic surface – a process termed succussion – was necessary. It has been said that Hahnemann came to this conclusion after deciding preparations subjected to agitation in transit, such as in saddle bags or in a carriage, were more "potent". Hahnemann had a saddle-maker construct a special wooden striking board covered in leather on one side and stuffed with horsehair. The process of dilution and succussion is termed "dynamization" or "potentization" by homeopaths. In industrial manufacture this may be done by machine. There are differences of opinion on the number and force of strikes, and some practitioners dispute the need for succussion at all. There are no laboratory assays and the importance and techniques for succussion cannot be determined with any certainty from the literature.

Potency Scales

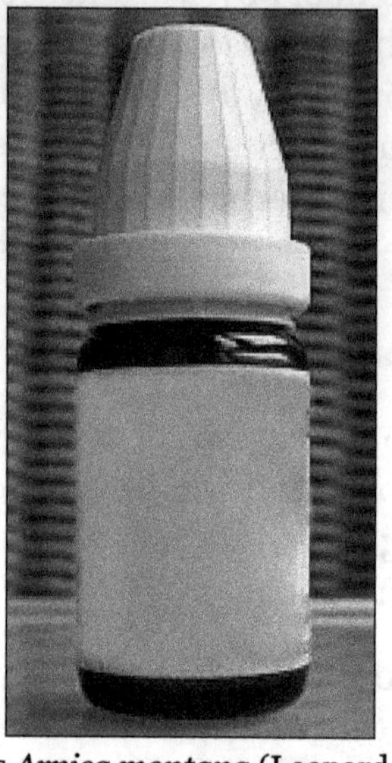

Figure: This bottle contains *Arnica montana* (Leopard›s Bane, Fallkraut) D6, i.e. the nominal dilution is one part in a million (10^6).

Three main logarithmic dilution scales are in regular use in homeopathy. Hahnemann created the "centesimal" or "C scale", diluting a substance by a factor of 100 at each stage. There is also a decimal dilution scale (notated as "X" or "D") in which the preparation is diluted by a factor of 10 at each stage. The centesimal scale was favoured by Hahnemann for most of his life, although in his last ten years Hahnemann developed a quintamillesimal (Q) scale which diluted the drug 1 part in 50,000. The greatest dilution reasonably likely to contain at least one molecule of the original substance is around 12C.

A 2C dilution requires a substance to be diluted to one part in one hundred, and then some of that diluted solution diluted by a further factor of one hundred. This works out to one part of the original substance in 10,000 parts of the solution. A 6C dilution repeats this process six times, ending up with the original material diluted by a factor of $100^{-6}=10^{-12}$. Higher dilutions follow the same pattern. In homeopathy, a solution that is more dilute is described as having a higher *potency*, and more dilute substances are considered by homeopaths to be stronger and deeper-acting. The end product is often so diluted that it is indistinguishable from the dilutant (typically ethanol or pure water for liquids, milk sugar for insoluble solids).

Hahnemann advocated 30C dilutions for most purposes (that is, dilution by a factor of 10). Hahnemann regularly used dilutions up to 300C but opined that "there must be a limit to the matter". A solution that is more dilute is described as having a higher "potency", and more dilute substances are considered by homeopaths to be stronger and deeper-acting. In

Hahnemann's time it was reasonable to assume that preparations could be diluted indefinitely, as the concept of the atom or molecule as the smallest possible unit of a chemical substance was just beginning to be recognized. We now know that the greatest dilution that is reasonably likely to contain one molecule of the original substance is 12C, if starting from 1 mole of original substance.

Some homeopaths developed a decimal scale (D or X), diluting the substance to ten times its original volume each stage. The D or X scale dilution is therefore half that of the same value of the C scale; for example, "12X" is the same level of dilution as "6C". Hahnemann never used this scale but it was very popular throughout the 19th century and still is in Europe. This potency scale appears to have been introduced in the 1830s by the American homeopath Constantine Hering. In the last ten years of his life, Hahnemann also developed a quintamillesimal (Q) or LM scale diluting the drug 1 part in 50,000 parts of diluent. A given dilution on the Q scale is roughly 2.35 times its designation on the C scale. For example, a preparation described as "20Q" has about the same concentration as one described with "47C".

Potencies of 1000C and above are usually labelled with Roman numeral M and with the centesimal 'C' indicator implied (since all such high potencies are centesimal dilutions): 1M = 1000C; 10M = 10,000C; CM = 100,000C; LM (which would indicate 50,000C) is typically not used because of confusion with the LM potency scale.

The following table is a synopsis comparing the X and C dilution scales and equating them by equivalent dilution. However, the homeopathic understanding of its principles is not explained by dilution but by "potentisation", hence one cannot assume that the different potencies can be equated on the basis of equivalence of dilution factors.

X Scale	C Scale	Ratio	Note
1X	–	1:10	Described as low potency
2X	1C	1:100	Called higher potency than 1X by homeopaths
6X	3C	10^{-6}	
8X	4C	10^{-8}	
12X	6C	10^{-12}	
24X	12C	10^{-24}	Has a 60% probability of containing one molecule of original material if one mole of the original substance was used.
26X	13C	10^{-26}	If pure water were used as the diluent, no molecules of the original solution remain in the water.
60X	30C	10^{-60}	Dilution advocated by Hahnemann for most purposes: on average, this would require giving two billion doses per second to six billion people for 4 billion years to deliver a single molecule of the original material to any patient.
400X	200C	10^{-400}	Dilution of popular homeopathic flu preparation Oscillococcinum

Common Homeopathic Medicines

These medicines should be taken in the 6th or 30th potency. Generally, if there is minor pain or discomfort, you should take the medicine three times a day, stopping once health has been restored. If there is more severe the pain, you can consider taking the medicine every one to three hours, decreasing the doses as symptoms are reduced. If you do not observe some improvement after 24 hours in an acute condition, the medicine is probably not the correct one. If symptoms persist, consider another medicine or seek professional homeopathic care.

It is generally recommended that people treat themselves for non-threatening acute conditions only and obtain professional care for chronic or potential dangerous health conditions.

- Allium cepa (onion): Because it is known to cause tearing of the eyes and dripping of the nose, it is a frequent remedy for the common cold and hay fever, especially when there is a thin, watery, and burning nasal discharge that irritates the nostrils. Typically, the person's symptoms are worse in a warm room and are relieved in a cool room or in the open air.

- Arnica (mountain daisy): This is the best remedy in sports medicine and first aid. It is used for shock and trauma from injury. It also helps to reduce pain from injury and to speed the healing process. Whether you're into competitive sports or exercise regularly or if you simply don't like to feel the pain of an injury, Arnica is the place to start.

- Arnica (topical): The above use of Arnica is for internal consumption, usually in pill or pellet form. Another way to use Arnica is in a topical external application in a gels, ointment, or spray form. This application of Arnica is great for healing sprains and strains as well as black and blue bruising (without broken skin).

- Chamomilla (chamomille): Many parents owe their sleep to homeopathy, not because it helps them directly, but because it is so good for their infant. Chamomilla is THE remedy for the irritable infant, especially from teething or colic. The infant cries incessantly, and nothing seems to provide any relief, except carrying them, and even then, the crying begins recurs as soon as the parent puts the child down.

- Hypericum (St. John's wort): This remedy is the first medicine to consider for injuries to the nerves or to parts of the body rich with them, including the fingers, toes, and back. Any injury with shooting pains should be given this remedy.

- Ignatia (St. Ignatius bean): One day this remedy will be used by the majority of psychiatrists. It is one of the leading homeopathic medicines for acute grief, anxiety, and depression, especially after a death or separation from a loved one. The person sighs frequently, has a lump in the throat, and may tremble.

- Magnesia phosphorica (phosphate of magnesia): This is the most effective remedy for cramps, including menstrual cramps. It has helped prevent many women turn from Dr. Jekkyl into Ms. Hyde as a result of menstrual cramps. It is particularly indicated when a woman's cramps cause her to bend over and when they experience some relief from warm applications.

- Nux vomica (poison nut): This is the premier medicine for ailments exacerbated by conventional or recreational drugs. It is also a common remedy for treating symptoms of overeating or from drinking too much alcohol. Considering how many people have these vices, this is an all too frequent medicine today.

- Pulsatilla (windflower): Perhaps the most common remedy given to children and women, this medicine is not indicated for a specific disease but for a specific pattern of physical symptoms and psychological characteristics. Physically, these people are warm-blooded: they wear fewer clothes than others, prefer open air, and don't feel as well in the heat. Psychologically, they are a gentle, mind, and yielding person, with a quickly changing emotional state and a strong tendency to want to please others.
- Rhus tox (poison ivy): This medicine is the most common remedy for sprains and strains. It is especially indicated when a person experiences a "rusty gate" syndrome, that is, pain on initial motion which is reduced the more the person continues to move. It is also often given to people with the flu or arthritis who experience this similar rusty gate syndrome.

References

- Understanding-of-Naturopathy-342643163: researchgate.net, Retrieved 02, August 2020
- Magnet-therapy: spineuniverse.com, Retrieved 18, February 2020
- Homeopathy-227861810: researchgate.net, Retrieved 20, May 2020
- Ten-common-homeopathic-medicines: homeopathic.com, Retrieved 16, March 2020

Chapter 6

Chiropractic Treatment

A form of alternative medicine that deals with the diagnosis and treatment of diseases related to the musculoskeletal system is referred to as chiropractic treatment. Some of the significant topics studied under chiropractic treatment are chiropractic treatment techniques, chiropractic criticism, spinal adjustment, etc. This chapter elaborates these topics in detail.

Chiropractic

Chiropractic is a form of alternative medicine concerned with the diagnosis and treatment of unproven mechanical disorders of the musculoskeletal system, especially the spine, under the belief that such a disorder affects general health via the nervous system. The main chiropractic treatment technique involves manual therapy, especially spinal manipulation therapy (SMT), manipulations of other joints and soft tissues. The "specific focus of chiropractic practice" is chiropractic subluxation, an unproven concept that has no scientific basis. Chiropractors often also offer conventional therapies such as physical therapy and lifestyle counseling, and it may for the lay person be difficult to distinguish the unscientific from the scientific. The underlying philosophy as well as certain practices employed by chiropractors are pseudoscience and anti-scientific.

Numerous controlled clinical studies of treatments used by chiropractors have been conducted, with conflicting results. Systematic reviews of this research have not found evidence that chiropractic manipulation is effective, with the possible exception of treatment for back pain. A critical evaluation found that collectively, spinal manipulation was ineffective at treating any condition. A Cochrane review found very low to moderate evidence that spinal manipulation therapy was any more effective than inert interventions, sham SMT or as an adjunct therapy for acute low back pain. Spinal manipulation may be cost-effective for sub-acute or chronic low back pain but the results for acute low back pain were insufficient. The efficacy and cost-effectiveness of maintenance chiropractic care are unknown. There is not sufficient data to establish the safety of chiropractic manipulations. The rate of adverse events is unknown as they are under–reported. It is frequently associated with mild to moderate adverse effects. The incidence of serious complications which can lead to permanent disability or death is probably rare. There is controversy regarding the degree of risk of vertebral artery dissection, which can lead to stroke and death, from cervical manipulation. Several deaths have been associated with this technique and it is suggested that the relationship is causative. This is disputed by many chiropractors who believe it is unproven.

Many chiropractors describe themselves as primary care providers, but the chiropractic clinical training does not support the requirements to be considered primary care providers, so their role on primary care is limited and disputed. Chiropractic is well established in the United States, Canada, and Australia. It overlaps with other manual-therapy professions, including massage therapy, osteopathy, and physical therapy. Most who seek chiropractic care do so for low back pain, and back and neck pain are considered the specialties of chiropractic, but many chiropractors treat ailments other than musculoskeletal issues. A considerable number of chiropractors fear that if they do not separate themselves from the traditional vitalistic concept of "innate intelligence", chiropractic will continue to be seen as a fringe profession. Chiropractic has two main groups: "straights", now the minority, emphasize vitalism, "innate intelligence" and spinal adjustments, and consider vertebral subluxations to be the cause of all disease; "mixers", the majority, are more open to mainstream views and conventional medical techniques, such as exercise, massage, and ice therapy.

D. D. Palmer founded chiropractic in the 1890s, and his son B. J. Palmer helped to expand it in the early 20th century. Throughout its history, chiropractic has been controversial. Its foundation is at odds with mainstream medicine, and has been sustained by pseudoscientific ideas such as subluxation and innate intelligence that are not based on sound science because they do not exist. Neither the concept of subluxation nor spinal manipulation has any scientific basis. It is classified as a field of pseudomedicine. Despite the overwhelming evidence that vaccination is an effective public health intervention, among chiropractors there are significant disagreements over the subject, which has led to negative impacts on both public vaccination and mainstream acceptance of chiropractic. The American Medical Association called chiropractic an "unscientific cult" in 1966 and boycotted it until losing an antitrust case in 1987. Chiropractic has had a strong political base and sustained demand for services; in recent decades, it has gained more legitimacy and greater acceptance among conventional physicians and health plans in the U.S., and evidence-based medicine has been used to review research studies and generate practice guidelines.

Conceptual Basis

Philosophy

Chiropractic is a form of alternative medicine which focuses on manipulation of the musculoskeletal system, especially the spine. Its founder, D.D. Palmer, called it "a science of healing without drugs".

Two chiropractic belief system constructs	
The testable principle	**The untestable metaphor**
Chiropractic adjustment ↓ Restoration of structural integrity ↓ Improvement of health status	Universal intelligence ↓ Innate intelligence ↓ Body physiology
Materialistic:	*Vitalistic:*
• Operational definitions possible • Lends itself to scientific inquiry	• Origin of holism in chiropractic • Cannot be proven or disproven
Taken from Mootz & Phillips 1997	

Chiropractic's origins lie in the folk medicine of bonesetting, and as it evolved it incorporated vitalism, spiritual inspiration and rationalism. Its early philosophy was based on deduction from irrefutable doctrine helped distinguish chiropractic from medicine, provided it with legal and political defenses against claims of practicing medicine without a license, and allowed chiropractors to establish themselves as an autonomous profession. This "straight" philosophy, taught to generations of chiropractors, rejects the inferential reasoning of the scientific method, and relies on deductions from vitalistic first principles rather than on the materialism of science. However, most practitioners tend to incorporate scientific research into chiropractic, and most practitioners are "mixers" who attempt to combine the materialistic reductionism of science with the metaphysics of their predecessors and with the holistic paradigm of wellness. A 2008 commentary proposed that chiropractic actively divorce itself from the straight philosophy as part of a campaign to eliminate untestable dogma and engage in critical thinking and evidence-based research.

Although a wide diversity of ideas exist among chiropractors, they share the belief that the spine and health are related in a fundamental way, and that this relationship is mediated through the nervous system. Some chiropractors claim spinal manipulation can have an effect of a variety of ailments such as irritable bowel syndrome and asthma.

Chiropractic Philosophy Includes The Following Perspectives:

Holism assumes that health is affected by everything in an individual's environment; some sources also include a spiritual or existential dimension. In contrast, reductionism in chiropractic reduces causes and cures of health problems to a single factor, vertebral subluxation. Homeostasis emphasizes the body's inherent self-healing abilities. Chiropractic's early notion of innate intelligence can be thought of as a metaphor for homeostasis.

A variant of chiropractic called naprapathy originated in Chicago in the early twentieth century. It holds that manual manipulation of soft tissue can reduce "interference" in the body and thus improve health.

Straights and Mixers

Range of belief perspectives in chiropractic		
Perspective attribute	**Potential belief endpoints**	
Scope of practice:	narrow ("straight") ←	→ broad ("mixer")
Diagnostic approach:	intuitive ←	→ analytical
Philosophic orientation:	vitalistic ←	→ materialistic
Scientific orientation:	descriptive ←	→ experimental
Process orientation:	implicit ←	→ explicit
Practice attitude:	doctor/model-centered ←	→ patient/situation-centered
Professional integration:	separate and distinct ←	→ integrated into mainstream
Taken from Mootz & Phillips 1997		

Straight chiropractors adhere to the philosophical principles set forth by D.D. and B.J. Palmer, and retain metaphysical definitions and vitalistic qualities. Straight chiropractors believe that vertebral subluxation leads to interference with an "innate intelligence" exerted via the human nervous system and is a primary underlying risk factor for many diseases. Straights view the medical diagnosis of patient complaints (which they consider to be the "secondary effects" of subluxations) to be unnecessary for chiropractic treatment. Thus, straight chiropractors are concerned primarily with the detection and correction of vertebral subluxation via adjustment and do not "mix" other types of therapies into their practice style. Their philosophy and explanations are metaphysical in nature and they prefer to use traditional chiropractic lexicon terminology (e.g., perform spinal analysis, detect subluxation, correct with adjustment). They prefer to remain separate and distinct from mainstream health care. Although considered the minority group, "they have been able to transform their status as purists and heirs of the lineage into influence dramatically out of proportion to their numbers."

Mixer chiropractors "mix" diagnostic and treatment approaches from chiropractic, medical and/or osteopathic viewpoints and make up the majority of chiropractors. Unlike straight chiropractors, mixers believe subluxation is one of many causes of disease, and hence they tend to be open to mainstream medicine. Many of them incorporate mainstream medical diagnostics and employ conventional treatments including techniques of physical therapy such as exercise, stretching, massage, ice packs, electrical muscle stimulation, therapeutic ultrasound, and moist heat. Some mixers also use techniques from alternative medicine, including nutritional supplements, acupuncture, homeopathy, herbal remedies, and biofeedback.

Although mixers are the majority group, many of them retain belief in vertebral subluxation as shown in a 2003 survey of 1100 North American chiropractors, which found that 88% wanted to retain the term "vertebral subluxation complex", and that when asked to estimate the percent of disorders of internal organs (such as the heart, the lungs, or the stomach) that subluxation significantly contributes to, the mean response was 62%. A 2008 survey of 6,000 American chiropractors demonstrated that most chiropractors seem to believe that a subluxation-based clinical approach may be of limited utility for addressing visceral disorders, and greatly favored non-subluxation-based clinical approaches for such conditions. The same survey showed that most chiropractors generally believed that the majority of their clinical approach for addressing musculoskeletal/biomechanical disorders such as back pain was based on subluxation.

Vertebral Subluxation

Palmer hypothesized that vertebral joint misalignments, which he termed *vertebral subluxations*, interfered with the body's function and its inborn ability to heal itself. D. D. Palmer repudiated his earlier theory that vertebral subluxations caused pinched nerves in the intervertebral spaces in favor of subluxations causing altered nerve vibration, either too tense or too slack, affecting the tone (health) of the end organ. D. D. Palmer, using a vitalistic approach, imbued the term *subluxation* with a metaphysical and philosophical meaning. He qualified this by noting that knowledge of innate intelligence was not essential to the competent practice of chiropractic. This concept was later expanded upon by his son, B. J. Palmer, and was instrumental in providing the legal basis of differentiating chiropractic from conventional medicine. In 1910, D. D. Palmer theorized that the nervous system controlled health:

> "Physiologists divide nerve-fibers, which form the nerves, into two classes, afferent and efferent. Impressions are made on the peripheral afferent fiber-endings; these create sensations that are transmitted to the center of the nervous system. Efferent nerve-fibers carry

impulses out from the center to their endings. Most of these go to muscles and are therefore called motor impulses; some are secretory and enter glands; a portion are inhibitory, their function being to restrain secretion. Thus, nerves carry impulses outward and sensations inward. The activity of these nerves, or rather their fibers, may become excited or allayed by impingement, the result being a modification of functionality—too much or not enough action—which is disease."

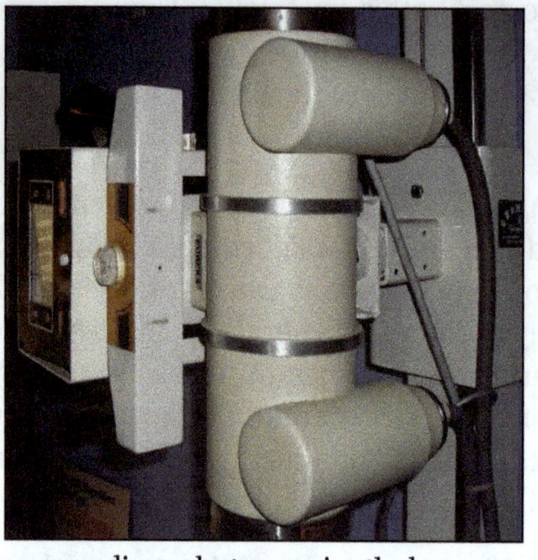

Chiropractors use x-ray radiography to examine the bone structure of a patient.

Vertebral subluxation, a core concept of traditional chiropractic, remains unsubstantiated and largely untested, and a debate about whether to keep it in the chiropractic paradigm has been ongoing for decades. In general, critics of traditional subluxation-based chiropractic (including chiropractors) are skeptical of its clinical value, dogmatic beliefs and metaphysical approach. While straight chiropractic still retains the traditional vitalistic construct espoused by the founders, evidence-based chiropractic suggests that a mechanistic view will allow chiropractic care to become integrated into the wider health care community. This is still a continuing source of debate within the chiropractic profession as well, with some schools of chiropractic still teaching the traditional/straight subluxation-based chiropractic, while others have moved towards an evidence-based chiropractic that rejects metaphysical foundings and limits itself to primarily neuromusculoskeletal conditions.

In 2005, the chiropractic subluxation was defined by the World Health Organization as "a lesion or dysfunction in a joint or motion segment in which alignment, movement integrity and/or physiological function are altered, although contact between joint surfaces remains intact. It is essentially a functional entity, which may influence biomechanical and neural integrity." This differs from the medical definition of subluxation as a significant structural displacement, which can be seen with static imaging techniques such as X-rays. The 2008 book *Trick or Treatment* states "X-rays can reveal neither the subluxations nor the innate intelligence associated with chiropractic philosophy, because they do not exist." Attorney David Chapman-Smith, Secretary-General of the World Federation of Chiropractic, has stated that "Medical critics have asked how there can be a subluxation if it cannot be seen on x-ray. The answer is that the chiropractic subluxation is essentially a functional entity, not structural, and is therefore no more visible on static x-ray than a limp or headache or any other functional problem." The General Chiropractic Council, the statutory regulatory body for chiropractors in the United Kingdom, states that the chiropractic vertebral subluxation complex "is not supported by any clinical research evidence that would allow claims to be made that it is the cause of disease."

As of 2014, the National Board of Chiropractic Examiners states "The specific focus of chiropractic practice is known as the chiropractic subluxation or joint dysfunction. A subluxation is a health concern that manifests in the skeletal joints, and, through complex anatomical and physiological relationships, affects the nervous system and may lead to reduced function, disability or illness."

Scope of Practice

Chiropractors emphasize the conservative management of the neuromusculoskeletal system without the use of medicines or surgery, with special emphasis on the spine. Back and neck pain are the specialties of chiropractic but many chiropractors treat ailments other than musculoskeletal issues. There is a range of opinions among chiropractors: some believed that treatment should be confined to the spine, or back and neck pain; others disagreed. For example, while one 2009 survey of American chiropractors had found that 73% classified themselves as "back pain/musculoskeletal specialists", the label "back and neck pain specialists" was regarded by 47% of them as a *least* desirable description in a 2005 international survey. Chiropractic combines aspects from mainstream and alternative medicine, and there is no agreement about how to define the profession: although chiropractors have many attributes of primary care providers, chiropractic has more of the attributes of a medical specialty like dentistry or podiatry. It has been proposed that chiropractors specialize in nonsurgical spine care, instead of attempting to also treat other problems, but the more expansive view of chiropractic is still widespread. Mainstream health care and governmental organizations such as the World Health Organization consider chiropractic to be complementary and alternative medicine (CAM); and a 2008 study reported that 31% of surveyed chiropractors categorized chiropractic as CAM, 27% as integrated medicine, and 12% as mainstream medicine. Many chiropractors believe they are primary care providers, including US and UK chiropractors, but the length, breadth, and depth of chiropractic clinical training do not support the requirements to be considered primary care providers, so their role on primary care is limited and disputed.

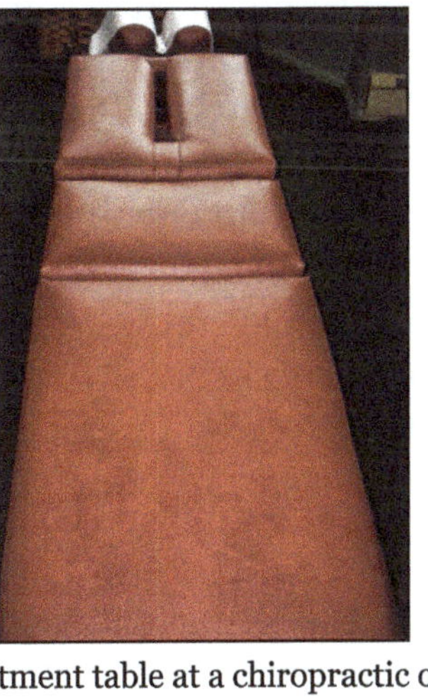

A treatment table at a chiropractic office.

Chiropractic overlaps with several other forms of manual therapy, including massage therapy, osteopathy, physical therapy, and sports medicine. Chiropractic is autonomous from and competitive with mainstream medicine, and osteopathy outside the US remains primarily a manual medical system; physical therapists work alongside and cooperate with mainstream medicine, and osteopathic medicine in the U.S. has merged with the medical profession. Practitioners may distinguish these competing approaches through claims that, compared to other therapists, chiropractors heavily emphasize spinal manipulation, tend to use firmer manipulative techniques, and promote maintenance care; that osteopaths use a wider variety of treatment procedures; and that physical therapists emphasize machinery and exercise.

Chiropractic diagnosis may involve a range of methods including skeletal imaging, observational and tactile assessments, and orthopedic and neurological evaluation. A chiropractor may also refer a patient to an appropriate specialist, or co-manage with another health care provider. Common patient management involves spinal manipulation (SM) and other manual therapies to the joints and soft tissues, rehabilitative exercises, health promotion, electrical modalities, complementary procedures, and lifestyle advice.

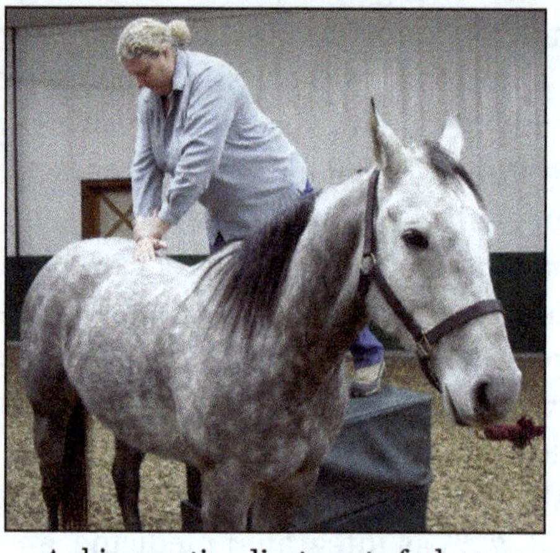

A chiropractic adjustment of a horse.

Chiropractors are not normally licensed to write medical prescriptions or perform major surgery in the United States, (although New Mexico has become the first US state to allow "advanced practice" trained chiropractors to prescribe certain medications.). In the US, their scope of practice varies by state, based on inconsistent views of chiropractic care: some states, such as Iowa, broadly allow treatment of "human ailments"; some, such as Delaware, use vague concepts such as "transition of nerve energy" to define scope of practice; others, such as New Jersey, specify a severely narrowed scope. US states also differ over whether chiropractors may conduct laboratory tests or diagnostic procedures, dispense dietary supplements, or use other therapies such as homeopathy and acupuncture; in Oregon they can become certified to perform minor surgery and to deliver children via natural childbirth. A 2003 survey of North American chiropractors found that a slight majority favored allowing them to write prescriptions for over-the-counter drugs. A 2010 survey found 72% of Switzerland chiropractors judged the current allowance in Switzerland to prescribing nonprescription medication as an advantage for chiropractic treatment.

A related field, veterinary chiropractic, applies manual therapies to animals and is recognized in 40 US states, but is not recognized by the American Chiropractic Association as being chiropractic. It remains controversial within certain segments of the veterinary, and chiropractic profession.

No single profession "owns" spinal manipulation and there is little consensus as to which profession should administer SM, raising concerns by chiropractors that other medical physicians could "steal" SM procedures from chiropractors. A focus on evidence-based SM research has also raised concerns that the resulting practice guidelines could limit the scope of chiropractic practice to treating backs and necks. Two U.S. states (Washington and Arkansas) prohibit physical therapists from performing SM, some states allow them to do it only if they have completed advanced training in SM, and some states allow only chiropractors to perform SM, or only chiropractors and physicians. Bills to further prohibit non-chiropractors from performing SM are regularly introduced into state legislatures and are opposed by physical therapist organizations.

Treatments

Spinal manipulation, which chiropractors call "spinal adjustment" or "chiropractic adjustment", is the most common treatment used in chiropractic care. Spinal manipulation is a passive manual maneuver during which a three-joint complex is taken past the normal range of movement, but not so far as to dislocate or damage the joint. Its defining factor is a dynamic thrust, which is a sudden force that causes an audible release and attempts to increase a joint's range of motion. High-velocity, low-amplitude spinal manipulation (HVLA-SM) thrusts have physiological effects that signal neural discharge from paraspinal muscle tissues, depending on duration and amplitude of the thrust are factors of the degree in paraspinal muscle spindles activation. Clinical skill in employing HVLA-SM thrusts depends on the ability of the practitioner to handle the duration and magnitude of the load. More generally, spinal manipulative therapy (SMT) describes techniques where the hands are used to manipulate, massage, mobilize, adjust, stimulate, apply traction to, or otherwise influence the spine and related tissues.

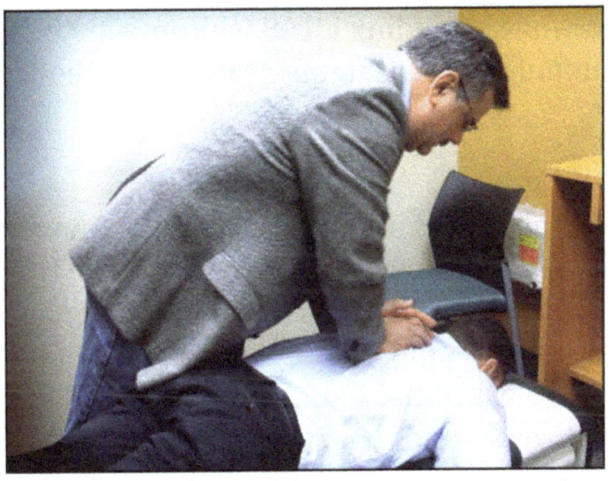

A chiropractor performs an adjustment on a patient.

There are several schools of chiropractic adjustive techniques, although most chiropractors mix techniques from several schools. The following adjustive procedures were received by more than 10% of patients of licensed U.S. chiropractors in a 2003 survey: Diversified technique (full-spine manipulation, employing various techniques), extremity adjusting, Activator technique (which uses a spring-loaded tool to deliver precise adjustments to the spine), Thompson Technique (which relies on a drop table and detailed procedural protocols), Gonstead (which emphasizes evaluating the spine along with specific adjustment that avoids rotational vectors), Cox/flexion-distraction (a gentle, low-force adjusting procedure which mixes chiropractic with osteopathic principles and utilizes specialized adjusting tables with movable parts), adjustive instrument, Sacro-Occipital Technique (which models the spine as a torsion bar), Nimmo Receptor-Tonus Technique, applied kinesiology (which emphasises "muscle testing" as a diagnostic tool), and cranial. Chiropractic biophysics technique uses inverse functions of rotations during spinal manipulation. Koren Specific Technique (KST) may use their hands, or they may use an electric device known as an "ArthroStim" for assessment and spinal manipulations. Insurers in the US and UK that cover other chiropractic techniques exclude KST from coverage because they consider it to be "experimental and investigational." Medicine-assisted manipulation, such as manipulation under anesthesia, involves sedation or local anesthetic and is done by a team that includes an anesthesiologist; a 2008 systematic review did not find enough evidence to make recommendations about its use for chronic low back pain.

Many other procedures are used by chiropractors for treating the spine, other joints and tissues, and general health issues. The following procedures were received by more than one-third of patients of licensed U.S. chiropractors in a 2003 survey: Diversified technique (full-spine manipulation; mentioned in previous paragraph), physical fitness/exercise promotion, corrective or therapeutic exercise, ergonomic/postural advice, self-care strategies, activities of daily living, changing risky/unhealthy behaviors, nutritional/dietary recommendations, relaxation/stress reduction recommendations, ice pack/cryotherapy, extremity adjusting (also mentioned in previous paragraph), trigger point therapy, and disease prevention/early screening advice.

A 2010 study describing Belgium chiropractors and their patients found chiropractors in Belgium mostly focus on neuromusculoskeletal complaints in adult patients, with emphasis on the spine. The diversified technique is the most often applied technique at 93%, followed by the Activator mechanical-assisted technique at 41%. A 2009 study assessing chiropractic students giving or receiving spinal manipulations while attending a U.S. chiropractic college found Diversified, Gonstead, and upper cervical manipulations are frequently used methods.

Practice Guidelines

Reviews of research studies within the chiropractic community have been used to generate practice guidelines outlining standards that specify which chiropractic treatments are "legitimate" (i.e. supported by evidence) and conceivably reimbursable under managed care health payment systems. Evidence-based guidelines are supported by one end of an ideological continuum among chiropractors; the other end employs antiscientific reasoning and makes unsubstantiated claims. Chiropractic remains at a crossroads, and that in order to progress it would need to embrace science; the promotion by some for it to be a cure-all was both "misguided and irrational". A 2007 survey of Alberta chiropractors found that they do not consistently apply research in practice, which may have resulted from a lack of research education and skills.

Effectiveness

There is no good evidence that chiropractic is effective for the treatment of any medical condition, except perhaps for certain kinds of back pain. Generally, the research carried out into the effectiveness of chiropractic has been of poor quality. Numerous controlled clinical studies of treatments used by chiropractors have been conducted, with conflicting results. Research published by chiropractors is distinctly biased. For reviews of SM for back pain chiropractic authors tend to have positive conclusions, while others did not show any effectiveness.

There is a wide range of ways to measure treatment outcomes. Chiropractic care, like all medical treatment, benefits from the placebo response. It is difficult to construct a trustworthy placebo for clinical trials of spinal manipulative therapy (SMT), as experts often disagree about whether a proposed placebo actually has no effect. The efficacy of maintenance care in chiropractic is unknown.

Available evidence covers the following conditions:

- Low back pain: A 2013 Cochrane review found very low to moderate evidence that SMT was no more effective than inert interventions, sham SMT or as an adjunct therapy for acute low back pain. The same review found that SMT appears to be no better than other recommended therapies. A 2012 overview of systematic reviews found that collectively, SM failed to show it is an effective intervention for pain. A 2011 Cochrane review found strong evidence that suggests there is no clinically meaningful difference between SMT and other treatments for reducing pain and improving function for chronic low back pain. A 2010 Cochrane review found no current evidence to support or refute a clinically significant difference between the effects of combined chiropractic interventions and other interventions for chronic or mixed duration low back pain. A 2010 systematic review found that most studies suggest SMT achieves equivalent or superior improvement in pain and function when compared with other commonly used interventions for short, intermediate, and long-term follow-up. Specific guidelines concerning the treatment of nonspecific (i.e. unknown cause) low back pain are inconsistent between countries.

- Radiculopathy: A 2013 systematic review and meta-analysis found a statistically significant improvement in overall recovery from sciatica following SM, when compared to usual care, and suggested that SM may be considered. There is moderate quality evidence to support the use of SM for the treatment of acute lumbar radiculopathy and acute lumbar disc herniation with associated radiculopathy. There is low or very low evidence supporting SM for chronic lumbar spine-related extremity symptoms and cervical spine-related extremity symptoms of any duration and no evidence exists for the treatment of thoracic radiculopathy.

- Whiplash and other neck pain: There is no consensus on the effectiveness of manual therapies for neck pain. A 2013 systematic review found that the data suggests that there are minimal short- and long-term treatment differences when comparing manipulation or mobilization of the cervical spine to physical therapy or exercise for neck pain improvement. A 2013 systematic review found that although there is insufficient evidence that thoracic SM is more effective than other treatments, it is a suitable intervention to treat some patients with non-specific neck pain. A 2011 systematic review found that thoracic SM may offer short-term improvement for the treatment of acute or subacute mechanical neck pain; although the body of literature is still weak. A 2010 Cochrane review found low quality evidence that suggests cervical manipulation may offer better short-term pain relief than a control for neck pain, and moderate evidence that cervical manipulation and mobilization produced similar effects on pain, function and patient satisfaction. A 2010 systematic review found low level evidence that suggests chiropractic care improves cervical range of motion and pain in the management of whiplash.

- Headache: A 2011 systematic review found evidence that suggests that chiropractic SMT might be as effective as propranolol or topiramate in the prevention of migraine headaches.

A 2011 systematic review found evidence that does not support the use of SM for the treatment of migraine headaches. A 2006 review found no rigorous evidence supporting SM or other manual therapies for tension headache. A 2005 review found that the evidence was weak for effectiveness of chiropractic manipulation for tension headache, and that it was probably more effective for tension headache than for migraine. A 2004 Cochrane review found evidence that suggests SM may be effective for migraine, tension headache and cervicogenic headache.

- Extremity conditions: A 2011 systematic review and meta-analysis concluded that the addition of manual mobilizations to an exercise program for the treatment of knee osteoarthritis resulted in better pain relief then a supervised exercise program alone and suggested that manual therapists consider adding manual mobilisation to optimise supervised active exercise programs. There is silver level evidence that manual therapy is more effective than exercise for the treatment of hip osteoarthritis, however this evidence could be considered to be inconclusive. A 2008 systematic review found that the addition of cervical spine mobilization to a treatment regimen for lateral epicondylosis (tennis elbow) resulted in significantly better pain relief and functional improvements in both the short and long-term. There is a small amount of research into the efficacy of chiropractic treatment for upper limbs, limited to low level evidence supporting chiropractic management of shoulder pain and limited or fair evidence supporting chiropractic management of leg conditions.

- Other: A 2012 systematic review found insufficient low bias evidence to support the use of spinal manipulation as a therapy for the treatment of hypertension. A 2011 systematic review found moderate evidence to support the use of manual therapy for cervicogenic dizziness. There is very weak evidence for chiropractic care for adult scoliosis (curved or rotated spine) and no scientific data for idiopathic adolescent scoliosis. A 2007 systematic review found that few studies of chiropractic care for nonmusculoskeletal conditions are available, and they are typically not of high quality; it also found that the entire clinical encounter of chiropractic care (as opposed to just SM) provides benefit to patients with cervicogenic dizziness, and that the evidence from reviews is negative, or too weak to draw conclusions, for a wide variety of other nonmusculoskeletal conditions, including ADHD/learning disabilities, dizziness, high blood pressure, and vision conditions. Other reviews have found no evidence of significant benefit for asthma, baby colic, bedwetting, carpal tunnel syndrome, fibromyalgia, gastrointestinal disorders, kinetic imbalance due to suboccipital strain (KISS) in infants, menstrual cramps, or pelvic and back pain during pregnancy.

Safety

There is not sufficient data to establish the safety of chiropractic manipulations. Manipulation is regarded as relatively safe but complications can arise, and it has known adverse effects, risks and contraindications. Absolute contraindications to spinal manipulative therapy are conditions that should not be manipulated; these contraindications include rheumatoid arthritis and conditions known to result in unstable joints. Relative contraindications are conditions where increased risk is acceptable in some situations and where low-force and soft-tissue techniques are treatments of choice; these contraindications include osteoporosis. Although most contraindications apply only to manipulation of the affected region, some neurological signs indicate referral to emergency medical services; these include sudden and severe headache or neck pain unlike that previously experienced. Indirect risks of chiropractic involve delayed or missed diagnoses through consulting a chiropractor.

Spinal manipulation is associated with frequent, mild and temporary adverse effects, including new or worsening pain or stiffness in the affected region. They have been estimated to occur in 33% to 61% of patients, and frequently occur within an hour of treatment and disappear within 24 to 48 hours; adverse reactions appear to be more common following manipulation than mobilization. Chiropractic is correlated with a very high incidence of minor adverse effects. Chiropractic are more commonly associated with serious related adverse effects than other professionals following manipulation. Rarely, spinal manipulation, particularly on the upper spine, can also result in complications that can lead to permanent disability or death; these can occur in adults and children. Estimates vary widely for the incidence of these complications, and the actual incidence is unknown, due to high levels of underreporting and to the difficulty of linking manipulation to adverse effects such as stroke, which is a particular concern. Adverse effects are poorly reported in recent studies investigating chiropractic manipulations. A 2016 systematic review concludes that the level of reporting is unsuitable and unacceptable. Reports of serious adverse events have occurred, resulting from spinal manipulation therapy of the lumbopelvic region. Estimates for serious adverse events vary from 5 strokes per 100,000 manipulations to 1.46 serious adverse events per 10 million manipulations and 2.68 deaths per 10 million manipulations, though it was determined that there was inadequate data to be conclusive. Several case reports show temporal associations between interventions and potentially serious complications. The published medical literature contains reports of 26 deaths since 1934 following chiropractic manipulations and many more seem to remain unpublished.

Vertebrobasilar artery stroke (VAS) is statistically associated with chiropractic services in persons under 45 years of age, but it is similarly associated with general practitioner services, suggesting that these associations are likely explained by preexisting conditions. Weak to moderately strong evidence supports causation (as opposed to statistical association) between cervical manipulative therapy (CMT) and VAS. There is insufficient evidence to support a strong association or no association between cervical manipulation and stroke. While the biomechanical evidence is not sufficient to support the statement that CMT causes cervical artery dissection (CD), clinical reports suggest that mechanical forces have a part in a substantial number of CDs and the majority of population controlled studies found an association between CMT and VAS in young people. It is strongly recommended that practitioners consider the plausibility of CD as a symptom, and people can be informed of the association between CD and CMT before administrating manipulation of the cervical spine. There is controversy regarding the degree of risk of stroke from cervical manipulation. Many chiropractors state that, the association between chiropractic therapy and vertebral arterial dissection is not proven. However, it has been suggested that the causality between chiropractic cervical manipulation beyond the normal range of motion and vascular accidents is probable or definite. There is very low evidence supporting a small association between internal carotid artery dissection and chiropractic neck manipulation. The incidence of internal carotid artery dissection following cervical spine manipulation is unknown. The literature infrequently reports helpful data to better understand the association between cervical manipulative therapy, cervical artery dissection and stroke. The limited evidence is inconclusive that chiropractic spinal manipulation therapy is not a cause of intracranial hypotension.

Chiropractors, like other primary care providers, sometimes employ diagnostic imaging techniques such as X-rays and CT scans that rely on ionizing radiation. Although there is no clear evidence for the practice, some chiropractors may still X-ray a patient several times a year. Practice guidelines aim to reduce unnecessary radiation exposure, which increases cancer risk in proportion to the amount of radiation received. Research suggests that radiology instruction given at chiropractic schools worldwide seem to be evidence-based. Although, there seems to be a disparity between some schools and available evidence regarding the aspect of radiography for patients with acute low back pain without an indication of a serious disease, which may contribute to chiropractic overuse of radiography for low back pain.

Risk-benefit

A 2012 systematic review concluded that no accurate assessment of risk-benefit exists for cervical manipulation. A 2010 systematic review stated that there is no good evidence to assume that neck manipulation is an effective treatment for any medical condition and suggested a precautionary principle in healthcare for chiropractic intervention even if a causality with vertebral artery dissection after neck manipulation were merely a remote possibility. The same review concluded that the risk of death from manipulations to the neck outweighs the benefits. Chiropractors have criticized this conclusion, claiming that the author did not evaluate the potential benefits of spinal manipulation. Edzard Ernst stated "This detail was not the subject of my review. I do, however, refer to such evaluations and should add that a report recently commissioned by the General Chiropractic Council did not support many of the outlandish claims made by many chiropractors across the world."

A 2009 review evaluating maintenance chiropractic care found that spinal manipulation is routinely associated with considerable harm and no compelling evidence exists to indicate that it adequately prevents symptoms or diseases, thus the risk-benefit is not evidently favorable.

Cost-effectiveness

A 2012 systematic review suggested that the use of spine manipulation in clinical practice is a cost-effective treatment when used alone or in combination with other treatment approaches. A 2011 systematic review found evidence supporting the cost-effectiveness of using spinal manipulation for the treatment of sub-acute or chronic low back pain; the results for acute low back pain were insufficient.

A 2006 systematic cost-effectiveness review found that the reported cost-effectiveness of spinal manipulation in the United Kingdom compared favorably with other treatments for back pain, but that reports were based on data from clinical trials without sham controls and that the specific cost-effectiveness of the treatment (as opposed to non-specific effects) remains uncertain. A 2005 American systematic review of economic evaluations of conservative treatments for low back pain found that significant quality problems in available studies meant that definite conclusions could not be drawn about the most cost-effective intervention. The cost-effectiveness of maintenance chiropractic care is unknown.

Analysis of a clinical and cost utilization data from the years 2003 to 2005 by an integrative medicine independent physician association (IPA) which looked the chiropractic services utilization found that the clinical and cost utilization of chiropractic services based on 70,274 member-months over a 7-year period decreased patient costs associate with the following use of services by 60.2% for in-hospital admissions, 59.0% for hospital days, 62.0% for outpatient surgeries and procedures, and 85% for pharmaceutical costs when compared with conventional medicine (visit to a medical doctor primary care provider) IPA performance for the same health maintenance organization product in the same geography and time frame.

Education, Licensing, and Regulation

Requirements vary between countries. In the U.S. chiropractors obtain a first professional degree in the field of chiropractic. Chiropractic education in the U.S. have been criticized for failing to meet generally accepted standards of evidence-based medicine. The curriculum content of North American chiropractic and medical colleges with regard to basic and clinical sciences has been more similar than not, both in the kinds of subjects offered and in the time assigned to each subject. Accredited chiropractic programs in the U.S. require that applicants have 90 semester hours of undergraduate education with a grade point average of at least 3.0 on a 4.0 scale. Many programs require at least three years of undergraduate education, and more are requiring a bachelor's degree. Canada requires a minimum three years of undergraduate education for applicants, and at least 4200 instructional hours (or the equivalent) of full□time chiropractic education for matriculation through an accredited chiropractic program. Graduates of the Canadian Memorial Chiropractic College (CMCC) are formally recognized to have at least 7–8 years of university level education. The World Health Organization (WHO) guidelines suggest three major full-time educational paths culminating in either a DC, DCM, BSc, or MSc degree. Besides the full-time paths, they also suggest a conversion program for people with other health care education and limited training programs for regions where no legislation governs chiropractic.

Upon graduation, there may be a requirement to pass national, state, or provincial board examinations before being licensed to practice in a particular jurisdiction. Depending on the location, continuing education may be required to renew these licenses. Specialty training is available through part-time postgraduate education programs such as chiropractic orthopedics and sports chiropractic, and through full-time residency programs such as radiology or orthopedics.

In the U.S., chiropractic schools are accredited through the Council on Chiropractic Education (CCE) while the General Chiropractic Council (GCC) is the statutory governmental body responsible for the regulation of chiropractic in the UK. The U.S. CCE requires a mixing curriculum, which means a straight-educated chiropractor may not be eligible for licensing in states requiring CCE accreditation. CCEs in the U.S., Canada, Australia and Europe have joined to form CCE-International (CCE-I) as a model of accreditation standards with the goal of having credentials portable internationally. Today, there are 18 accredited Doctor of Chiropractic programs in the U.S., 2 in Canada, 6 in Australasia, and 5 in Europe. All but one of the chiropractic colleges in the U.S. are privately funded, but in several other countries they are in government-sponsored universities and colleges. Of the two chiropractic colleges in Canada, one is publicly funded (UQTR) and one is privately funded (CMCC). In 2005, CMCC was granted the privilege of offering a professional health care degree under the Post-secondary Education Choice and Excellence Act, which sets the program within the hierarchy of education in Canada as comparable to that of other primary contact health care professions such as medicine, dentistry and optometry.

Regulatory colleges and chiropractic boards in the U.S., Canada, Mexico, and Australia are responsible for protecting the public, standards of practice, disciplinary issues, quality assurance and maintenance of competency. There are an estimated 49,000 chiropractors in the U.S. (2008), 6,500 in Canada (2010), 2,500 in Australia (2000), and 1,500 in the UK (2000).

Chiropractors often argue that this education is as good as or better than medical physicians', but most chiropractic training is confined to classrooms with much time spent learning theory, adjustment, and marketing. The fourth year of chiropractic education persistently showed the highest stress levels. Every student, irrespective of year, experienced different ranges of stress when studying. The chiropractic leaders and colleges have had internal struggles. Rather than cooperation, there has been infighting between different factions. A number of actions were posturing due to the confidential nature of the chiropractic colleges in an attempt to enroll students.

Ethics

The chiropractic oath is a modern variation of the classical Hippocratic Oath historically taken by physicians and other healthcare professionals swearing to practice their professions ethically. The American Chiropractic Association (ACA) has an ethical code "based upon the acknowledgement that the social contract dictates the profession's responsibilities to the patient, the public, and the profession; and upholds the fundamental principle that the paramount purpose of the chiropractic doctor's professional services shall be to benefit the patient." The International Chiropractor's Association (ICA) also has a set of professional canons.

A 2008 commentary proposed that the chiropractic profession actively regulate itself to combat abuse, fraud, and quackery, which are more prevalent in chiropractic than in other health care professions, violating the social contract between patients and physicians. According to a 2015 Gallup poll of U.S. adults, the perception of chiropractors is generally favourable; two-thirds of American adults agree that chiropractors have their patient's best interest in mind and more than half also agree that most chiropractors are trustworthy. Less than 10% of US adults disagreed with the statement that chiropractors were trustworthy.

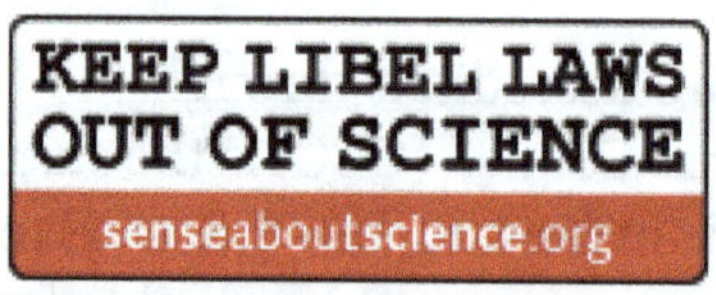

The charity Sense About Science launched a campaign to draw attention to this particular legal case against science writer Simon Singh. In 2009, a number of organizations and public figures signed a statement entitled "The law has no place in scientific disputes".

Chiropractors, especially in America, have a reputation for unnecessarily treating patients. In many circumstances the focus seems to be put on economics instead of health care. Sustained chiropractic care is promoted as a preventative tool, but unnecessary manipulation could possibly present a risk to patients. Some chiropractors are concerned by the routine unjustified claims chiropractors have made. A 2010 analysis of chiropractic websites found the majority of chiropractors and their associations made claims of effectiveness not supported by scientific evidence, while 28% of chiropractor websites advocate lower back pain care, which has some sound evidence.

In 2009, a backlash to the libel suit filed by the British Chiropractic Association (BCA) against Simon Singh, has inspired the filing of formal complaints of false advertising against more than 500 individual chiropractors within one 24-hour period, prompting the McTimoney Chiropractic Association to write to its members advising them to remove leaflets that make claims about whiplash and colic from their practice, to be wary of new patients and telephone inquiries, and telling their members: "If you have a website, take it down NOW." and "Finally, we strongly suggest you do NOT discuss this with others, especially patients." An editorial in *Nature* has suggested that the BCA may be trying to suppress debate and that this use of British libel law is a burden on the right to freedom of expression, which is protected by the European Convention on Human Rights. The libel case ended with the BCA withdrawing its suit in 2010.

Reception

Chiropractic is established in the US, Canada, and Australia, and is present to a lesser extent in many other countries. It is viewed as a marginal complementary and alternative medicine health care profession.

Australia

In Australia, most private health insurance funds cover chiropractic care, and the federal government funds chiropractic care when the patient is referred by a medical practitioner.

United Kingdom

In the United Kingdom chiropractic is available on the National Health Service in some areas, such as Cornwall where the treatment is only available for neck or back pain.

A 2010 study by questionnaire presented to UK chiropractors indicated only 45% of chiropractors disclosed with patients the serious risk associated with manipulation of the cervical spine and that 46% believed there was possibility of patient would refuse treatment if risk correctly explained. However 80% acknowledged the ethical/moral responsibility to disclose risk to patient.

United States and Canada

The percentage of the population that utilizes chiropractic care at any given time generally falls into a range from 6% to 12% in the U.S. and Canada, with a global high of 20% in Alberta in 2006. In 2008, chiropractors were reported to be the most common CAM providers for children and adolescents, consuming up to 14% of all visits to chiropractors. In 2002–03, the majority of those who sought chiropractic did so for relief from back and neck pain and other neuromusculoskeletal complaints; most do so specifically for low back pain. The majority of U.S. chiropractors participate in some form of managed care. Although the majority of U.S. chiropractors view themselves as specialists in neuroleptic malignant syndrome conditions, many also consider chiropractic as a type of primary care. In the majority of cases, the care that chiropractors and physicians provide divides the market, however for some, their care is complementary.

In the U.S., chiropractors perform over 90% of all manipulative treatments. Satisfaction rates are typically higher for chiropractic care compared to medical care, with a 1998 U.S. survey reporting

83% of respondents satisfied or very satisfied with their care; quality of communication seems to be a consistent predictor of patient satisfaction with chiropractors.

Utilization of chiropractic care is sensitive to the costs incurred by the co-payment by the patient. The use of chiropractic declined from 9.9% of U.S. adults in 1997 to 7.4% in 2002; this was the largest relative decrease among CAM professions, which overall had a stable use rate. As of 2007 7% of the U.S. population is being reached by chiropractic. Employment of U.S. chiropractors is expected to increase 14% between 2006 and 2016, faster than the average for all occupations.

In the U.S., most states require insurers to cover chiropractic care, and most HMOs cover these services.

History

Early chiropractors believed that all disease was caused by interruptions in the flow of innate intelligence, a vitalistic nervous energy or life force that represented God's presence in man; chiropractic leaders often invoked religious imagery and moral traditions. D.D. and B.J. both seriously considered declaring chiropractic a religion, which might have provided legal protection under the U.S. constitution, but decided against it partly to avoid confusion with Christian Science. Early chiropractors also tapped into the Populist movement, emphasizing craft, hard work, competition, and advertisement, aligning themselves with the common man against intellectuals and trusts, among which they included the American Medical Association (AMA).

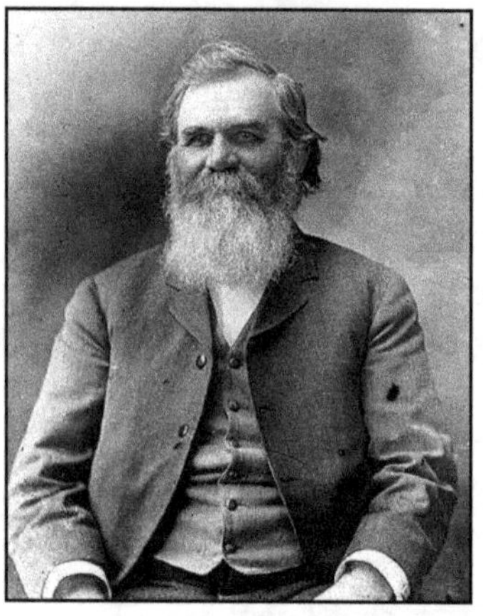

D.D. Palmer, founder of chiropractic.

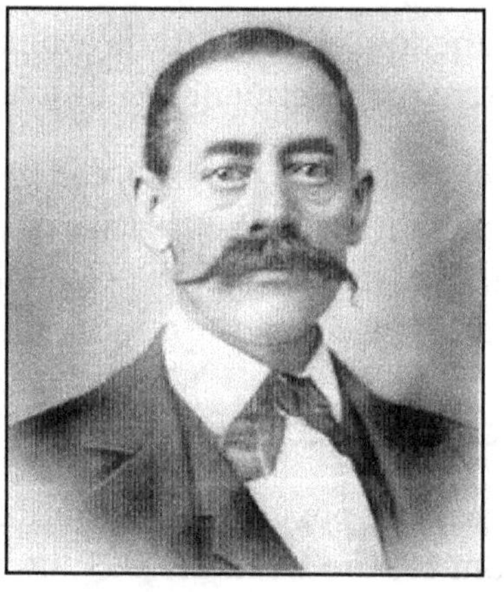

Harvey Lillard, first chiropractic patient.

Chiropractic has seen considerable controversy and criticism. Although D.D. and B.J. were "straight" and disdained the use of instruments, some early chiropractors, whom B.J. scornfully called "mixers", advocated the use of instruments. In 1910 B.J. changed course and endorsed X-rays as necessary for diagnosis; this resulted in a significant exodus from the Palmer School of the more conservative faculty and students. The mixer camp grew until by 1924 B.J. estimated that only 3,000 of the U.S.'s 25,000 chiropractors remained straight. That year, B.J.'s invention and promotion of the neurocalometer, a temperature-sensing device, was highly controversial among B.J.'s fellow straights. By the 1930s chiropractic was the largest alternative healing profession in the U.S.

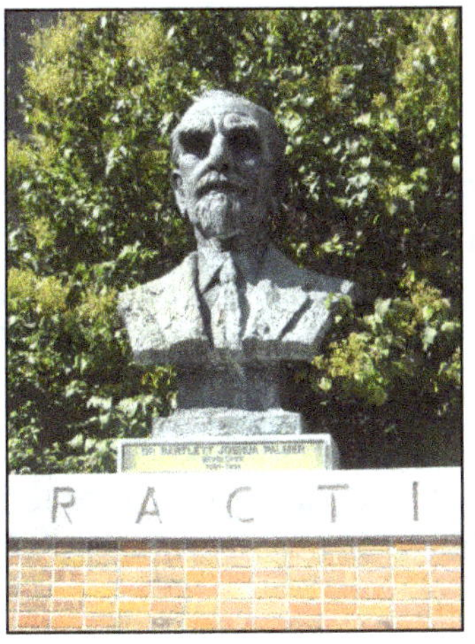

B. J. Palmer, early developer of chiropractic.

Chiropractors faced heavy opposition from organized medicine. Thousands of chiropractors were prosecuted for practicing medicine without a license, and D.D. and many other chiropractors were jailed. To defend against medical statutes B.J. argued that chiropractic was separate and distinct from medicine, asserting that chiropractors "analyzed" rather than "diagnosed", and "adjusted" subluxations rather than "treated" disease. B.J. cofounded the Universal Chiropractors' Association (UCA) to provide legal services to arrested chiropractors. Although the UCA won their first test case in Wisconsin in 1907, prosecutions instigated by state medical boards became increasingly common and in many cases were successful. In response, chiropractors conducted political campaigns to secure separate licensing statutes, eventually succeeding in all fifty states, from Kansas in 1913 through Louisiana in 1974. The longstanding feud between chiropractors and medical doctors continued for decades. The AMA labeled chiropractic an "unscientific cult" in 1966, and until 1980 advised its members that it was unethical for medical doctors to associate with "unscientific practitioners". This culminated in a landmark 1987 decision, *Wilk v. AMA*, in which the court found that the AMA had engaged in unreasonable restraint of trade and conspiracy, and which ended the AMA's de facto boycott of chiropractic.

Serious research to test chiropractic theories did not begin until the 1970s, and is continuing to be hampered by antiscientific and pseudoscientific ideas that sustained the profession in its long battle with organized medicine. By the mid 1990s there was a growing scholarly interest in chiropractic, which helped efforts to improve service quality and establish clinical guidelines that recommended manual therapies for acute low back pain. In recent decades chiropractic gained legitimacy and greater acceptance by medical physicians and health plans, and enjoyed a strong political base and sustained demand for services. However, its future seemed uncertain: as the number of practitioners grew, evidence-based medicine insisted on treatments with demonstrated value, managed care restricted payment, and competition grew from massage therapists and other health professions. The profession responded by marketing natural products and devices more aggressively, and by reaching deeper into alternative medicine and primary care.

Public Health

Some chiropractors oppose vaccination and water fluoridation, which are common public health practices. Within the chiropractic community there are significant disagreements about vaccination, one of the most cost-effective public health interventions available. Most chiropractic writings on vaccination focus on its negative aspects, claiming that it is hazardous, ineffective, and unnecessary. Some chiropractors have embraced vaccination, but a significant portion of the profession rejects it, as original chiropractic philosophy traces diseases to causes in the spine and states that vaccines interfere with healing. The extent to which anti-vaccination views perpetuate the current chiropractic profession is uncertain. The American Chiropractic Association and the International Chiropractors Association support individual exemptions to compulsory vaccination laws, and a 1995 survey of U.S. chiropractors found that about a third believed there was no scientific proof that immunization prevents disease. The Canadian Chiropractic Association supports vaccination; a survey in Alberta in 2002 found that 25% of chiropractors advised patients for, and 27% against, vaccinating themselves or their children.

Early opposition to water fluoridation included chiropractors, some of whom continue to oppose it as being incompatible with chiropractic philosophy and an infringement of personal freedom. Other chiropractors have actively promoted fluoridation, and several chiropractic organizations have endorsed scientific principles of public health. In addition to traditional chiropractic opposition to water fluoridation and vaccination, chiropractors' attempts to establish a positive reputation for their public health role are also compromised by their reputation for recommending repetitive lifelong chiropractic treatment.

Controversy

Throughout its history chiropractic has been the subject of internal and external controversy and criticism. According to Daniel D. Palmer, the founder of chiropractic, subluxation is the sole cause of disease and manipulation is the cure for all diseases of the human race. A 2003 profession-wide survey found "most chiropractors (whether "straights" or "mixers") still hold views of Innate Intelligence and of the cause and cure of disease (not just back pain) consistent with those of the Palmers." A critical evaluation stated "Chiropractic is rooted in mystical concepts. This led to an internal conflict within the chiropractic profession, which continues today." Chiropractors, including D.D. Palmer, were jailed for practicing medicine without a license. For most of its existence, chiropractic has battled with mainstream medicine, sustained by antiscientific and pseudoscientific ideas such as subluxation. Collectively, systematic reviews have not demonstrated that spinal manipulation, the main treatment method employed by chiropractors, is effective for any medical condition, with the possible exception of treatment for back pain. Chiropractic remains controversial, though to a lesser extent than in past years.

Chiropractic Treatment Techniques

Chiropractors primarily use manipulation ("adjustment") of the spine as a treatment. Such treatments trace back to ancient China, Greece and Egypt. It gained popularity in the late 19th century, with the development of osteopathic and chiropractic medicine in North America.

Spinal manipulation (*SMT*) became more popular in the 1980s. It includes manipulation and massage to "adjust" the spine and related tissues, and is a primary basis of chiropractic. Systematic reviews have not found evidence that chiropractic manipulation is effective for any medical condition, with the possible exception of treatment for lower back pain. The safety of manipulation, particularly on the cervical spine has been debated. Adverse results, including death, are rare. Chiropractors may use exercise and other treatments and advice.

Interventions

Skilled, specific hands-on techniques, including manipulation and mobilization, are used to diagnose and treat soft tissues and joint structures, to reduce pain and to increase range of motion and general health.

The approach is generally conservative, and treatment may include:

- Manual procedures, including spinal or joint manipulation or mobilization, soft-tissue and reflex techniques.
- Exercise, and other active care.
- Psychosocial aspects of patient management.
- Patient education on spinal health, posture, nutrition and lifestyle modifications.
- Emergency treatment and acute pain management.
- Other supportive measures, including the use of back supports and orthotics.
- Recognition of the limitations of chiropractic care, and of the need for referral to other health professionals.

Chiropractors may also use exercise and other conservative treatments and advice.

Manual and Manipulative Therapy

The Chinese used such techniques more than 3000 years ago. Hippocrates also used such techniques as did the ancient Egyptians and other cultures.

In the late 19th century in North America, therapies including osteopathy and chiropractic became popular. Spinal manipulation gained mainstream recognition during the 1980s.

In this system, hands are used to manipulate, massage or otherwise influence the spine and related tissues. It is the most common and primary intervention used in chiropractic care.

Effectiveness

Neuromusculoskeletal Disorders

Treatment is usually for neck or low back pain and related disorders.

For acute low back pain, low quality evidence has suggested no difference between real and sham spine manipulation, and moderate quality evidence has suggested no difference between spine manipulation and other commonly used treatments, such as medication and physical therapy.

National guidelines vary; some recommend the therapy for those who do not improve with other treatment. It may be effective for lumbar disc herniation with radiculopathy, as effective as mobilization for neck pain, some forms of headache, and some extremity joint conditions. A 2011 Cochrane review found strong evidence that suggests there is no clinically meaningful difference between spinal manipulation therapy and other treatments for reducing pain and improving function for chronic low back pain. A 2008 review found that with the possible exception of back pain, chiropractic manipulation has not been shown to be effective for any medical condition.

Non-musculoskeletal Disorders

The use of spinal manipulation for non-musculoskeletal is controversial. It has not been shown to be effective for asthma, headache, hypertension, or dysmenorrhea. There is no scientific data that supports the use of SMT for idiopathic adolescent scoliosis.

Cost-effectiveness

Spinal manipulation is generally regarded as cost-effective treatment of musculoskeletal conditions when used alone or in combination with other treatment approaches. Evidence supports the cost-effectiveness of using spinal manipulation for the treatment of sub-acute or chronic low back pain whereas the results for acute low back pain were inconsistent.

Safety

All treatments need a thorough medical history, diagnosis and plan of management. Chiropractors, must rule out contraindications to any treatments, including adverse events.

Relative contraindications, such as osteoporosis are conditions where increased risk is acceptable in some situations and where mobilization and soft-tissue techniques may be treatments of choice. Most contraindications apply to the manipulation of the affected region.

While safety has been debated, and serious injuries and deaths can occur and may be under-reported, these are generally rare and spinal manipulation is relatively safe when employed skillfully and appropriately.

Adverse events are believed to be under-reported and appear to be more common following high velocity/ low amplitude manipulation than mobilization. Mild, frequent and temporary adverse events occur in SMT which include temporary increase in pain, tenderness and stiffness. These effects generally are reduced within 24–48 hours Serious injuries and fatal consequences, especially to SM in the upper cervical region, can occur. but are regarded as rare when spinal manipulation is employed skillfully and appropriately.

The relationship to stroke has been debated. Stroke is statistically associated with both general practitioner and chiropractic services in persons under 45 years of age, and these associations may be related to preexisting conditions. Weak to moderately strong evidence supports causation (as opposed to statistical association) between cervical manipulative therapy and vertebrobasilar artery stroke. A 2012 review found that there is not enough evidence to support a strong association or no association between cervical manipulation and stroke. A 2008 review found chiropractic are more commonly associated with serious related adverse effects than other professionals following manipulation and concluded that the risk of death from manipulations to the neck outweighs the benefits.

Techniques

According to the American Chiropractic Association the most frequently used techniques by chiropractors are Diversified technique 95.9%, Extremity manipulating/adjusting 95.5%, Activator Methods 62.8%, Gonstead technique 58.5%, Cox Flexion/Distraction 58.0%, Thompson 55.9%, Sacro Occipital Technique [SOT] 41.3%, Applied Kinesiology 43.2%, NIMMO/Receptor Tonus 40.0%, Cranial 37.3%, Manipulative/Adjustive Instruments 34.5%, Palmer upper cervical [HIO] 28.8%, Logan Basic 28.7%, Meric 19.9%, and Pierce-Stillwagon 17.1%. Koren Specific Technique (KST) is a chiropractic technique was created around 2004. There are about 200 chiropractic technique, but there is a mostly overlap between them, and many techniques involve slight changes of other techniques.

Diversified Technique

Diversified technique is a non-proprietary and eclectic approach to spinal manipulation that is commonly used by chiropractors. The technique, as it is applied today, is largely attributed to the work of Joe Janse, D.C. Diversified is the most common spine manipulation technique used by chiropractors, with approximately 96% of chiropractors using it for approximately 70% of their patients. Diversified is also the technique most preferred for use during future practice by chiropractic students. Diversified is the only spine manipulation technique taught in Canadian chiropractic programs. Like many chiropractic and osteopathic manipulative techniques, Diversified is characterized by a high-velocity, low-amplitude thrust. is considered the most generic chiropractic manipulative technique and is differentiated from other techniques in that its objective is to restore proper movement and alignment of spine and joint dysfunction.

Atlas Orthogonal Technique

Atlas Orthogonal Technique is an upper cervical chiropractic treatment technique created by Roy Sweat, DC. It is a technique which uses a percussion instrument in attempts to adjust what is perceived to be a subluxation of the atlas vertebra, the top vertebra in the cervical spine. It is based on the teachings of B. J. Palmer, who advocated the Hole-In-One version of spinal adjustment. It is primarily used by straight chiropractors. Referring to the origins of upper cervical techniques, Dan Murphy, DC, DABCO, wrote: “Over the past 100 years, the practice of chiropractic has branched into dozens of specialty techniques. However, historically, for a third of this time, from the 1930s into the 1960s, the predominant practice of chiropractic involved primarily the upper cervical spine.”

Extremity Manipulating/Adjusting

Activator Methods

The Activator Method Chiropractic Technique (AMCT) is a chiropractic treatment method and device created by Arlan Fuhr as an alternative to manual manipulation of the spine or extremity joints. The device is categorized as a mechanical force manual assisted (MFMA) instrument which is generally regarded as a softer chiropractic treatment technique.

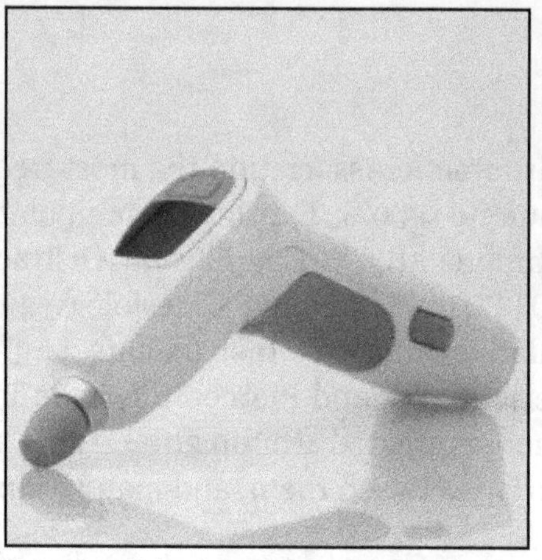

Activator V Chiropractic Adjusting Instrument.

The activator is a small handheld spring-loaded instrument which delivers a small impulse to the spine. It was found to give off no more than 0.3 J of kinetic energy in a 3-millisecond pulse. The aim is to produce enough force to move the vertebrae but not enough to cause injury.

The AMCT involves having the patient lie in a prone position and comparing the functional leg lengths. Often one leg will seem to be shorter than the other. The chiropractor then carries out a series of muscle tests such as having the patient move their arms in a certain position in order to activate the muscles attached to specific vertebrae. If the leg lengths are not the same, that is taken as a sign that the problem is located at that vertebra. The chiropractor treats problems found in this way moving progressively along the spine in the direction from the feet towards the head.

Although prone "functional leg length" is a widely used chiropractic tool, it is not a recognized anthropometric technique, since legs are often of unequal length, and measurements in the prone position are not entirely valid estimates of standing X-ray differences. Measurements in the standing position are far more reliable. Another confounding factor is that simply moving the two legs held together and leaning them imperceptibly to one side or the other produces different results. Fuhr claims that properly trained doctors show good interexaminer reliability.

In 2003, the National Board of Chiropractic Examiners found that 69.9% of chiropractors used the technique, and 23.9% of patients received it. The majority of U.S. chiropractic schools and some schools in other countries teach the AMCT method, and an estimated 45,000 chiropractors worldwide use AMCT or some part of the technique.

There have been a number of studies of AMCT, including case reports, clinical studies and randomized controlled trials, but there are still unanswered questions. A few studies suggest that the activator may be as effective as manual adjustment in treatment of back pain.

Graston Technique

Graston Technique (GT) is a trademarked therapeutic method for diagnosing and treating disorders of the skeletal muscles and related connective tissue. The method employs a collection of six stainless steel instruments of particular shape and size, which are used by practitioners to rub patients' muscles in order to detect and resolve adhesions in the muscles and tendons. Practitioners must be licensed by the parent corporation (Graston Technique, LLC.) in order to use the Graston Technique trademark or the patented instruments.

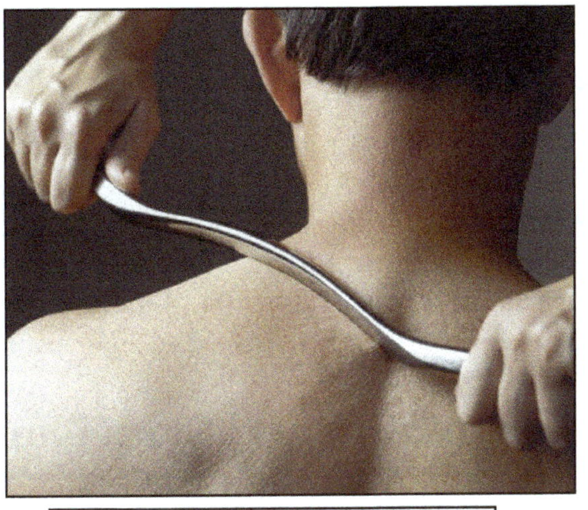

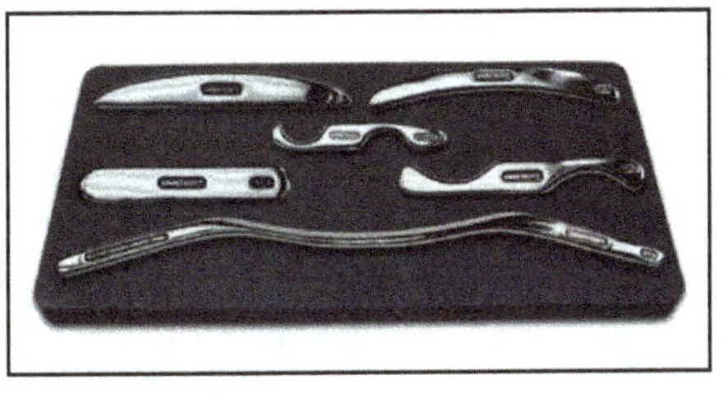

Several examples of Graston treatment have been used in contact sports where scars and contusions are common. However, the Graston Technique has not been rigorously scientifically tested and its evidence basis and assumptions are considered questionable at best. There are no high quality clinical trials that validate the efficacy of the Graston Techniques.

Koren Specific Technique

Koren specific technique (KST) is a technique developed by Tedd Koren. While the technique is associated with chiropractic techniques, Koren has variously described it as an "analysis protocol" or "healthcare protocol". KST may use their hands, or they may use an electric device known as an "ArthroStim" for assessment and adjustments. KST can use different postures. The insurers Aetna, NHS Leeds West CCG, North Dakota Department of Human Services, and The Ohio State University cover other chiropractic techniques but exclude KST from coverage because they consider it to be "experimental and investigational." Aetna's policy states there is a lack of efficacy regarding this method.

Cox Flexion/Distraction

Gonstead Technique

The Gonstead technique is chiropractic method that had been developed by Clarence Gonstead since 1923. The technique focuses on hands-on adjustment and is claimed to expand "*standard diversified technique*" by implementing additional instrumentation including X-rays, Gonstead

Radiographic Parallel, a measuring device, and the development of Nervo-Scope, a device said to detect the level of neurophysiologic activity due to the existence of vertebral subluxation based on changes in skin temperature. Heat detector devices are unreliable and lack scientific evidence. The technique gained popularity in the 1960s. About 28.9% of patients have been treated with the Gonstead technique.

Trigenics Technique

Trigenics is a neurological-based manual or instrument-assisted assessment and treatment system developed and patented by Allan Oolo Austin, DC, DO, CCSP, CCRD. The technique originally began as a chiropractic technique, but is now practiced by osteopaths, physiotherapists and massage therapists. The technique is relatively infrequently used by chiropractors compared to other chiropractic techniques such as Diversified, Trigger point therapy and Activator.

Chiropractic Controversy and Criticism

Throughout its history chiropractic has been the subject of internal and external controversy and criticism. According to magnetic healer Daniel D. Palmer, the founder of chiropractic, "vertebral subluxation" was the sole cause of all diseases and manipulation was the cure for all diseases of the human race. A 2003 profession-wide survey found "most chiropractors (whether 'straights' or 'mixers') still hold views of Innate Intelligence and of the cause and cure of disease (not just back pain) consistent with those of the Palmers." A critical evaluation stated "Chiropractic is rooted in mystical concepts. This led to an internal conflict within the chiropractic profession, which continues today." Chiropractors, including D.D. Palmer, were jailed for practicing medicine without a license. D.D. Palmer considered establishing chiropractic as a religion to resolve this problem. For most of its existence, chiropractic has battled with mainstream medicine, sustained by antiscientific and pseudoscientific ideas such as subluxation.

Chiropractic researchers have documented that fraud, abuse and quackery are more prevalent in chiropractic than in other health care professions. Unsubstantiated claims about the efficacy of chiropractic have continued to be made by individual chiropractors and chiropractic associations. The core concept of traditional chiropractic, vertebral subluxation, is not based on sound science. Collectively, systematic reviews have not demonstrated that spinal manipulation, the main treatment method employed by chiropractors, was effective for any medical condition, with the possible exception of treatment for back pain. Although rare, spinal manipulation, particularly of the upper spine, can also result in complications that can lead to permanent disability or death; these can occur in adults and children.

In 2008, Simon Singh was sued for libel by the British Chiropractic Association (BCA) for criticizing their activities in a column in *The Guardian*. A preliminary hearing took place at the Royal Courts of Justice in front of judge David Eady. The judge held that merely using the phrase "happily promotes bogus treatments" meant that he was stating, as a matter of fact, that the British Chiropractic Association was being consciously dishonest in promoting chiropractic for treating the children's ailments in question. An editorial in *Nature* has suggested that the BCA may be trying to suppress debate and that this use of British libel law is a burden on the right to freedom of expression, which is protected by the European Convention on Human Rights. The libel case ended with the BCA withdrawing its suit in 2010.

Chiropractors historically were strongly opposed to vaccination based on their belief that all diseases were traceable to causes in the spine, and therefore could not be affected by vaccines. Some chiropractors continue to be opposed to vaccination. Early opposition to water fluoridation included chiropractors in the U.S. Some chiropractors opposed water fluoridation as being incompatible with chiropractic philosophy and an infringement of personal freedom. Recently, other chiropractors have actively promoted fluoridation, and several chiropractic organizations have endorsed scientific principles of public health.

Historical Controversy and Critical Elements

The birth of chiropractic was on September 18, 1895. There is controversy over what happened with several different accounts. Daniel D. Palmer later claimed that on that day he manipulated the spine of Harvey Lillard, a man who was nearly deaf, allegedly curing him of deafness. Palmer said *"there was nothing accidental about this, as it was accomplished with an object in view, and the expected result was obtained. There was nothing 'crude' about this adjustment; it was specific so much so that no chiropractor has equaled it."*

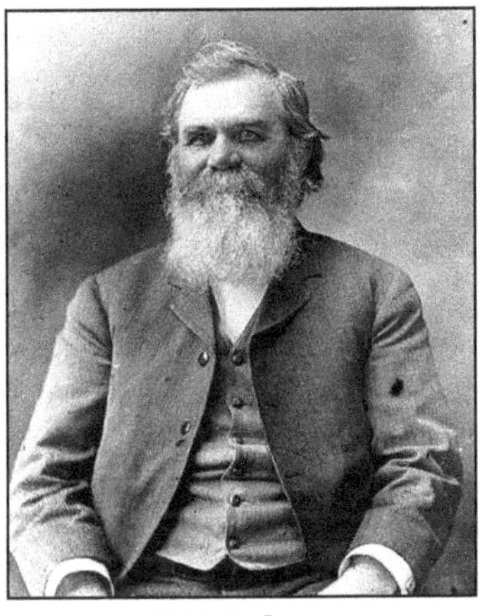

D.D Palmer.

However, this version was disputed by Lillard's daughter, Valdeenia Lillard Simons. She said that her father told her that he was telling jokes to a friend in the hall outside Palmer's office and Palmer, who had been reading, joined them. When Lillard reached the punch line, Palmer, laughing heartily, slapped Lillard on the back with the hand holding the heavy book he had been reading. A few days later, Lillard told Palmer that his hearing seemed better. Palmer then decided to explore manipulation as an expansion of his magnetic healing practice. Simons said "the compact was that if they can make [something of] it, then they both would share. But, it didn't happen."

In spite of the fact that Lillard could hear well enough to tell jokes, B.J. Palmer claimed under sworn testimony that Lillard had been "thoroughly deaf". Since 1895, the story of Palmer's curing a man of deafness has been a part of chiropractic tradition. Palmer's account differs significantly from what actually happened, in that, according to Lillard's daughter, his improved hearing was likely caused by an accidentally fortuitous jarring of Lillard's body and not, as claimed by D.D. Palmer, caused by a "specific" adjustment. It was after this event that Palmer began to experiment with manipulation. He also claimed that his second patient, a man with heart disease, was also cured by spinal manipulation.

Chiropractic included vitalistic ideas of Innate Intelligence with religious attributes of Universal Intelligence as substitutes for science. Evidence suggests that D.D. Palmer had acquired knowledge of manipulative techniques from Andrew Taylor Still, the founder of osteopathy. Although D.D. Palmer combined bonesetting to give chiropractic its method, and "magnetic healing" for the theory, he acknowledged a special relation to magnetic healing when he wrote, "chiropractic was not evolved from medicine or any other method, except that of magnetic." He also "claimed that his profession had nothing to do with medicine, that he healed by the laying on of hands;... He also said that he had a diploma from no earthly school but from High Heaven."

According to D.D. Palmer, subluxation was the sole cause of all diseases and manipulation was the cure for all diseases of the human race. A 2003 profession-wide survey found "most chiropractors (whether "straights" or "mixers") still hold views of Innate and of the cause and cure of disease (not just back pain) consistent with those of the Palmers. On the one hand, modern promotional brochures make a bid for medical legitimacy by describing Innate and adjustments using more scientific-sounding terms such as "inherent" and "nerve force.""

Chiropractic has had a strong salesmanship element since it was started by D.D. Palmer. His son, B.J. Palmer, asserted that their chiropractic school was founded on "...a business, not a professional basis. We manufacture chiropractors. We teach them the idea and then we show them how to sell it". D.D. Palmer established a magnetic healing facility in Davenport, Iowa, styling himself 'doctor'. Not everyone was convinced, as a local paper in 1894 wrote about him:

> "A crank on magnetism has a crazy notion that he can cure the sick and crippled with his magnetic hands. His victims are the weak-minded, ignorant and superstitious, those foolish people who have been sick for years and have become tired of the regular physician and want health by the short-cut method...he has certainly profited by the ignorance of his victims...His increase in business shows what can be done in Davenport, even by a quack."

Before adopting the term "chiropractic" in about 1896, his advertising used the term "magnetic". In 1891-92, a city business directory stated: "Dr. Palmer can cure with his Magnetic Hands Diseases of the Head, Throat, Heart, Lungs, Stomach, Liver, Spleen, Kidneys, Nerves, and Muscles, ten times quicker than any one can with medicines."

The following remark by D.D. Palmer implied that naivety is required to accept the implausibility of the chiropractic concepts.:

> "Give me a simple mind that thinks along single tracts, give me 30 days to instruct him, and that individual can go forth on the highways and byways and get more sick people well than the best, most complete, all around, unlimited medical education of any medical man who ever lived."

Chiropractic was rooted in mystical concepts, leading to internal conflicts between straights and mixers which continue to this day. It has two main groups: "straights", now the minority, emphasize vitalism, innate intelligence and spinal adjustments, and consider subluxations to be the leading cause of all disease; "mixers" are more open to mainstream and alternative medical techniques such as exercise, massage, nutritional supplements, and acupuncture. The straights adhere religiously to the gospel of its founders while mixers are more open. There is a lack of uniformity and consensus among chiropractors in regard to their role. Depending upon whose point of view, chiropractors are, for example, subluxation-correctors, primary care physicians, neuromusculoskeletal specialists, or holistic health specialists. Straights have claimed mixers are not real chiropractors because they do not acknowledge Palmer's foundation of chiropractic therapy.

In 1906, D.D. Palmer was the first of hundreds of chiropractors who went to jail. Chiropractors were jailed for practicing medicine without a license. In the 1920s hundreds of unlicensed chiropractors chose jail rather than fines. Herbert Reaver was the most jailed chiropractor in the U.S. Chiropractors were charged with not complying with the medical practice act. California chiropractors adopted the motto, "Go to jail for chiropractic." 450 chiropractors were jailed in a single year at the peak of the controversy. Many chiropractors treated fellow prisoners and visiting patients while in jail.

D.D. Palmer defined chiropractic as "a science of healing without drugs" and considered establishing chiropractic as a religion as a means to use religious "exemption clauses" to resolve legal difficulties presented by restrictive "chiro laws". In 1911, he stated:

> "You ask, what I think will be the final outcome of our law getting. It will be that we will have to build a boat similar to Christian Science and hoist a religious flag. I have received chiropractic from the other world, similar as did Mrs. Eddy. No other one has lad claim to that, NOT EVEN B.J."

> "Exemption clauses instead of chiro laws by all means, and LET THAT EXEMPTION BE THE RIGHT TO PRACTICE OUR RELIGION. But we must have a religious head, one who is the founder, as did Christ, Mohamed, Jo. Smith, Mrs. Eddy, Martin Luther and other who have founded religions. I am the fountain head. I am the founder of chiropractic in its science, in its art, in its philosophy and in its religious phase. Now, if chiorpractors desire to claim me as their head, their leader, the way is clear. My writings have been gradually steering in that direction until now it is time to assume that we have the same right to as has Christian Scientists."

Chiropractors have struggled with survival and identity during its formative years, including internal struggles between its leaders and colleges. For much of the history of the chiropractic profession chiropractors showed little interest in scientific research and regarded their principles and practices as valid. Despite heavy opposition by mainstream medicine, by the 1930s chiropractic was the largest alternative healing profession in the U.S. Long-standing American Medical Association (AMA) policies against chiropractic contributed to a lack of acceptance within mainstream public health. The AMA created the Committee on Quackery "to contain and eliminate chiropractic." Using the Committee on Quackery, efforts were made to prevent the participation of chiropractic in organized health care. In 1966 a policy passed by the AMA House of Delegates stating: "It is the position of the medical profession that chiropractic is an unscientific cult whose practitioners lack the necessary training and background to diagnose and treat human disease. Chiropractic constitutes a hazard to rational health care in the United States because of its substandard and unscientific education of its practitioners and their rigid adherence to an irrational, unscientific approach to disease causation." The longstanding feud between chiropractors and medical doctors continued for decades. The AMA labeled chiropractic an "unscientific cult" in 1966, and until 1980 held that it was unethical for medical doctors to associate with "unscientific practitioners". This culminated in a landmark 1987 decision, *Wilk v. AMA*, in which the court found that the AMA had engaged in unreasonable restraint of trade and conspiracy, and which ended the AMA's de facto boycott of chiropractic. The rivalry was not solely with conventional medicine; many osteopaths proclaimed that chiropractic was a bastardized form of osteopathy.

Serious research to test chiropractic theories did not begin until the 1970s, and is continuing to be hampered by antiscientific and pseudoscientific ideas that sustained the profession in its long battle with organized medicine. By the mid-1990s there was a growing scholarly interest in chiropractic, which helped efforts to improve service quality and establish clinical guidelines that recommended manual therapies for acute low back pain. Some people believe chiropractic has little more than a placebo effect, while some randomized trials of spinal manipulation have verified its effectiveness for the treatment of (specifically) low back pain. There are several barriers between primary care physicians and chiropractors for having positive referral relationships which includes a lack of good communication. The medical establishment has not entirely accepted chiropractic care as mainstream. After 100 years, the chiropractic profession has failed to define a message that is understandable, credible, and scientifically valid. The future of chiropractic is uncertain due to the economic struggles and restrictions of the science and methods in chiropractic.

Chiropractic has seen considerable controversy within the profession over its philosophy. In connection with a controversial and divisive 2015 organizational split in the Australian chiropractic community, an article described the profession's long standing and current problems:

> "The chiropractic profession is notorious for its infighting, with quarrels over the value of vaccination, the evidence or lack thereof to support the theory of subluxation and whether spinal adjustments should be performed on children."

Allegations of Patricide Connected With The Death Of D.D. Palmer

The 2008 book *Trick or Treatment* states that in 1913 B.J. Palmer ran over his father, D.D. Palmer, at a homecoming parade during the Palmer School of Chiropractic. Weeks later D.D. Palmer died. The official cause of death was recorded as typhoid. The book *Trick or Treatment* indicated "it seems more likely that his death was a direct result of injuries caused by his son. Indeed there is speculation that this was not an accident, but rather a case of patricide." A 1999 documentary study suggests D.D. Palmer's widow may have also played a role in the patricide controversy. D.D. Palmer's attending physicians were persuaded to change their opinions about the main cause of death. Chiropractic historian Joseph C. Keating, Jr. has described the attempted patricide of D.D. Palmer as a "myth" and "absurd on its face" and cites an eyewitness who recalled that D.D. was not struck by B.J.'s car, but rather, had stumbled. He also says that "Joy Loban, DC, executor of D.D.'s estate, voluntarily withdrew a civil suit claiming damages against B.J. Palmer, and that several grand juries repeatedly refused to bring criminal charges against the son." A 1969 article stated that in July 1913 at the Palmer School of Chiropractic B.J. Palmer "insisted on leading the alumni procession, but was prohibited from doing so by the marshal of the parade, who was a student at the school. An altercation ensued. B.J. drove up in his automobile. Words passed between father and son. What happened after that depends on whom you believe. Daniel David claimed that B.J. struck him with his automobile, and D.D's friends and allies later produced affidavits of witnesses to prove it. B.J. flatly denied it, and produced many more affidavits to this effect than D.D.'s cohorts were able to muster."

Ethics and Claims

A study of California disciplinary statistics during 1997–2000 reported 4.5 disciplinary actions per 1000 chiropractors per year, compared to 2.27 for medical doctors, and the incident rate for fraud was 9 times greater among chiropractors (1.99 per 1000 chiropractors per year) than among medical doctors (0.20). According to a 2006 Gallup Poll of U.S. adults, when asked how they would "rate the honesty and ethical standards of people in these different fields", chiropractic compared unfavorably with mainstream medicine. When chiropractic was rated, it "rated dead last amongst healthcare professions". While 84% of respondents considered nurses' ethics "very high" or "high," only 36% felt that way about chiropractors. Other healthcare professions ranged from 38% for psychiatrists, to 62% for dentists, 69% for medical doctors, 71% for veterinarians, and 73% for druggists or pharmacists. Similar results were found in the 2003 Gallup Poll. Chiropractic authors have placed these results in perspective in articles, with one writing that "we were the least trusted and least believed health care discipline", and another writing that chiropractors who use unethical marketing methods "poison the well" for others in the profession, and that they "might be responsible for the negative opinion people have about the ethics of the chiropractic profession." Many chiropractors have sought to address their minor status within the U.S. medical community by attending practice-building seminars to assist chiropractors to persuade their patients of the efficacy of their treatments, increase their revenue, and boost their morale as unorthodox medical practitioners.

Historically the profession has often been accused of quackery, with the profession often responding negatively to such accusations. In its early days, the accusation of quackery was voiced in a 1913 editorial in the *Journal of the American Medical Association*:

> "Chiropractic is a freak offshoot from osteopathy. Disease, say the chiropractors, is due to pressure on the spinal nerves; ergo it can be cured by "adjusting" the spinal column. It is the sheerest quackery, and those who profess to teach it make their appeal to the cupidity of the ignorant. Its practice is in no sense a profession but a trade - and a trade that is potent for great harm. It is carried on almost exclusively by those of no education, ignorant of anatomy, ignorant even of the fundamental sciences on which the treatment of disease depends." (p. 29)

The view that chiropractic was a trade, rather than a profession, was stated clearly by B.J. Palmer, who asserted that chiropractic was founded on "...a business, not a professional basis. We manufacture chiropractors. We teach them the idea and then we show them how to sell it".

In more modern times (1991), when the president of the ACA called accusations of quackery a "myth", chiropractic historian, Joseph C. Keating, Jr. responded by calling his comments "absurd" and stated:

> "The so-called 'quackery myth about chiropractic' is no myth.....the kernels of quackery (i.e., unsubstantiated and untested health remedies offered as "proven") are ubiquitous in this profession. I dare say that health misinformation (if not quackery) can be found in

> just about any issue of any chiropractic trade publication and much of the promotional materials chiropractors disseminate to patients. The recent unsubstantiated claims of the ACA are exemplary *[examples provided]*...It escapes me entirely how Dr. Downing, the ACA, MPI, and Dynamic Chiropractic can suggest that there is no quackery in chiropractic. Either these groups and individuals do not read the chiropractic literature or have no crap-detectors. I urge a reconsideration of advertising and promotion policies in chiropractic."

In an article on quackery, W.T. Jarvis has stated that "Non-scientific health care (e.g., acupuncture, ayurvedic medicine, chiropractic, homeopathy, naturopathy) is licensed by individual states. Practitioners use unscientific practices and deception on a public who, lacking complex health-care knowledge, must rely upon the trustworthiness of providers. Quackery not only harms people, it undermines the scientific enterprise and should be actively opposed by every scientist."

In a 2008 commentary, the chiropractic authors proposed that "the chiropractic profession has an obligation to actively divorce itself from metaphysical explanations of health and disease as well as to actively regulate itself in refusing to tolerate fraud, abuse and quackery, which are more rampant in our profession than in other healthcare professions," a situation which violates the social contract between patients and physicians. Such self-regulation "will dramatically increase the level of trust in and respect for the profession from society at large." Another chiropractic study documented that the largest chiropractic associations in the U.S. and Canada distributed patient brochures which contained unsubstantiated claims. Chiropractors, especially in America, have a reputation for unnecessarily treating patients. Sustained chiropractic care is promoted as a preventative tool but unnecessary manipulation could possibly present a risk to patients. Some chiropractors are concerned by the routine unjustified claims chiropractors have made. In English speaking countries the majority of chiropractors and their associations appear to make efficacy claims that are unsupported by scientific evidence. Claims not supported by solid evidence were made about asthma, ear infection, earache, otitis media, and neck pain.

A 2009 chiropractic spinal manipulation review for infant colic stated "Some chiropractors claim that spinal manipulation is an effective treatment for infant colic but the "evidence fails to demonstrate the effectiveness of this treatment. It is concluded that the above claim is not based on convincing data from rigorous clinical trials."

Some New Zealand chiropractors appeared to have used the title 'Doctor' in a New Zealand Yellow pages telephone directory in a way that implied they are registered medical practitioners, when no evidence was presented it was true. In New Zealand, chiropractors are allowed to use the title 'doctor' when it is qualified to show that the title refers to their chiropractic role. A representative from the NZ Chiropractic Board states that entries in the Yellow Pages under the heading of 'Chiropractors' fulfills this obligation when suitably qualified. If a chiropractor is not a registered medical practitioner, then the misuse of the title 'Doctor' while working in healthcare will not comply with the Health Practitioners Competence Assurance Act 2003.

UK chiropractic organizations and their members make numerous claims which are not supported by scientific evidence. Many chiropractors adhere to ideas which are against science and most seemingly violate important principles of ethical behaviour on a regular basis. The advice chiropractors gave to their patients is often misleading and dangerous. This situation, coupled with a backlash to the libel suit filed against Simon Singh, has inspired the filing of formal complaints of false advertising against more than 500 individual chiropractors within one 24-hour period, prompting the McTimoney Chiropractic Association to write to its members advising them to remove leaflets that make claims about whiplash and colic from their practice, to be wary of new patients and telephone inquiries, and telling their members: "If you have a website, take it down NOW." and "Finally, we strongly suggest you do NOT discuss this with others, especially patients."

On 19 April 2008, Simon Singh wrote a cautionary article about chiropractic therapies in *The Guardian* which resulted in him being sued for libel by the British Chiropractic Association. Singh wrote in *The Guardian* criticising the claims made by chiropractors about the efficacy of spinal manipulation in treating childhood ailments, among other things. He suggested there was "not a jot" of evidence to support such interventions for these ailments, and argued that the British Chiropractic Association "happily promotes bogus treatments". Singh stated that he would "contest the action vigorously... There is an important issue of freedom of speech at stake." The article developed the theme of Singh's recently published book *Trick or Treatment? Alternative Medicine on Trial*, making various claims about the usefulness of chiropractic. Commentators suggested this ruling could set a precedent to restrict freedom of speech to criticise alternative medicine. The charity Sense About Science launched a campaign to draw attention to this particular case. They issued a statement entitled "The law has no place in scientific disputes", which was signed by myriad signers representing science, journalism, publishing, arts, humanities, entertainment, skeptics, campaign groups and law. As of April 16, 2010, over 50,000 had signed. On 1 April 2010, Simon Singh won his court appeal for the right to rely on the defence of fair comment. On 15 April 2010, the BCA officially withdrew its lawsuit, thus ending the case.

Efficacy

Not all criticism originated from critics in the medical profession. Some chiropractors are cautiously calling for reform. Evidence-based guidelines are supported by one end of an ideological continuum among chiropractors; the other end employs antiscientific reasoning and unsubstantiated claims, that are ethically suspect when they let practitioners maintain their beliefs to patients' detriment. Samuel Homola writes that the bottom line is "A good chiropractor can do a lot to help you when you have mechanical-type back pain and other musculoskeletal problems. But until the chiropractic profession cleans up its act, and its colleges uniformly graduate properly limited chiropractors who specialize in neuromusculoskeletal problems, you'll have to exercise caution and informed judgment when seeking chiropractic care."

Vertebral subluxation, the core concept of chiropractic, is not based on solid science. A 2008 review found that with the possible exception of back pain, chiropractic manipulation has not been shown to be effective for any medical condition. Commenting on a famous 'systematic' review by Bronfort et al., Edzard Ernst stated that it was a notorious example of a pseudo-systematic review that omitted evidence, for instance, of negative primary studies. The concept of subluxation remains unsubstantiated and largely untested, and has been debated about whether to keep it in the chiropractic paradigm for decades. The dogma of subluxation is the biggest single barrier to professional development for chiropractors. Vertebral subluxation skews the practice of legitimacy in ways that bring ridicule from the scientific community and uncertainty among the general public.

Commitment to the subluxation dogma undermines the desire for scientific investigation of subluxation as hypothesis, and further perpetuates a cycle of a marketing tradition, inevitably bringing charges of quackery. The cost, effectiveness, and safety, of spinal manipulation are uncertain. Edzard Ernst stated "the best evidence available to date fails to demonstrate clinically relevant benefits of chiropractic for paediatric patients, and some evidence even suggests that chiropractors can cause serious harm to children". A 2007 survey of Alberta chiropractors found that they do not consistently apply research in practice, which may have resulted from a lack of research education and skills though the chiropractic profession has research-focused professional training encouraged by professional association incentives which provide time and support for research. According to David Colquhoun, chiropractic is no more effective than conventional treatment at its best, and has a disadvantage of being "surrounded by gobbledygook about 'subluxations'", and, more seriously, it does kill patients occasionally. Neck spinal manipulation has a risk of stroke or death. Although rare, spinal manipulation, particularly of the upper spine, can also result in complications that can lead to permanent disability or death; these can occur in adults and children. Most of the adverse events were benign, however, there are complications that were life-threatening. A 2010 systematic review found that numerous deaths since 1934 have been recorded after chiropractic neck manipulation typically associated with vertebral artery dissection. Some chiropractic proponents seem to think that a critical evaluation of the research is tantamount to a 'scare story' or to 'puffing up (the evidence) out of all proportion'. A reasonable approach to serious risk from chiropractic therapy, however, requires an open examination.

The 2008 book *Trick or Treatment* states that "chiropractors may X-ray the same patient several times a year, even though there is no clear evidence that X-rays will help the therapist treat the patient. X-rays can reveal neither the subluxations nor the innate intelligence associated with chiropractic philosophy, because they do not exist. There is no conceivable reason at all why X-raying the spine should help a straight chiropractor treat an ear infection, asthma or period pains. Most worrying of all, chiropractors generally require a full spine X-ray, which delivers a significant higher radiation dose than most other X-ray procedures". Practice guidelines aim to reduce unnecessary radiation exposure, which increases cancer risk in proportion to the amount of radiation received. Research suggests that radiology instruction given at chiropractic schools worldwide seem to be evidence-based. Although, there seems to be a disparity between some schools and available evidence regarding the aspect of radiography for patients with acute low back pain without an indication of a serious disease, which may contribute to chiropractic overuse of radiography for low back pain.

Quackwatch is critical of chiropractic; its founder, Stephen Barrett, has written that it is "absurd" to think that chiropractors are qualified to be primary care providers and considers applied kinesiology to be a "term most commonly used to identify a pseudoscientific system of muscle-testing and therapy".

A 2009 perspective stated there is consistent evidence that manual therapies such as chiropractic manipulations are "helpful and generally produce moderate but significant and sustained improvement for back pain in populations" and writes that the suggestion that chiropractic does more harm than good as "specious". The author went on to write that the more serious suggestion is that chiropractic treatment can kill people, and it is often claimed that chiropractic manipulation causes strokes.

Lon Morgan, DC, a reform chiropractor, expressed his view of Innate Intelligence this way: "Innate Intelligence clearly has its origins in borrowed mystical and occult practices of a bygone era. It remains untestable and unverifiable and has an unacceptably high penalty/benefit ratio for the chiropractic profession. The chiropractic concept of Innate Intelligence is an anachronistic holdover from a time when insufficient scientific understanding existed to explain human physiological processes. It is clearly religious in nature and must be considered harmful to normal scientific activity."

Chiropractic historian Joseph C. Keating, Jr. articulated that "So long as we propound the "One cause, one cure" rhetoric of Innate, we should expect to be met by ridicule from the wider health science community. Chiropractors can't have it both ways. Our theories cannot be both dogmatically held vitalistic constructs and be scientific at the same time. The purposiveness, consciousness and rigidity of the Palmers' Innate should be rejected."

William T. Jarvis, Ph.D. has stated: "Chiropractic is a controversial health-care system that has been legalized throughout the United States and in several other countries. In the United States in 1984, roughly 10.7 million people made 163 million office visits to 30,000 chiropractors. More than three fourths of the states require insurance companies to include chiropractic services in health and accident policies. The federal government pays for limited chiropractic services under Medicare, Medicaid, and its vocational rehabilitation program, and the Internal Revenue Service allows a medical deduction for chiropractic services. Chiropractors cite such facts as evidence of "recognition." However, these are merely business statistics and legal arrangements that have nothing to do with chiropractic's scientific validity."

Vaccination and Water Fluoridation

Many forms of alternative medicine are based on philosophies that oppose vaccination and have practitioners who voice their opposition. These include some elements of the chiropractic community. The reasons for this negative vaccination view are complicated and rest, at least in part, on the early philosophies which shape the foundation of these professions. Chiropractors historically were strongly opposed to vaccination based on their belief that all diseases were traceable to causes in the spine, and therefore could not be affected by vaccines; D.D. Palmer wrote, "It is the very height of absurdity to strive to 'protect' any person from smallpox or any other malady by inoculating them with a filthy animal poison." Some chiropractors continue to be opposed to vaccination, one of the most effective public health measures in history.

Some chiropractic groups still oppose attempts to limit or eliminate nonmedical exemptions to vaccination. In March 2015, the Oregon Chiropractic Association invited Andrew Wakefield, chief author of a fraudulent research paper, to testify against Senate Bill 442, "a bill that would eliminate nonmedical exemptions from Oregon's school immunization law." The California Chiropractic Association lobbied against a 2015 bill ending belief exemptions for vaccines. They had also opposed a 2012 bill related to vaccination exemptions. On April 24, 2015, Wakefield received two standing ovations from the students at Life Chiropractic College West when he told them to oppose Senate Bill SB277, a bill which proposes limits on non-medical vaccine exemptions. Responding to his critics, he stated that "[i]t doesn't matter if I go to the grave discredited. I don't care what they say about me. In fact, I have nothing to lose now. This is such an important issue." Wakefield had previously been a featured speaker at a 2014 "California Jam" gathering of chiropractors, as well as a 2015 "California Jam" seminar, with continuing education credits, sponsored by Life Chiropractic College West.

In response to threatening activities by anti-vaccination activists, the California Medical Association (CMA) sent a warning letter to California Chiropractic Association President Brian Stenzler, whom they could document had encouraged the stalking of lobbyists who supported Senate Bill SB277. The CMA also filed a police report.

Early opposition to water fluoridation included chiropractors in the U.S. Some chiropractors oppose water fluoridation as being incompatible with chiropractic philosophy and an infringement of personal freedom. Recently, other chiropractors have actively promoted fluoridation, and several chiropractic organizations have endorsed scientific principles of public health.

Ownership of Spinal Manipulation

While no single profession "owns" spinal manipulation (SM), and there is little consensus as to which profession should administer SM, chiropractors have expressed concern that orthodox medical physicians and physical therapists could "steal" SM procedures from chiropractors. Chiropractors regularly introduce bills into state legislatures to further prohibit non-chiropractors from performing SM, and they are opposed by physical therapist organizations. Two U.S. states (Washington and Arkansas) prohibit physical therapists from performing SM, some states allow them to do it only if they have completed advanced training in SM. In the most restrictive states, SM is limited to chiropractors and medical physicians.

A focus on evidence-based SM research has also raised concerns that the resulting tighter practice guidelines could limit the scope of chiropractic practice to treating backs and necks.

Chiropractic Professional Ethics

Various organizations of practicing chiropractors have outlined formal codes of professional ethics. Actual practice has revealed a wide range of behaviors which may or may not conform to these standards.

Official Positions

The American Chiropractic Association (ACA) has a "Code of Ethics" "based upon the acknowledgement that the social contract dictates the profession's responsibilities to the patient, the public, and the profession; and upholds the fundamental principle that the paramount purpose of the chiropractic doctor's professional services shall be to benefit the patient." The smaller International Chiropractor's Association (ICA) also has a detailed set of professional canons.

Reports of Actual Practice

Various situations have occurred in which the ethics of chiropractors and chiropractic organizations have been called into question.

A 2008 commentary proposed that the chiropractic profession actively regulate itself to combat abuse, fraud, and quackery, which are more prevalent in chiropractic than in other health care professions, violating the social contract between patients and physicians.

Gleberzon *et al.* identify "deliberate fraud" as a notably harmful element of the chiropractic profession, finding that dubious practice techniques can translate into "outlandish billing and utilization rates". Those at the "fringe of ethical behavior" present the profession with a challenge, they believe, and must be weeded out.

A study of California disciplinary statistics during 1997–2000 reported 4.5 disciplinary actions per 1000 chiropractors per year, compared to 2.27 for medical doctors, and the incident rate for fraud was nine times greater among chiropractors (1.99 per 1000 chiropractors per year) than among medical doctors (0.20). According to a 2006 Gallup poll of U.S. adults, when asked how they would "rate the honesty and ethical standards of people in these different fields", chiropractic compared unfavorably with mainstream medicine. When chiropractic was rated, it "rated dead last amongst healthcare professions". While 84% of respondents considered nurses' ethics "very high" or "high," only 36% felt that way about chiropractors. Other healthcare professions ranged from 38% for psychiatrists, to 62% for dentists, 69% for medical doctors, 71% for veterinarians, and 73% for druggists or pharmacists. Similar results were found in the 2003 Gallup Poll.

In 2001, the largest chiropractic associations in the U.S. and Canada were reported to have distributed patient brochures which contained unsubstantiated claims. Chiropractors, especially in America, have a reputation for unnecessarily treating patients. In many circumstances the focus seems to be put on economics instead of health care. Sustained chiropractic care is promoted as a preventative tool, but unnecessary manipulation could possibly present a risk to patients. Some chiropractors are concerned by the routine unjustified claims chiropractors have made. A 2010 analysis of chiropractic websites found the majority of chiropractors and their associations made claims of effectiveness not supported by scientific evidence, while 28% of chiropractic websites advocate lower back pain care, which has some sound evidence.

Although in the vast majority of US States chiropractors are considered physicians pursuant to statute (exceptions are *inter alia*, New York and California). The Joint Commission recognizes chiropractors as physicians as well. In some jurisdictions, like New Zealand, chiropractors appeared to have used the title 'doctor' in a New Zealand yellow pages telephone directory in a way that implied they are registered medical practitioners, when no evidence was presented it was true. In New Zealand, chiropractors are allowed to use the title 'doctor' when it is qualified to show that the title refers to their chiropractic role. A representative from the NZ Chiropractic Board states that entries in the yellow pages under the heading of 'Chiropractors' fulfills this obligation when suitably qualified. If a chiropractor is not a registered medical practitioner, then the misuse of the title 'doctor' while working in healthcare will not comply with the Health Practitioners Competence Assurance Act 2003.

UK chiropractic organizations and their members make numerous claims which are not supported by scientific evidence. Many chiropractors adhere to ideas which are against science and most seemingly violate important principles of ethical behaviour on a regular basis. The advice chiropractors gave to their patients is often misleading and dangerous. In 2009, a backlash to the libel suit filed by the British Chiropractic Association (BCA) against Simon Singh, has inspired the filing of formal complaints of false advertising against more than 500 individual chiropractors within one 24-hour period, prompting the McTimoney Chiropractic Association to write to its members advising them to remove leaflets that make claims about whiplash and colic from their practice, to be wary of new patients and telephone inquiries, and telling their members: "If you have a website, take it down NOW." and "Finally, we strongly suggest you do NOT discuss this with others, especially patients." An editorial in *Nature* has suggested that the BCA may be trying to suppress debate and that this use of British libel law is a burden on the right to freedom of expression, which is protected by the European Convention on Human Rights. The libel case ended with the BCA withdrawing its suit in 2010.

Tenets

- ACA's Page on Ethical Practice.
- ICA Ethics.

Spinal Adjustment

Spinal adjustment and chiropractic adjustment are terms used by chiropractors to describe their approaches to spinal manipulation, as well as some osteopaths, who use the term adjustment.

Spinal adjustments were among many chiropractic techniques invented in the 19th century by Daniel David Palmer, the founder of Chiropractic. Claims made for the benefits of spinal adjustments range from temporary, palliative (pain relieving) effects to long term wellness and preventive care. Despite anecdotal success, there is not yet scientific evidence that spinal adjustment is effective against disease.

Adjustment/Manipulation

In a section titled "Spinal Manipulation: The Chiropractic Adjustment", chiropractic authors and researchers Meeker and Haldeman write that the core clinical method that all chiropractors agree upon is spinal manipulation, although chiropractors much prefer to use the term spinal "adjustment", a term which reflects "their belief in the therapeutic and health-enhancing effect of correcting spinal joint abnormalities." (p. 218)

Defined as Unique to Chiropractic

The International Chiropractor's Association (ICA) states that the "chiropractic spinal adjustment is unique and singular to the chiropractic profession", and that it "is characterized by a specific thrust applied to the vertebra utilizing parts of the vertebra and contiguous structures as levers to directionally correct articular malposition. Adjustment shall be differentiated from spinal manipulation in that the adjustment can only be applied to a vertebral malposition with the express intent to improve or correct the subluxation, whereas any joint, subluxated or not, may be manipulated to mobilize the joint or to put the joint through its range of motion... Chiropractic is a specialized field in the healing arts, and by prior rights, the spinal adjustment is distinct and singular to the chiropractic profession." One author claims that this concept is now repudiated by mainstream chiropractic. The definition of this procedure describes the use of a load (force) to specific body tissues with therapeutic intent. This 'load' is traditionally supplied by hand, and can vary in its velocity, amplitude, duration, frequency, and body location (p. 218) and is usually abbreviated HVLA (high velocity low amplitude) thrust.

Intention: To Correct Vertebral Subluxations

The intention of a chiropractic adjustment is to affect or correct the alignment, motion and/or function of a vertebral joint. Specifically, they are intended to correct "vertebral subluxations", the term given to the signs and symptoms that are said by chiropractors to result from abnormal alignment of vertebrae. (p. 218) This intention forms the legal and philosophical foundation of the profession, and US Medicare law formulates it in this manner:

> "Coverage of chiropractic services is specifically limited to manual manipulation of the spine to correct a subluxation... Medicare will not pay for treatment unless it is 'manual manipulation of the spine to correct a subluxation'."

Adjustment Methods

As the chiropractic profession grew, individual practitioners and institutions proposed and developed various proprietary techniques and methods. While many of these techniques did not endure, hundreds of different approaches remain in chiropractic practice today. Not all of them involve HVLA thrust manipulation. Most cite case studies, anecdotal evidence, and patient testimonials as evidence for effectiveness. These techniques include:

- Toggle Drop – this is when the chiropractor, using crossed hands, presses down firmly on a particular area of the spine. Then, with a quick and precise thrust, the chiropractor adjusts the spine. This is done to improve mobility in the vertebral joints.
- Lumbar Roll (aka side posture) – the chiropractor positions the patient on his or her side, then applies a quick and precise manipulative thrust to the misaligned vertebra, returning it to its proper position.
- Release Work – the chiropractor applies gentle pressure using his or her fingertips to separate the vertebrae.
- Table adjustments – The patient lies on a special table with sections that drop down. The chiropractor applies a quick thrust at the same time the section drops. The dropping of the table allows for a lighter adjustment without the twisting positions that can accompany other techniques.
- Instrument adjustments – often the gentlest methods of adjusting the spine. The patient lies on the table face down while the chiropractor uses a spring-loaded activator instrument to perform the adjustment. This technique is often used to perform adjustments on animals as well.
- Manipulation under anesthesia (MUA) – this is performed by a chiropractor certified in this technique in a hospital outpatient setting when the patient is unresponsive to traditional adjustments.

Techniques

There are many techniques which chiropractors can specialize in and employ in spinal adjustments. Some of the most notable techniques include:

- Activator Methods – uses the Activator Adjusting Instrument instead of by-hand adjustments to give consistent mechanical low-force, high-speed impulses to the body. Utilizes a leg-length analysis to determine segmental aberration.
- Active Release Techniques – soft tissue system/movement based technique that treats problems with muscles, tendons, ligaments, fascia and nerves.

- Bio-Geometric Integration – a framework for understanding the body's response to force dynamics. Can be utilized with many techniques. Focuses on the body's full integration of forces and on assessment for choosing the most appropriate adjustive force application, ranging from light pressure to traditional joint cavitation, for each particular case presentation.

- Blair Upper Cervical Technique – an objective upper cervical technique focusing primarily on misalignments in the first bone of the spine (Atlas) as it comes into contact with the head (Occiput).

- Chiropractic Biophysics (CBP) - a research and evidence based technique which aims to correct improper curvatures of the spine with traditional chiropractic manipulation (SMT), focused rehabilitation exercises, and a unique form of spinal traction which utilizes mechanically assisted and focused stretching to stretch and remodel the ligaments and related tissues of the spine.

- Cox Flexion-Distraction – a decompression focused procedure which utilizes specialized adjusting tables with movable parts; these tables stretch and decompress the facets and ligaments of the spine in a gentle rocking motion.

- Directional Non-Force Technique – utilizes a diagnostic system for subluxation analysis consisting of gentle challenging and a unique leg check allowing the body to indicate the directions of misalignment of structures that are producing nerve interference. A gentle but directionally specific thumb impulse provides a long lasting correction to bony and soft tissue structures.

- Diversified – the classic chiropractic technique, developed by D.D. Palmer, DC. Uses specific manual thrusts focused on restoring normal biomechanical function. Has been developed to adjust extremity joints as well.

- Gonstead Technique – Developed by an automotive engineer turned chiropractor, this technique uses a very specific method of analysis by the use of nervoscopes, full spine x-rays and precise adjusting techniques that condemns "torquing" of the spine, which may harm the Intervertebral disc.

- Hole-in-one Technique/Toggle Recoil Technique – Synonyms for the upper cervical technique developed by B.J. Palmer which utilizes a quick thrust and release, and later incorporated a drop table as seen in modern practice.

- Kale Technique (Specific Chiropractic) – gentle technique which utilizes a special adjusting table that helps adjust and stabilize the upper cervical region surrounding the brain stem.

- Logan Basic Technique – a light touch technique that works to "level the foundation" or sacrum. Its concept employs the use of heel lifts and specific contacts.

- NUCCA Technique – manual method of adjusting the atlas subluxation complex based on 3D x-ray studies which determine the correct line of drive or vector of force.

- Orthospinology Procedure – is a method of analyzing and correcting the chiropractic upper cervical subluxation complex based on vertebral alignment measurements on neck x-rays taken from three different directions. The adjustment can be delivered by hand, hand-held or table mounted instruments along a pre-calculated vector using approximately 1 to 7 pounds of force. The patient is in a side-lying posture with a solid mastoid support. The procedure is based on the work of the late John F. Grostic, D.C.

- Thompson Terminal Point Technique (Thompson Drop-Table Technique) – uses a precision adjusting table with a weighing mechanism which adds only enough tension to hold the patient in the "up" position before the thrust is given.

Over the years, many variations of these techniques have been delivered, most as proprietary techniques developed by individual practitioners. WebMD has made a partial list:

<table>
<tr>
<td>• Activator technique
• Advanced BioStructural Correction
• Applied Kinesiology
• Atlas Orthogonal
• Auricular
• Barge Analysis
• Bio Magnetic
• Bio-Energetic Synchronization
• Bio-Geometric Integration
• Biomechanics</td>
<td>• Blair
• Body Restoration Technique
• Carver Technique
• Cervical Care
• Cervical Drop
• Chiropractic Biophysics (CBP)
• Clinical Kinesiology
• Concept Therapy
• Contact Reflex Analysis
• Cox</td>
<td>• Craniosacral Therapy
• Directional Non-Force
• Diversified technique
• Flexion-Distraction
• Gonstead
• Grostic
• Hole in one [HIO]
• Kale
• Leander
• Logan Basic</td>
<td>• Manual Adjusting
• Meric
• Motion Palpation
• Network
• Neural Organization Technique
• Neuro Emotional Technique
• Neuro Muscular Technique
• Neuro Vascular Technique
• Nimmo
• Nutrition Response Testing
• Palmer Package</td>
<td>• Pettibon
• Pierce
• Pierce Stillwagon
• Pro-Adjuster
• Receptor Tonus
• Sacral Occipital Technique (SOT)
• Soft Tissue Orthopedics
• Spinal Biomechanics
• Spinal Biomedical Engineering
• Spinal Biophysics</td>
<td>• Thompson
• Thompson Terminal Point
• Toftness
• Toggle Recoil
• Torque Release
• Total Body Modification
• Traction
• Upper Cervical
• Vector Point Therapy
• Versendaal</td>
</tr>
</table>

Effects

The effects of spinal adjustment vary depending on the method performed. All techniques claim effects similar to other manual therapies, ranging from decreased muscle tension to reduced stress. Studies show that most patients go to chiropractors for musculoskeletal problems: 60% with low back pain, and the rest with head, neck and extremity symptoms. (p. 219) Also the article "Chiropractic: A Profession at the Crossroads of Mainstream and Alternative Medicine" states that, "chiropractic was to be a revolutionary system of healing based on the premise that neurologic dysfunction caused by 'impinged' nerves at the spinal level was the cause of most disease". (p. 218) The mechanisms that are claimed to alter nervous system function and affect overall health are seen as speculative in nature, however, clinical trials have been conducted that include "placebo-controlled comparisons [and] comparisons with other treatments". (p. 220) The American Chiropractic Association promotes chiropractic care of infants and children under the theory that "poor posture and physical injury, including birth trauma, may be common primary causes of illness in children and can have a direct and significant impact not only on spinal mechanics, but on other bodily functions".

The effects of spinal manipulation have been shown to include: temporary relief of musculoskeletal pain, increased range of joint motion, changes in facet joint kinematics, increased pain tolerance and increased muscle strength. (p. 222) Common side effects of spinal manipulative therapy (SMT) are characterized as mild to moderate and may include: local discomfort, headache, tiredness, or radiating discomfort. (p. 222)

Safety

The World Health Organization states that when "employed skillfully and appropriately, chiropractic care is safe and effective for the prevention and management of a number of health problems." As with all interventions, there are risks associated with spinal manipulative therapy (SMT). Common, but nonserious side effects include: discomfort, headache, and fatigue which will go away after 24 to 48 hours. Extremely rare, but potentially serious side effects include: strokes, spinal disc herniation, vertebral and rib fractures and cauda equina syndrome. (p. 222).

Vertebral Subluxation

In chiropractic, vertebral subluxation is a supposed misalignment of the spinal column leading to a set of set of signs and symptoms sometimes termed vertebral subluxation complex. It has no biomedical basis and is categorized as pseudoscientific by leading authorities. Traditionally, the "specific focus of chiropractic practice" is the chiropractic subluxation and historical chiropractic practice assumes that a vertebral subluxation or spinal joint dysfunction interferes with the body's function and its innate intelligence, as promulgated by D. D. Palmer, the inventor of chiropractic.

The chiropractic subluxation is the heart of the split between "straight" and "mixer" chiropractors. Straight chiropractors continue to follow Palmer's vitalistic tradition, claiming that subluxation has considerable health effects and also adding a visceral component to the definition, while mixers, as exemplified by the United Kingdom's General Chiropractic Council, consider it a historical concept with no evidence identifying it as the cause of disease.

Within the chiropractic tradition, a vertebral subluxation complex is believed to be a dysfunctional biomechanical spinal segment which actively alters neurological function, which in turn, is believed to lead to neuromusculoskeletal and visceral disorders. The WHO acknowledges this difference between the medical and chiropractic definitions of a subluxation: medical doctors only refer to "significant structural displacements" as subluxations, whereas chiropractors suggest that a dysfunctional segment, whether displaced significantly or not, should be referred to as a subluxation. This difference has been noted in the proceedings of the chiropractic profession's *Mercy Center Consensus Conference*: "The chiropractic profession refers to this concept as a 'subluxation'. This use of the word *subluxation* should not be confused with the term's precise anatomic usage, which considers only the anatomical relationships."

The chiropractic vertebral subluxation complex has been a source of controversy since its inception in 1895 due to the lack of empirical evidence for its existence, its metaphysical origins, and claims of its far reaching effects on health and disease. Although some chiropractic associations and colleges support the concept of subluxation, many in the chiropractic profession reject it and shun the use of this term as a diagnosis. In the United States and in Canada the term *nonallopathic lesion* may be used in place of *subluxation.*

A 2009 review concluded that epidemiologic evidence does not support the chiropractic subluxation, concluding:

> "No supportive evidence is found for the chiropractic subluxation being associated with any disease process or of creating suboptimal health conditions requiring intervention. Regardless of popular appeal, this leaves the subluxation construct in the realm of unsupported speculation. This lack of supportive evidence suggests the subluxation construct has no valid clinical applicability."

In 2015, 8 internationally accredited chiropractic colleges: AECC, WIOC, IFEC-Paris, IFEC-Toulouse, USD-Odense, UZ-Zurich, UJ-Johannesburg and Durban University of Technology made an open statement which included: "The teaching of the vertebral subluxation complex as a vitalistic construct that claims that it is the cause of disease is unsupported by evidence. Its inclusion in a modern chiropractic curriculum in anything other than an historic context is therefore inappropriate and unnecessary".

History

In 1909 B.J. Palmer wrote that:

> "Chiropractors have found in every disease that is supposed to be contagious, *a cause in the spine*. In the spinal column we *will* find a subluxation that corresponds to every type of disease. If we had one hundred cases of small-pox, I can prove to you where, in one, you *will* find a subluxation and you will find the *same conditions* in the other ninety-nine. I adjust one and return his functions to normal... . There is no contagious disease... . There is no infection... . There is a cause internal to man that makes of his body in a certain spot, more or less a breeding ground [for microbes]. It is a place where they can multiply, propagate, and then because they become so many they are classed as a cause." -- B.J. Palmer, *The Philosophy of Chiropractic*, V. Davenport, IA: Palmer School of Chiropractic; 1909.

Definitions, Official Status and ICD Coding

Definitions and Status

The WHO definition of the chiropractic vertebral subluxation is:

> "A lesion or dysfunction in a joint or motion segment in which alignment, movement integrity and/or physiological function are altered, although contact between joint surfaces remains intact. It is essentially a functional entity, which may influence biomechanical and neural integrity."

The purported displacement is not necessarily visible on X-rays. This is in contrast to the medical definition of spinal subluxation which, according to the WHO, is a *"significant structural displacement"*, and therefore visible on X-rays.

As of 2014, the National Board of Chiropractic Examiners states:

> "The specific focus of chiropractic practice is known as the chiropractic subluxation or joint dysfunction. A subluxation is a health concern that manifests in the skeletal joints, and, through complex anatomical and physiological relationships, affects the nervous system and may lead to reduced function, disability or illness."

In 1996 an official consensus definition of subluxation was formed. Cooperstein and Gleberzon have described the situation: "... although many in the chiropractic profession reject the concept of "subluxation" and shun the use of this term as a diagnosis, the presidents of at least a dozen chiropractic colleges of the Association of Chiropractic Colleges (ACC) developed a consensus definition of "subluxation" in 1996. It reads:

> "Chiropractic is concerned with the preservation and restoration of health, and focuses particular attention on the subluxation. A subluxation is a complex of functional and/or structural and/or pathological articular changes that compromise neural integrity and may influence organ system function and general health. A subluxation is evaluated, diagnosed, and managed through the use of chiropractic procedures based on the best available rational and empirical evidence."

In 2001 the World Federation of Chiropractic, representing the national chiropractic associations in 77 countries, adopted this consensus statement which reaffirms belief in the vertebral subluxation.

The ACC paradigm has been criticized by chiropractic authors:

> "All in all, the ambiguities that permeate the ACC's statements on subluxation render it inadequate as a guide to clinical research... Whether the ACC's subluxation claims have succeeded as a political statement is beyond our concern here. These assertions were published as a priori truths (what many chiropractors have traditionally referred to as "principle"), and are exemplary of scientifically unjustified assertions made in many corners of the profession. It matters not whether unsubstantiated assertions are offered for clinical, political, scientific, educational, marketing or other purposes; when offered without acknowledgment of their tentative character, they amount to dogmatism. We contend that attempts to foster unity (among the schools or in the wider profession) at the expense of scientific integrity is ultimately self-defeating. To be sure, the profession's lack of cultural authority is based in part upon our characteristic disunity. However, attempts to generate unity by adoption of a common dogma can only bring scorn and continued alienation from the wider health care community and the public we all serve."

In May 2010 the General Chiropractic Council, the statutory regulatory body for chiropractors in the United Kingdom, issued guidance for chiropractors stating that the chiropractic vertebral subluxation complex "is an historical concept" and "is not supported by any clinical research evidence that would allow claims to be made that it is the cause of disease or health concerns."

ICD Coding

The differences between a medical subluxation and a chiropractic "vertebral subluxation" create confusion and difficulties when it comes to following official ICD-9 and ICD-10 coding. In a 2014 article in *Dynamic Chiropractic* by a chiropractor who is a certified professional coder, these difficulties were discussed in detail. He noted that the WHO recognizes the differences between the two types of "subluxations", and also pointed out certain difficulties for chiropractors:

> "...the official definition of 739 codes is "nonallopathic lesions, not elsewhere classified.... In other words, 739 is a code that does not describe a subluxation. It does not even say what the patient has; it says that there is no code to describe what the patient has.... [T]he elusive "vertebral subluxation complex" I learned about in school has no place in the ICD-9 code set. All we get is 739, which is a code for conditions that do not have a code."
>
> "ICD-9 has never provided a code that truly describes this and differentiates between the chiropractic subluxation and the allopathic subluxation. Chiropractors have been compelled to try to fit a square peg into a round hole for many years."

At the time of writing (August 2014) it was still uncertain which codes in the newer ICD-10 would be useful for chiropractors and how they would be interpreted.

Components

Traditionally there have been 5 components that form the chiropractic subluxation. The vertebral subluxation complex is differentiated by the fifth component, general systemic disturbances secondary to the spinal misalignment (vertebral subluxation).

- Spinal Kinesiopathology.
- Neuropathophysiology/Neuropathology.
- Myopathology.
- Histopathology.
- Pathophysiology/Pathology.

Examination

Historically, the detection of spinal misalignments (subluxations) by the chiropractic profession has relied on X-ray findings and physical examination. At least 2 of the following 4 physical signs and/or symptoms must be documented to qualify for reimbursement:

- Pain and tenderness.
- Asymmetry/misalignment.
- Range of motion abnormality.
- Tissue/tone changes.

Background

It has been proposed that a vertebral subluxation can negatively affect general health by altering the neurological communication between the brain, spinal cord and peripheral nervous system.

Although individuals may not always be symptomatic, straight chiropractors believe that the presence of vertebral subluxation is in itself justification for correction via spinal adjustment.

Chiropractic treatment of vertebral subluxation focuses on delivering a chiropractic adjustment which is a high velocity low amplitude (HVLA) thrust to the dysfunctional spinal segments to help correct the chiropractic subluxation complex. Spinal adjustment is the primary procedure used by chiropractors in the adjustment. Adjustment/manipulation has been shown to help with low back pain, neck pain and tension type headaches, but further studies are inconclusive on the use of spinal manipulation outside the treatment of neuromusculoskeletal disorders.

Rationale and Disagreements

In 1910, D.D. Palmer, the founder of chiropractic, wrote:

> "Physiologists divide nerve-fibers, which form the nerves, into two classes, afferent and efferent. Impressions are made on the peripheral afferent fiber-endings; these create sensations which are transmitted to the center of the nervous system. Efferent nerve-fibers carry impulses out from the center to their endings. Most of these go to muscles and are therefore called motor impulses; some are secretory and enter glands; a portion are inhibitory their function being to restrain secretion. Thus, nerves carry impulses outward and sensations inward. The activity of these nerves, or rather their fibers, may become excited or allayed by impingement, the result being a modification of functionating — too much or not enough action — which is dis-ease."

Chiropractors use and have used various terms to express this concept: subluxation, vertebral subluxation (VS), vertebral subluxation complex (VSC), "killer subluxations," and the "silent killer."

They, along with some physical therapists and osteopathic physicians, have also used another term, BOOP, meaning "bone out of place."

Some chiropractors have described the disagreements within the profession about the concept, and have written skeptically about BOOP as an antiquated idea. In 1992 one wrote:

> "The main problem we often run into is the bone out of place (BOOP) concept. It seems we somehow step on toes when we describe the spine as a functioning entity instead of a stack of bones that can be shifted back and forth into the ideal configuration. The BOOP concept will eventually fade, and we are grateful for its contribution to chiropractic. For many decades, it offered a model to work from. This model has been updated by the rest of the healing profession, but chiropractors have been hesitant to let this antiquated model go. Some within our profession hold onto this model with a religious fervor. The chiropractic profession has moved into a new age. The BOOP concept has been updated and science is ever upon us in the 90s. Let's start asking questions again and drive the chiropractic profession kicking and screaming into the 21st century."

One wrote in 1994 about the "brutal civil war":

> "According to various gossip columnists in chiropractic, our profession appears to be currently enmeshed in a brutal civil war between BOOP (bone-out-of-place) practitioners and low back pain practitioners. It should be known that the BOOPers incorrectly call them-

> selves subluxation-based practitioners. My experience has demonstrated that the BOOPers do not know enough about subluxation to call themselves subluxation-based chiropractors. We would all do well to not be subluxation-based in the BOOP sense. It should also be known that this so-called war is really an over-dramatized skirmish between vocal BOOPers and a theoretical group of anti-chiropractic DCs. I have yet to meet any of these anti-chiropractic DCs. Unfortunately, the BOOPers seem to think that those who do not embrace the totality of BOOP philosophy are merely non-BOOPers who are still very pro-chiropractic and appreciate the philosophy of chiropractic from a contemporary and nondogmatic perspective."

Ten years later (in 2004) he openly disparaged the idea still propounded by "modern-day advocates of this concept":

> "... it is essentially impossible to have nerve interference. To summarize, nerve interference is described, by modern-day advocates of this concept, as a reduction of neural or mental impulses, which occurs in response to a bone-out-of-place (BOOP) subluxation... Clearly, the BOOP subluxation model fails miserably when considered in the light of basic neuroscience facts... BOOP subluxationists become angry and defensive when the BOOP model of subluxation is criticized... The reactionary nature of certain BOOP subluxationists is to accuse those who don't buy into the BOOP model of being anti-chiropractic – an astonishing leap of ignorance, to say the least. Furthermore, anyone who does not buy into the model is trying to "medicalize chiropractic" - another example of low-IQ thinking. And if tears do not well up in your eyes when you hear the phrase, "The power that made the body, heals the body," you are accused of having no passion for chiropractic – still another example of depressed, frontal-lobe activity. Even worse, if you don't buy into every bizarre, New Age, tree-hugging notion that comes down the pike and is circularly attached to subluxation, you will be accused of being an atheist – an excellent example of the need for psychiatrists and the drugs they prescribe."

Functional Hypotheses

V. Strang, D.C., describes several hypotheses on how a misaligned vertebra may cause interference to the nervous system in his book, *Essential Principles of Chiropractic*:

- Nerve compression hypothesis: suggests that when the vertebrae are out of alignment, the nerve roots and/or spinal cord can become pinched or irritated. While the most commonly referenced hypothesis, and easiest for a patient to understand, it may be the least likely to occur.
- Proprioceptive insult hypothesis: focuses on articular alterations causing hyperactivity of the sensory nerve fibers.
- Somatosympathetic reflex hypothesis: all the visceral organ functions can be reflexly affected by cutaneous or muscular stimulation.
- Somatosomatic reflex hypothesis: afferent impulses from one part of the body can result in reflex activity in other parts of the body.

- Viscerosomatic reflex hypothesis: visceral afferent fibers cause reflex somatic problems.
- Somatopsychic hypothesis: the effects of a subluxation on the ascending paths of the reticular activating system.
- Neurodystrophic hypothesis: focuses on lowered tissue resistance that results from abnormal innervation.
- Dentate ligament-cord distortion hypothesis: upper cervical misalignments can cause the dentate ligaments to put a stress on the spinal cord.
- Psychogenic hypothesis: emotions, such as stress, causing contraction in skeletal muscles.

The vertebral subluxation has been described as a syndrome with signs and symptoms which include: altered alignment; aberrant motion; palpable soft tissue changes; localized/referred pain; muscle contraction or imbalance; altered physiological function; reversible with adjustment/manipulation; focal tenderness.

Scientific Investigation

Investigation by chiropractors attempting to confirm the existence of vertebral subluxations has been ongoing since it was first postulated in 1895. The early practitioners used palpation and the anatomy of the nervous system as a guide (meric system). In their efforts to be more specific, they seized the newly discovered X-ray technology and introduced the neurocalometer (a heat sensing device). It was during those early years that the medical establishment first criticized the chiropractic profession, saying that the conditions that those early chiropractors were treating were only psychophysiologic disorders. To prove that chiropractic patients had real conditions, BJ Palmer opened a research clinic as a part of the Palmer College of Chiropractic. When a patient entered the clinic, they were first examined by medical doctors and a diagnosis was formulated. They were then sent to the chiropractic part of the clinic, treated, and sent back to the medical doctors for evaluation. Since then, chiropractors have sought a greater understanding of the mechanisms and effects of the vertebral subluxation. Today we see motion x-rays, surface EMG, and digital thermography though none of these methods have been proven to be reliable or valid in the detection of vertebral subluxations.

A 2004 research team at the National University of Health Sciences evaluated changes of the lumbar vertebral column following fixation (immobility) by surgically fusing spinal joints in experimental rats. The fixated joints showed significant degeneration compared to the mobile joints, confirming that surgical fixation results in time-dependent degenerative changes of the zygapophysial joints.

Believers within the chiropractic tradition assert that spinal health and function are directly related to general health and well-being. David Seaman reviewed the work of several researchers concerning autonomic nervous system relationship to the somatic tissues of the spine. He noted that Feinstein *et al.* were the first to clearly describe some symptoms associated with noxious irritation of spinal tissues. They injected hypertonic saline into interspinous tissues and paraspinal muscles of normal volunteers for the purpose of characterizing local and referred pain patterns that might develop. His observations included:

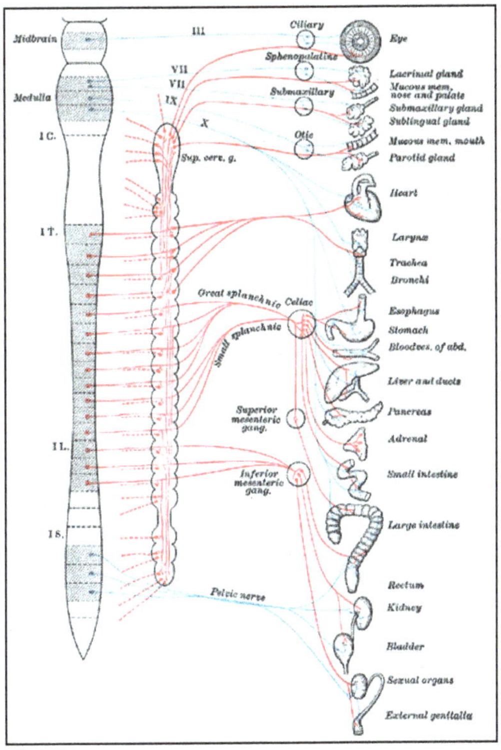

Autonomic nervous system
Blue = parasympathetic
Red = sympathetic

> "The pain elicited from muscles was accompanied by a characteristic group of phenomena which indicated involvement of other than segmental somatic mechanisms ... The manifestations were pallor, sweating bradycardia, fall in blood pressure, subjective faintness, and nausea, but vomiting was not observed. Syncope occurred in two early procedures in the series of paravertebral injections and was subsequently avoided by quickly depressing the subject's head or by having him lie down at the first sign of faintness. These features were not proportional to the severity of or to the extent of radiation; on the contrary, they seemed to dominate the experience of subjects who complained of little pain, but who were overwhelmed by this distressing complex of symptoms."

Feinstein referred to these symptoms as autonomic concomitants. It is likely that these autonomic concomitants were caused by nociceptive stimulation of autonomic centers in the brainstem, particularly the medulla. Feinstein indicated that "this is an example of the ability of deep noxious stimulation to activate generalized autonomic responses independently of the relay of pain to conscious levels." In other words, pain may not be the symptomatic outcome of nociceptive stimulation of spinal structures. Such a conclusion has profound implications for the chiropractic profession. Clearly, patients do not need to be in pain to be candidates for spinal adjustments.

The efficacy and validity of spinal manipulation to address visceral disorders systems remains a source of controversy within the chiropractic profession. Although research is ongoing on this topic, conclusions that support the usefulness of spinal manipulation for organic disorders remains to be seen. Additionally, to complicate matters, chiropractic professors and researchers, Nansel and Szlazak, found that:

> "the proper differential diagnosis of somatic (musculoskeletal) vs. visceral (organ) dysfunction represents a challenge for both the medical and chiropractic physician. The afferent convergence mechanisms, which can create signs and symptoms that are virtually indistinguishable with respect to their somatic vs. visceral etiologies, suggest it is not unreasonable that this somatic visceral-disease mimicry could very well account for the "cures" of presumed organ disease that have been observed over the years in response to various somatic therapies (e.g., spinal manipulation, acupuncture, Rolfing, Qi Gong, etc.) and may represent a common phenomenon that has led to "holistic" health care claims on the part of such clinical disciplines."

Considering this phenomenon, Seaman suggests that the chiropractic concept of joint complex (somatic) dysfunction should be incorporated into the differential diagnosis of pain and visceral symptoms because these dysfunctions often generate symptoms similar to those produced by true visceral disease and notes that this mimicry leads to unnecessary surgical procedures and medications.

Other chiropractic researchers have also questioned some of the claimed effects of vertebral subluxation:

> "The literature supports the existence of somatovisceral and viscerosomatic reflexes, but there is little or no evidence to support the notion that the spinal derangements (often referred to as subluxations by chiropractors) can cause prolonged aberrant discharge of these reflexes. Equally unsupported in the literature is the notion that the prolonged activation of these reflexes will manifest into pathological state of tissues, and most relevantly, that the application of spinal manipulative therapy can alter the prolonged reflex discharge or be associated with a reversal of the pathological degeneration of the affected reflexes or tissues. The evidence that has been amassed is largely anecdotal or case report based and it has attracted much intra disciplinary debate because of its frequent association with certain approaches to management (largely described as being traditional or "philosophical" in nature)."

Still other chiropractic researchers state quite directly:

> "... early chiropractic philosophy ... considered disease the result of spinal nerve dysfunction caused by misplaced (subluxated) vertebrae. Although rejected by medical science, this concept is still [2000] accepted by a minority of chiropractors... Indeed, many progressive chiropractors have rejected the historical concept of the chiropractic subluxation in favor of ones that more accurately describe the nature of the complex joint disfunctions they treat."

Researchers at the RMIT University-Japan, Tokyo studied reflex effects of vertebral subluxation with regards to the autonomic nervous system. They found that "recent neuroscience research supports a neurophysiologic rationale for the concept that aberrant stimulation of spinal or paraspinal structures may lead to segmentally organized reflex responses of the autonomic nervous system, which in turn may alter visceral function."

Professor Philip S. Bolton of the School of Biomedical Sciences at University of Newcastle, Australia writes in Journal of Manipulative and Physiological Therapeutics, "The traditional chiropractic vertebral subluxation hypothesis proposes that vertebral misalignment cause illness, disease, or both. This hypothesis remains controversial." His objective was, "To briefly review and update experimental evidence concerning reflex effects of vertebral subluxations, particularly concerning peripheral nervous system responses to vertebral subluxations. Data source: Information was obtained from chiropractic or, scientific peer-reviewed literature concerning human or animal studies of neural responses to vertebral subluxation, vertebral displacement or movement, or both." He concluded, "Animal models suggest that vertebral displacements and putative vertebral subluxations may modulate activity in group I to IV afferent nerves. However, it is not clear whether these afferent nerves are modulated during normal day-to-day activities of living and, if so, what segmental or whole-body reflex effects they may have."

Conclusions: Monitoring mixed-nerve root discharges in response to spinal manipulative thrusts *in vivo* in human subjects undergoing lumbar surgery is feasible. Neurophysiologic responses appeared sensitive to the contact point and applied force vector of the spinal manipulative thrust. Further study of the neurophysiologic mechanisms of spinal manipulation in humans and animals is needed to more precisely identify the mechanisms and neural pathways involved.

Researchers at the Department of Physiology, University College London studied the effects of compression upon conduction in myelinated axons. Using pneumatic pressure of varying degrees on the sciatic nerves of frog specimens, the study supported the idea of nerve conduction failure as a result of compression.

Critiques

Edzard Ernst has stated that the "core concepts of chiropractic, subluxation and spinal manipulation, are not based on sound science."

An area of debate among chiropractors is whether "vertebral subluxation" is a metaphysical concept (as posited in B. J. Palmer's philosophy of chiropractic) or a real phenomenon.

In an article on vertebral subluxation, the chiropractic authors wrote:

> "Subluxation syndrome is a legitimate, potentially testable, theoretical construct for which there is little experimental evidence. Acceptable as hypothesis, the widespread assertion of the clinical meaningfulness of this notion brings ridicule from the scientific and health care communities and confusion within the chiropractic profession. We believe that an evidence-orientation among chiropractors requires that we distinguish between subluxation dogma vs. subluxation as the potential focus of clinical research. We lament efforts to generate unity within the profession through consensus statements concerning subluxation dogma, and believe that cultural authority will continue to elude us so long as we assert dogma as though it were validated clinical theory."

Since its inception, the concept of *vertebral subluxation* has been a source of definitional debate. Tedd Koren, DC offers this explanation as a possible cause of the confusion:

The vertebral subluxation cannot be precisely defined because it is an abstraction, an intellectual construct used by chiropractors, chiropractic researchers, educators and others to explain the success of the chiropractic adjustment.

This is not a unique state of affairs, abstract entities populate many branches of science...

Subluxations, genes, gravity, the ego and life are all heuristic devices, "useful fictions" that are used to explain phenomenon that are far larger than our understanding. We use them as long as they work for us and discard or limit their application when they become unwieldy or unable to account for new observations...

Critics of chiropractic have incorrectly assumed that chiropractic is based on the theory or principle that vertebral subluxations cause "pinched" nerves that cause disease. They have it backwards. Chiropractic is based on the success of the spinal adjustment. The theory attempting to explain the success of the adjustment (nerve impingement, disease, subluxations) followed its clinical discovery.

Examples of such erroneous criticisms based on this straw man argument abound in the medical literature. Some examples: "The teachers, research workers and practitioners of medicine reject the so-called principle on which chiropractic is based and correctly and bluntly label it a fraud and hoax on the human race." "The basis of chiropractic is completely unscientific." The theory on which chiropractic is based [is false], namely that a "subluxation" of a spinal vertebra presses on a nerve interfering with the passage of energy down that nerve causing disease to organs supplied by that nerve, and that chiropractic "adjustments" can alleviate the pressure thereby treating or preventing such disease. There is no scientific evidence for the validity of this theory."

To be fair, statements by some chiropractors have tended to perpetuate this misunderstanding: "Pressure on nerves causes irritation and tension with deranged functions as a result."

When chiropractors declare that "pinched nerves" "nerve impingement" "spinal fixations" or others mechanisms of action explain how subluxations affect the person and how chiropractic works they are making the same mistake medical critics make – assuming chiropractic is based on theory. Mechanisms and theories are useful tools, but their limitations should always be kept in mind.

Other chiropractors have declared its unproven status as an area that needs reform:

> "Some may suggest that chiropractors should promote themselves as the experts in "correcting vertebral subluxation." However, the scientific literature has failed to demonstrate the very existence of the subluxation. Until and unless sound research published in credible journals demonstrates the existence and reliable identification of vertebral subluxation, and vertebral subluxation is found to be an important public health problem, society at large will not care about its correction. Thus, "subluxation correction" alone is not a viable option for chiropractic's future."

A Beth Israel Deaconess Medical Center article describes the mainstream understanding of vertebral subluxation theory:

Since its origin, chiropractic theory has based itself on "subluxations," or vertebrae that have shifted position in the spine. These subluxations are said to impede nerve outflow and cause disease in various organs. A chiropractic treatment is supposed to "put back in" these "popped out" vertebrae. For this reason, it is called an "adjustment."

However, no real evidence has ever been presented showing that a given chiropractic treatment alters the position of any vertebrae. In addition, there is as yet no real evidence that impairment of nerve outflow is a major contributor to common illnesses, or that spinal manipulation changes nerve outflow in such a way as to affect organ function.

In 2009, four scholarly chiropractors concluded that epidemiologic evidence does not support chiropractic's most fundamental theory. Since its inception, the vast majority of chiropractors have postulated that "subluxations" (misalignments) are the cause or underlying cause of ill health and can be corrected with spinal "adjustments." After searching the scientific literature, the chiropractic authors concluded:

> "No supportive evidence is found for the chiropractic subluxation being associated with any disease process or of creating suboptimal health conditions requiring intervention. Regardless of popular appeal, this leaves the subluxation construct in the realm of unsupported speculation. This lack of supportive evidence suggests the subluxation construct has no valid clinical applicability."

References

- Keating JC Jr (2005). "A brief history of the chiropractic profession". In Haldeman S; Dagenais S; Budgell B; et al. Principles and Practice of Chiropractic (3rd ed.). McGraw-Hill. pp. 23–64. ISBN 0-07-137534-1
- Robert Cooperstein, Brian J. Gleberzon. Technique systems in chiropractic. Elsevier Health Sciences, 2004, ISBN 0-443-07413-5, ISBN 978-0-443-07413-4
- Anderson M. D. Robert Anderson M. D.; Robert Anderson (October 2009). The Back Door to Medicine: An Embedded Anthropologist Tells All. iUniverse. pp. 59–. ISBN 978-1-4401-7289-2
- Singh S, Ernst E (2008). "The truth about chiropractic therapy". Trick or Treatment: The Undeniable Facts about Alternative Medicine. W.W. Norton. pp. 145–90. ISBN 978-0-393-06661-6
- WHO guidelines on basic training and safety in chiropractic, World Health Organization, Geneva, 2005. ISBN 92-4-159371-7. available online
- David Chapman-Smith (2000). The Chiropractic Profession: Its Education, Practice, Research and Future Directions. NCMIC Group. p. 160. ISBN 1-892734-02-8
- Chapman-Smith D (2000). "Current status of the profession". The Chiropractic Profession: Its Education, Practice, Research and Future Directions. West Des Moines, IA: NCMIC. ISBN 1-892734-02-8
- World Health Organization (2005). "WHO guidelines on basic training and safety in chiropractic" (PDF). ISBN 92-4-159371-7. Retrieved 29, February 2020
- David Chapman-Smith (2000). "Principles and Goals of Chiropractic Care". The Chiropractic Profession: Its Education, Practice, Research and Future Directions. NCMIC Group. p. 160. ISBN 1-892734-02-8

Chapter 7

Osteopathy

Osteopathy is a type of alternative medicine that is concerned with the physical manipulation of the bones and muscle tissues of the body. It is attempted to diagnose and treat somatic dysfunction by manipulating the muscles and bones of the person. The topics explained in this chapter are crucial for a complete understanding of osteopathy.

There are two main distinctions between osteopathic and allopathic physicians. The first, more obvious difference lies in the osteopathic physicians' use of osteopathic manipulative medicine (OMM). While OMM is most commonly known by the general public to treat neuromusculoskeletal injury, DOs may utilize it in their diagnosis and treatment of disease involving internal organs and all other parts of the body as well. The other, more subtle – and arguably more important – distinction between the two professions is that osteopathic medicine offers a concise philosophy on which all clinical practice is based. Central to this philosophy is the belief that the body has an inherent healing mechanism that allows it to maintain health, resist illness, and recover from disease processes. The goal of osteopathic medical treatment is to provide patients with the tools they need to restore and maintain their natural, self-healing state. The four major tenets of the osteopathic medical philosophy are listed and briefly explained below:

- The body is completely united; the person is a fully integrated being of body, mind and spirit. No single part of the body functions independently. Each separate part is interconnected with all others and serves to benefit the collective whole of the person. Alterations in any part of the system, including an individual's mental and spiritual health, affect the function of the body as a whole and all other parts therein.
- The body is capable of self-regulation, self-healing, and health-maintenance. Health is the natural state of the body, and the body possesses complex, homeostatic, self-regulatory mechanisms that it uses to heal itself from injury. In times of disease, when a part of the body is functioning sub-optimally, other parts of the body come out of their natural state of health in order to compensate for the dysfunction. During this compensatory process, however, new dysfunctions may arise. Osteopathic physicians must work to adjust the body so as to realign its parts back to normal. Osteopathic manipulative medicine aims to restore the body's self-healing capacity by decreasing allostatic load, or the physiologic effects of chronic bodily stresses, and enhancing the immune system.
- Structure and function are reciprocally interrelated. The structure of a body part governs its function, and thus abnormal structure manifests as dysfunction. Function also governs structure. In addition, if the body's overall structure is suboptimal, its functioning and capacity for self-healing will be inhibited as well.
- Rational treatment is based on an understanding of these three aforementioned principles.

These basic osteopathic tenets permeate all aspects of health maintenance and disease prevention and treatment. The osteopathic physician examines, diagnoses, and treats patients according to these principles.

Difference between Physiotherapist and Osteopath and Chiropractor

While they may seem similar at a glance, the three professions take very different approaches to health, so it is important to understand what sets each one apart from the others.

Physiotherapist

Probably the most well-known of the three job titles, it is worth starting off by drawing a distinction between a physiotherapist and the similar-but-distinct title of physical therapist. While both can be legitimate careers, it is important to know that only physiotherapists require a university degree, while physical therapists receive a narrower range of training over a shorter period of time.

In comparison to osteopaths and chiropractors, one of the primary distinctions of physiotherapy is its use of an all-encompassing approach that looks beyond the purely physical elements of an issue, also taking both psychological and social factors into account when treating patients. This means that if a patient were to present themselves to a physiotherapist complaining of back pain, rather than simply identifying the problem area and treating the symptoms, a physiotherapist will attempt to identify why the problem manifested in the first place, and prevent it from recurring in the future. This means looking at the physical side of things, such as posture and movement patterns, as well as psychological aspects such as stress or anxiety, and social factors such as work habits and hobbies.

Chiropractor

Of the three job titles, chiropractors are definitely the most commonly associated with back problems, although some claim it can help with issues such as asthma or sexual dysfunction. But at the same time, chiropractors are also among the most controversial in medical circles. The main feature of chiropractic treatment that sets it apart from physiotherapy and osteopathy is its focus on manipulation, which is when joints are pushed and pulled to their farthest possible range of motion. The belief is that physical pain can be resolved by getting a chiropractor to manually put everything "back in the right place".

Chiropractors are somewhat controversial for a number of reasons. Firstly, their techniques are seen as unnecessarily risky, with chiropractors having some of the highest instances of adverse patient reactions. They are also looked down upon from a scientific perspective, with one of their main theories having no evidence to even support its existence. "Chiropractic subluxation" is claimed to cause organ problems by disrupting the nerves along the spine, but this has never been shown to actually exist, meaning their attempts to treat it for both back pain and organ problems is viewed by many as not only ineffective, but meaningless and irresponsible.

Osteopath

Osteopaths are quite similar to chiropractors in that they also place a lot of importance on manual manipulation, although they tend to be a lot gentler. The prevailing theory of osteopathy is that the body is at its best when all of its tissues are moving how they are supposed to. Osteopaths therefore assess a patient's health by feeling their tissues, and attempt to stimulate movement where they believe it is lacking.

As osteopathic manipulation is so much gentler than chiropractic manipulation, many see it as harmless, or even beneficial when combined with other medical treatment. However, some studies have shown osteopathy to be ineffective in achieving its claims, while others show evidence to support it. The general consensus is that while osteopathy may have science to back up some of its claims, other claims are simply not true, and further research is needed.

Osteopathic Manipulative Medicine

A distinct component of osteopathic medical practice is a collection of treatment modalities called Osteopathic Manipulative Medicine (OMM), also referred to as "Osteopathic Manipulative Treatment" (or formerly "Osteopathic Manipulative Therapy") (OMT). Osteopathic physicians use OMM as a key treatment option in their care for patients. It involves the use of the hands as the primary diagnostic, treatment, and therapeutic tool. DOs utilize screening and scanning for visual and palpatory TART (see sidebar) changes to identify areas of somatic dysfunction in the bones, muscles, joints, ligaments, and tendons, which can then be treated with a wide array of manual techniques. The goal of OMM is to address the somatic dysfunction either by directly treating the lesion, or by manipulating the body in such a way that allows the musculoskeletal system to correct itself – this would be called an "indirect" technique. Oftentimes, OMM is used as an adjunct to traditional medical care and has been shown to reduce such clinical variables as pain, need for and extent of pharmaceutical drug use, and recovery time.

There are more than 500 different OMM techniques. Some are similar to those used by chiropractors, physical therapists, and/or massage therapists, while other methods are completely unique to osteopathic medicine. Below is a list of the major OMM techniques (both direct and indirect) that DOs are trained to use:

Direct Treatment Modalities

- Soft Tissue Techniques: Direct lateral or linear stretching of muscle and fascia (connective tissue that surrounds the muscles, organs and other structures), frequently used to prepare for or conclude overall treatment.
- Articulatory Treatment System: Low velocity, moderate- to high-amplitude springing focused on joint functioning.
- High Velocity Low Amplitude (HVLA): Use of fast, short thrusts through restrictive articulatory barriers; a technique with which most people are familiar (also known as the "cracking" or "popping" technique).

- Muscle Energy: Uses post-isometric relaxation to stretch muscles and increase range of motion. With the targeted muscle stretched to its barrier, the patient is instructed to move toward ease (away from restriction) while the physician resists by using an isometric counterforce.
- Inhibition: Slow, direct application of steady pressure to relax muscles or reduce muscle contraction.

Indirect Treatment Modalities

- Strain/Counterstrain: Focused on specific tender points on the body those are held in a position of ease for 90 seconds, after which the tenderness is relieved.
- Facilitated Positional Release: Patient's spine is placed at neutral position while the isolated segment for treatment is placed at ease. Compression or traction is then added to release muscle, fascia, and/or joints.

Both Direct and Indirect Treatment Modalities

- Myofascial Release: Encompasses many of the modalities mentioned above and is used to treat restrictions of muscle and fascia. This technique is generally not as aggressive as others and can thus be applied to a wider population.
- Osteopathic Cranial Manipulative Medicine: A system of treatment that utilizes the intrinsic motion of the cranial and neurological system to treat the whole body; one of the most difficult techniques for physicians to master, and for this reason, one of the more controversial within the medical field.
- Ligamentous Articulatory Release: Ligaments or joints are placed into a state of balanced tension until a release is felt.
- Still Technique: Patient held at position of ease until release, and then passively moved through the barrier quickly.

Treatment Modalities that are neither Direct nor Indirect

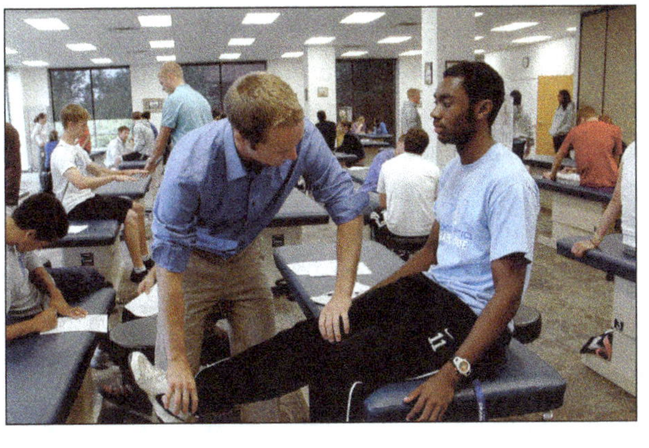

- Chapman's Reflexes: Chapman's points are points on the body that, if tender, indicate visceral dysfunction. These can be treated in a variety of ways, including muscle energy and myofascial release.

- Lymphatic Techniques: Rhythmic, usually passive, movement of patient to increase flow of lymphatic fluid.

OMM and Chronic Pain

Chronic pain mechanisms encompass a complicated array of different processes (eg, biomechanics, genetics, neurophysiology, psychology), each capable of contributing to clinical manifestations and symptoms. For OMM to be effective, similar symptoms in different patients may require dissimilar treatment plans that focus on various local, spinal, and supraspinal targets. For example, chronic pain initiated by peripheral trauma may result when supraspinal structures continue to respond as if peripheral tissues were actively injured. In such chronic conditions as fibromyalgia, the pathologic process may reflect an autonomic dysregulatory phenomenon or a dysfunction of descending antinociception pathways. Conditions involving myofascial trigger points (MTrPs) demonstrate specific peripheral dysfunction at a spinal level perpetuated by nonspecific biomechanical factors (eg, untreated postural strain, viscerosomatic reflexes).

In many cases, chronic pain pathways involving allodynia (generalized lowered thresholds to pain) develop when changing gene expression allows silent receptors to become active in the spinal cord, or when facilitatory modulation results in "spinal cord learning." In such cases, the patient may simply present with persistent pain.

The rational application of OMT for patients with persistent pain cannot have a singular focus, nor can it be considered a static phenomenon (i.e., effects on gene expression as well as the changing face of pain and pain perceptions as chronicity alters the body unit). In formulating multimodal treatment plans, approaches based on OMM embrace principles of body unity and integrate palpation and OMT techniques into each patient's prescription. Physician choices concerning OMT techniques and goals depend on each patient's unique pain presentation, suspected pathways involved in that presentation, and those body regions diagnosed as containing somatic dysfunction.

Pain Management Algorithm: Applying Osteopathic Principles and Practice

When patients present with chronic pain, especially pain that persists despite seemingly appropriate care, referring to an osteopathic algorithm can suggest approaches and rationale for applying OPP and OMT to patient care. The pain management algorithm is structured to identify frequently overlooked underlying etiologies included in an osteopathic differential diagnosis, as well as to address the persistent tangible and holistic impact of pain on the body unit. Evaluation of two main factors guide the osteopathic physician's timing for implementing OMM treatment strategies: the patient's capability to mount a homeostatic response and the patient's underlying pathophysiologic status as interpreted by components of palpated somatic dysfunction.

Treatment protocols formulated from this algorithm incorporate the interdependence of all tenets of osteopathic medicine, resulting in an individually designed prescription to address each patient who has persistent pain. In applying this algorithm to patient care, osteopathic physicians may also choose to use some or all of the mainstream and/or complementary treatment modalities used by other healthcare professionals.

Structure-Function Considerations: Somatic Causes of Persistent Pain

Certain somatic findings have been consistently documented in various persistent pain conditions. Depending on the particular situation, somatic dysfunction may be causative, reflexive, reactive, or perpetuating (or some combination of these pathophysiologic mechanisms). Thus, differential diagnoses and treatment considerations depend on both the specific body region and underlying pathophysiologic mechanism involved. The algorithm contains generalities taking these factors and structure function interrelationships into consideration.

An osteopathic palpatory examination often provides clues to the underlying mechanism(s) of a patient's injury. Such palpatory insights can lead to further questions, examinations, and tests, each designed to identify structural factors associated with specific pain generators or factors that interfere with certain self-healing mechanisms. The resulting findings, in turn, can lead the physician to explore functional demand issues associated with potential mechanisms of repeated injury or cumulative microtrauma caused by habitual, occupational, or postural ergonomic stresses.

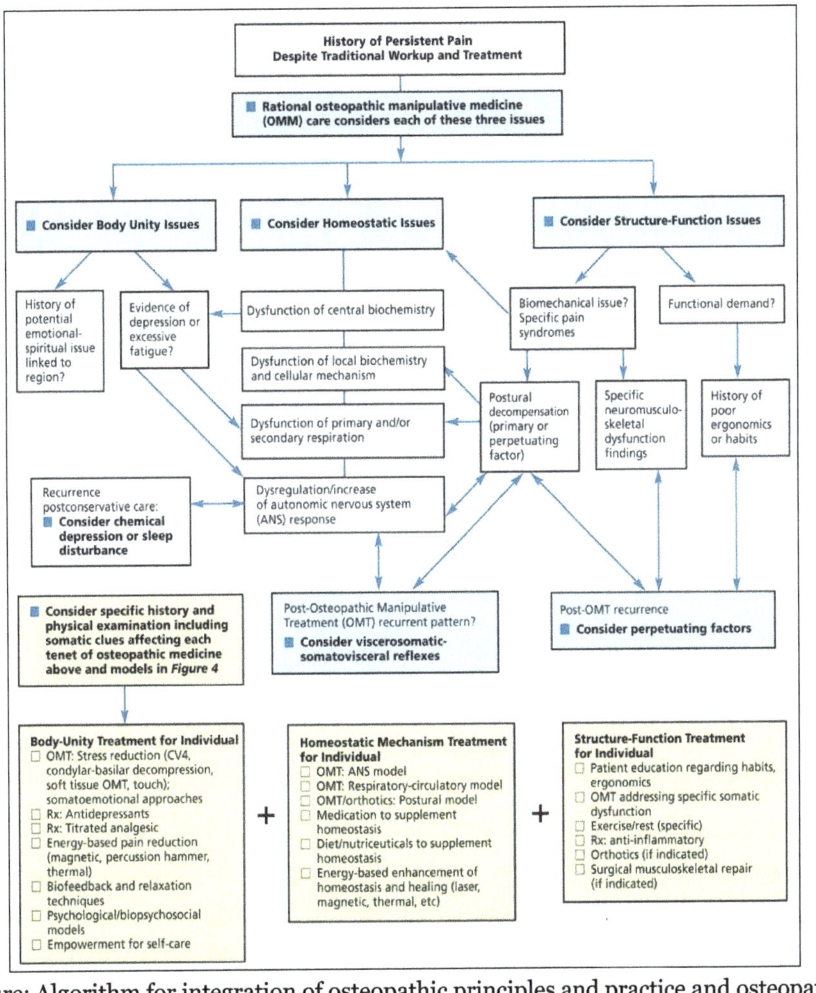

Figure: Algorithm for integration of osteopathic principles and practice and osteopathic manipulative medicine in diagnosis and management of persistent pain.

One way to determine whether a given structure or somatic dysfunction is a primary cause of significant discomfort in a patient is to determine if it is a "pain generator" tissue. Comparing the anatomic location, quality, and unique referral distribution of a patient's pain symptoms with known myotomal, neurologic, and sclerotomal pain maps increases the likelihood of locating pain generators. In many cases, such diagnoses can be confirmed by an effective therapeutic response—albeit even temporary—to local anesthetic injection or manual correction of dysfunction.

Sclerotomal tissues (ie, skeletal, arthrodial, and ligamentous generators) typically mediate pain described by patients as "deep, dull, and toothachelike." Sclerotomal pain patterns are frequently overlooked because they may project some distance from their pain generators. In addition, these pain patterns are infrequently taught to physicians. The "Glossary of Osteopathic Terminology" contains sclerotomal maps relating spinal segmental levels to sclerotomal appendicular pain.

Figure below illustrates segmentally related sclerotomal examples of ligamentous pain patterns commonly seen in patients with low back pain (LBP). Patients with ligamentous pain generators often cannot find a comfortable position and are continuously shifting position—a presentation sometimes referred to as "theater-cocktail party syndrome."

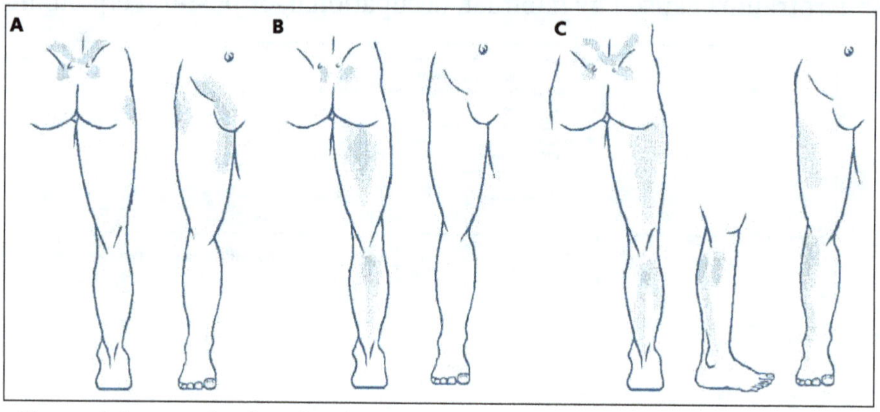

Figure: Sclerotomal pain referral regions from ligaments: (A) iliolumbar ligament, (B) sacrospinous and sacrotuberous ligaments, (C) posterior sacroiliac ligament.

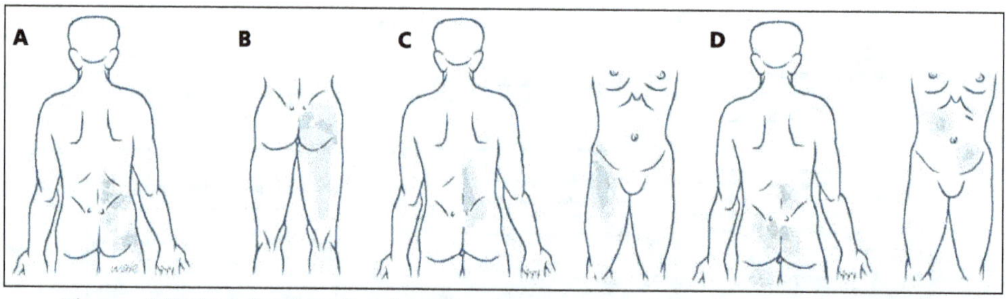

Figure: Myotomal pain referral regions from muscle trigger points: (A) quadratus lumborum, (B) piriformis, (C) iliopsoas, (D) rotatores and multifidi muscles.

Myotomal (muscle) pain is poorly localized, and the patient may describe symptoms located at a substantial distance from the actual lesion. Patients typically describe myotomal pain as "crampy" or "stiff," with the pain suddenly "grabbing" them during a particular motion. Muscle dysfunction may include latent and active MTrPs that, when overused, refer pain in recognizable patterns. Antigravity (postural) muscles harboring MTrPs are frequently hypertonic, whereas postural antagonist muscles harboring MTrPs demonstrate weakness upon strength testing.

Both antigravity and postural antagonist muscles are likely to contain taut bands that demonstrate a local twitch response within the affected muscle during perpendicularly applied snapping palpatory examination. This phenomenon has been linked to the presence of segmentally related spinal reflexes (i.e., segmental facilitation).

Peripheral myotomal pain generators can originate in a single muscle. Alternatively, multiple peripheral inputs may establish more complex patterns of muscle dysfunction. Peripheral input can also produce a central imprint that persists as a primary source of pain-modifying peripheral referral patterns (ie, somatosomatic reflex). Common myotomal patterns also include muscles sharing the same radicular innervation (as occurs in patients with discogenic disease) and muscles contributing to the same general function (as in the myotatic unit pattern occurring in patients with overuse syndromes).

In structure-function considerations, osteopathic physicians using osteopathic diagnostic palpation seek to identify "any impaired or altered skeletal, arthrodial, and/or myofascial function" (viz "somatic dysfunction") that adds to the nociceptive load, and to recognize any related lymphatic, neural, and/or vascular elements that might complicate underlying pathophysiologic conditions. The palpatory characteristics sought by osteopathic physicians include sensitivity to measured palpation (S), tissue texture changes (T), asymmetry (A), and restricted motion (R) (together known as STAR characteristics). Tissue texture changes often provide the most important information concerning the underlying pathophysiologic status of the patient's periphery and homeostatic response status.

After weighing risk-to-benefit ratios associated with the tentative diagnosis of a patient's condition, OMT may be delivered to reduce or remove the identified somatic dysfunction or to modulate central and peripheral mechanisms involved in pain generation.

Muscle Energy Technique

Muscle Energy Technique (MET) is a technique that was developed in 1948 by Fred Mitchell, Sr, D.O. It is a form of manual therapy, widely used in Osteopathy that uses a muscle's own energy in the form of gentle isometric contractions to relax the muscles via autogenic or reciprocal inhibition and lengthen the muscle. As compared to static stretching which is a passive technique in which the therapist does all the work, MET is an active technique in which the patient is also an active participant. MET is based on the concepts of Autogenic Inhibition and Reciprocal Inhibition. If a sub-maximal contraction of the muscle is followed by stretching of the same muscle it is known as Autogenic Inhibition MET, and if a submaximal contraction of a muscle is followed by stretching of the opposite muscle then this is known as Reciprocal Inhibition MET.

Autogenic and Reciprocal Inhibition

Autogenic and reciprocal inhibition both occur when certain muscles are inhibited from contracting due to the activation of the Golgi tendon organ (GTO) and the muscle spindles. These two musculotendinous proprioceptors located in and around the joints and muscles respond to changes in muscle tension and length, which helps manage muscular control and coordination.

The GTO, located between the muscle belly and its tendon, senses increased tension when the muscle contracts or stretches. When the muscle contracts, the GTO are activated and respond by inhibiting this contraction (reflex inhibition) and contracting the opposing (antagonist) muscle group. This process is known as autogenic inhibition.

The GTO response plays an important role in flexibility. When the GTO inhibits the (agonist) muscle's contraction and allows the antagonist muscle to contract more readily, the muscle can be stretched further and easier. Autogenic inhibition is often seen during static stretching, such as during a low-force, long-duration stretch. After 7 to 10 seconds, muscle tension increases and activates the GTO response, causing the muscle spindle in the stretched muscle to be inhibited temporarily, which makes it possible to stretch the muscle further.

The muscle spindle is located within the muscle belly and stretches along with the muscle itself. When this occurs, the muscle spindle is activated and causes a reflexive contraction in the agonist muscle (known as the stretch reflex) and relaxation in the antagonist muscle. This process is known as reciprocal inhibition.

Types of MET

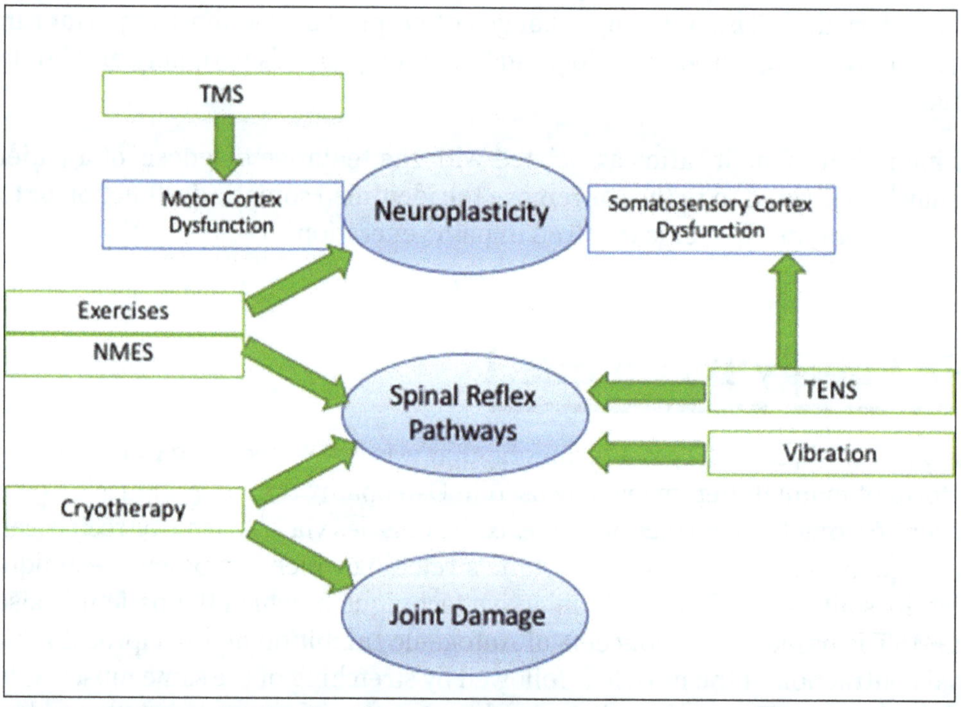

Figure showing the reflex neuro-muscular inhibition phenomenon.

- Autogenic Inhibition MET.
    - Post Isometric Relaxation (PIR).
    - Post Facilitation Stretching (PFS).
- Reciprocal Inhibition MET.

Autogenic Inhibition MET

Autogenic Inhibition METs work on the principle of autogenic inhibition. The two major and well-known types of MET that are based on the concept of autogenic inhibition are Post Isometric Relaxation (PIR) and Post facilitation Stretching (PFS).

Post Isometric Relaxation (PIR)

Post Isometric Relaxation is a technique that was later developed by Karel Lewitt. Post Isometric Relaxation (PIR) is the effect of the decrease in muscle tone in a single or group of muscles, after a brief period of submaximal isometric contraction of the same muscle. PIR works on the concept of autogenic inhibition.

The PIR technique is performed as follows:

- The hypertonic muscle is taken to a length just short of pain, or to the point where resistance to movement is first noted.
- A submaximal (10-20%) contraction of the hypertonic muscle is performed away from the barrier for between 5 and 10 seconds and the therapist applies resistance in the opposite direction. The patient should inhale during this effort.
- After the isometric contraction, the patient is asked to relax and exhale while doing so. Following this, a gentle stretch is applied to take up the slack till the new barrier.
- Starting from this new barrier, the procedure is repeated two or three times.

Post Facilitation Stretch (PFS)

This technique is more aggressive than PIR but is also based on the concept of autogenic inhibition.

The PFS technique is performed as follows:

- The hypertonic and shortened muscle is placed between a fully stretched and a fully relaxed state.
- The patient is asked to contract the agonist using a maximum degree of effort for 5–10 seconds while the therapist resists the patient's force.
- The patient is then asked to relax and release the effort, whereas the therapist applies a rapid stretch to a new barrier and is held for 10 seconds.
- The patient relaxes for approximately 20 seconds and the procedure is repeated between three to five times and five times more.
- Instead of starting from a new barrier, the muscle is placed between a fully stretched and a fully relaxed state before every repetition.

Reciprocal Inhibition MET

Reciprocal Inhibition MET is different from the above two techniques in that it involves the contraction of one muscle followed by stretching of the opposite muscle, because contrary to PIR and PFS, Reciprocal Inhibition MET as the name implies is based on the concept of Reciprocal Inhibition.

The Reciprocal Inhibition MET technique is performed as follows:

- The affected muscle is placed in a mid-range position.
- The patient pushes towards the restriction/barrier whereas the therapist completely resists this effort (isometric) or allows a movement towards it (isotonic).
- This is followed by relaxation of the patient along with exhalation, and the therapist applies a passive stretch to the new barrier.
- The procedure is repeated between three to five times and five times more.

Indication

Muscle Energy Techniques can be used for any condition in which the goal is to cause relaxation and lengthening of the muscles and improve range of motion (ROM) in joints. Muscle energy techniques can be applied safely to almost any joint in the body. Many athletes use MET as a preventative measure to guard against future injury of muscles and joints. It is mainly used by individuals who have a limited ROM due to facet joint dysfunction in the neck and back, and for broader areas such as shoulder pain, scoliosis, sciatica, asymmetrical legs, hips or arms, or to treat chronic muscle pain, stiffness or injury.

All Muscle Energy Techniques have essential steps to be followed:

- Accurate diagnosis of somatic dysfunction (SD) must be made.
- The restrictive barrier must be engaged in all planes of motion for any given joint. In the spine those motions should be flexion or extension, side-bending right or left, and rotation right or left.
- The operator must apply a distinct counterforce.
- The patient applies an appropriate amount of muscle contraction, in the correct direction, and for a correct duration of time.
- Complete relaxation of the patient's effort following muscle contraction, while the operator maintains the joint position.
- The operator repositions the restrictive barriers in all planes while always palpably monitoring the joint.
- Steps 3 to 6 are repeated one or two times.
- Always recheck the findings to make certain the dysfunction is corrected.

Joint Mobilization and Manipulation

Joint mobilization is a treatment technique used to manage musculoskeletal dysfunction. Most manipulative and mobilization techniques are performed by physical therapists, and fall under the category of manual therapy.

In most cases, at the end of a long bone there is a joint or articulation. The long bone is attached or joined to another bone by a joint. For example, the femur is attached to the tibia at the knee joint. The knee joint is made up of the surface of the tibia, femur, ligaments, and capsule. Thus, the knee joint is stable and yet mobile. When an individual is sitting in a chair and freely kicks his leg out (knee extension), the tibia moves, while the femur is stationary. However, at the surface of the articulating bones (tibia and femur), there is other movement. This movement is known as slide or glide; some have termed it "joint play." When an individual kicks his leg out, the lower leg or tibia is not only moving forward, but also gliding across the end of the femur. Mobilization is the treatment technique that involves the clinician applying a force to mimic the gliding that occurs between bones. It is a passive movement, the goal of which is to produce a slide or glide. Mobilizations are usually completed at slow speed, sometimes with oscillations, and even with a "hold" or stretch. Manipulations are more aggressive, high velocity techniques, or thrusts. They occur very fast, and at the end of available joint play.

Purpose

Mobilizations are used to restore joint play that has been lost due to injury or disease. In order for an individual to kick his leg out, there must be sufficient joint play, or freedom for the tibia to move on the femur. Thus, mobilizations are used when range of motion or mobility is lacking. Furthermore, gentle oscillations within the available joint play range, is a technique used to decrease pain. Manipulations are quick movements that occur beyond the available joint play range. The purpose of manipulations, or joint thrusts, is to increase the available range if it is not full. Secondly, manipulations are done to break adhesions that disrupt joint movement.

Precautions

Mobilizations and manipulations should not be done in the following circumstances:

- To the spine if there is severe osteoarthritis or osteoporosis.
- If there is any tumor or malignancy in the area.
- To the cervical region if there is dysfunction with the flow of blood within the vertebral artery.
- If there is bleeding in a joint.
- If there is a loose body in the joint.
- To total joint replacements.
- To joints near a growth plate.

- If the joint is degenerative.
- Until a full diagnosis is reached.

Description

Peripheral joint mobilization means mobilizing the joints of the periphery or limbs. There is a grading system for completing mobilizations. The grading system is based on how much joint play is available. Thus, the clinician must know what the total range is by examination through passive movement. Furthermore, there are stretching mobilizations used for pain management and stretching. The first common mobilization techniques are sustained joint play movements that have three grades. These mobilizations aid in decreasing pain and increasing mobility.

- Grade 1: The clinician applies passive movement in a very small range, approximately 15-25% of the available joint play range.
- Grade 2: Bone is passively moved in a moderate range to 50% or half of the available joint play range.
- Grade 3: Passive force by the clinician causes one bone to move on the other to the end of the available joint play range.

Within these three grades the stretch or "hold" is approximately five to seven seconds.

The other common mobilization technique is termed oscillatory mobilization. These mobilizations have five grades associated with them. Grades one to two are used to help decrease pain within a joint. Grades three to five are used to increase mobility of joint play. Interestingly, a grade five mobilization is really a manipulation. The following are grades for oscillatory mobilizations:

- Grade 1: Slow oscillations within the first 20-25% of the available joint play range.
- Grade 2: Slow oscillations within 45-55% of the available joint play range or from the beginning to the middle of available joint play range.
- Grade 3: Slow oscillations from the middle of the available joint play range to the end of available joint play range.
- Grade 4: Slow oscillations at the end of the available joint play range.
- Grade 5: Bone is passively moved to the end-range, and a fast thrust is performed. This is manipulation.

Preparation

The clinician should be aware of the following prior to performing manipulations:

- The clinician must use good body mechanics and be comfortable with the patient and the technique.
- The clinician must understand the patient's pain and not proceed if the patient has pain.

- The patient must be comfortable with the clinician, and the procedure must be explained fully to the patient.
- The patient must be relaxed.

Aftercare

Individuals with a chronic joint problem may have Grade 1 and Grade 2 techniques used at the beginning of treatment to decrease pain. Then, after treatment, the patient progresses to more aggressive rehabilitation such as therapeutic exercise. At the end of a rehabilitation session, Grades 3 and 4 can be used in conjunction with stretching to increase mobility. In an acute joint pathology, only Grades 1 and 2 should be used. Grades 1 and 2 mobilizations can be used at the beginning of therapy to reduce pain in an effort to increase performance during therapeutic exercise. Grades 1 and 2 mobilizations can be used again at the end of the treatment before cryotherapy to help alleviate pain.

Complications

Some complications associated with mobilizations, but more so with manipulations are:

- Fracture.
- Dislocation.
- Joint capsule tearing.
- Ligamentous tearing.
- Muscle or tendon injury.
- Nerve damage.

Results

If done appropriately, mobilizations can help reduce pain and restore joint play, which is critical for normal mobility. Manipulations are beneficial for releasing adhesions and are usually done under anesthesia by a medical physician.

References

- Whats-the-difference-between-a-physio-a-chiropracter-and-an-osteopath: thephysiocompany.com, Retrieved 22, June 2020
- Applying-osteopathic-principles-to-formulate-treatment-for-patients-with-chronic-pain-5859463: researchgate.net, Retrieved 26, April 2020
- Muscle-Energy-Technique: physio-pedia.com, Retrieved 01, July 2020
- BASIC-PRINCIPLES-OF-MUS: ymaws.com, Retrieved 19, January 2020

Permissions

All chapters in this book are published with permission under the Creative Commons Attribution Share Alike License or equivalent. Every chapter published in this book has been scrutinized by our experts. Their significance has been extensively debated. The topics covered herein carry significant information for a comprehensive understanding. They may even be implemented as practical applications or may be referred to as a beginning point for further studies.

We would like to thank the editorial team for lending their expertise to make the book truly unique. They have played a crucial role in the development of this book. Without their invaluable contributions this book wouldn't have been possible. They have made vital efforts to compile up to date information on the varied aspects of this subject to make this book a valuable addition to the collection of many professionals and students.

This book was conceptualized with the vision of imparting up-to-date and integrated information in this field. To ensure the same, a matchless editorial board was set up. Every individual on the board went through rigorous rounds of assessment to prove their worth. After which they invested a large part of their time researching and compiling the most relevant data for our readers.

The editorial board has been involved in producing this book since its inception. They have spent rigorous hours researching and exploring the diverse topics which have resulted in the successful publishing of this book. They have passed on their knowledge of decades through this book. To expedite this challenging task, the publisher supported the team at every step. A small team of assistant editors was also appointed to further simplify the editing procedure and attain best results for the readers.

Apart from the editorial board, the designing team has also invested a significant amount of their time in understanding the subject and creating the most relevant covers. They scrutinized every image to scout for the most suitable representation of the subject and create an appropriate cover for the book.

The publishing team has been an ardent support to the editorial, designing and production team. Their endless efforts to recruit the best for this project, has resulted in the accomplishment of this book. They are a veteran in the field of academics and their pool of knowledge is as vast as their experience in printing. Their expertise and guidance has proved useful at every step. Their uncompromising quality standards have made this book an exceptional effort. Their encouragement from time to time has been an inspiration for everyone.

The publisher and the editorial board hope that this book will prove to be a valuable piece of knowledge for students, practitioners and scholars across the globe.

Index

www.ingramcontent.com/pod-product-compliance
Lightning Source LLC
LaVergne TN
LVHW080906210926
848485LV00004B/604